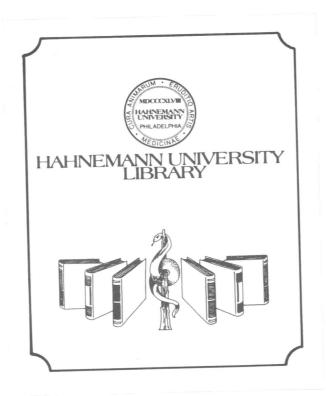

SECTIONAL ANATOMY BY MRI/CT

SECTIONAL ANATOMY BY MRI / CT

GEORGES Y. EL-KHOURY, M.D.

Professor
Departments of Radiology and Orthopaedic Surgery
University of Iowa College of Medicine
Iowa City, Iowa

RONALD A. BERGMAN, Ph.D.

Professor
Department of Anatomy
University of Iowa College of Medicine
Iowa City, Iowa

WILLIAM J. MONTGOMERY, M.D.

Formerly, Assistant Professor
Department of Radiology
University of Iowa College of Medicine
Iowa City, Iowa

CHURCHILL LIVINGSTONE
New York, Edinburgh, London, Melbourne

Library of Congress Cataloging-in-Publication Data

El-Khoury, Georges Y.
 Sectional anatomy by MRI/CT / Georges Y. El-Khoury, Ronald A.
Bergman, William J. Montgomery.
   p. cm.
  Includes bibliographical references.
  ISBN 0-443-08543-9
   1. Anatomy, Human — Atlases. 2. Magnetic resonance imaging —
Atlases. 3. Tomography — Atlases. I. Bergman, Ronald A., date
  II. Montgomery, William J. III. Title.
   [DNLM: 1. Anatomy, Regional — atlases. 2. Magnetic Resonance
Imaging — atlases. 3. Tomography, X-Ray Computed — atlases.   QS 17
E44s]
QM25.E38 1990
611′.9′0222 — dc20
DNLM/DLC
for Library of Congress   89-23857
                                                                                    CIP

© **Churchill Livingstone Inc. 1990**

Distributed in the United Kingdom by Churchill Livingstone, Robert Stevenson House, 1 – 3 Baxter's Place, Leith Walk, Edinburgh EH1 3AF, and by associated companies, branches, and representatives throughout the world.

Accurate indications, adverse reactions, and dosage schedules for drugs are provided in this book, but it is possible that they may change. The reader is urged to review the package information data of the manufacturers of the medications mentioned.

The cover illustrations are by Leonardo da Vinci and were made available by the Windsor Castle, Royal Library. © They are used by the gracious permission of Her Majesty, Queen Elizabeth II.

Copy Editor: *Kamely Dahir*
Book Designer: *Gloria Brown*
Production Supervisor: *Christina Hippeli*

Printed in the United States of America

First published in 1990

CONTRIBUTORS

CHARLES N. APRILL, M.D.
Spine Treatment Center
St. Charles General Hospital and Imaging Center,
New Orleans, Louisiana

GEORGE S. BISSET III, M.D.
Associate Professor
Department of Pediatric Radiology
University of Cincinnati College of Medicine
  and Children's Hospital Medical Center
Cincinnati, Ohio

HIROSHI HONDA, M.D.
Assistant Professor
Department of Radiology
Kyushu University Faculty of Medicine
Fukouka, Japan

WILLIAM STANFORD, M.D.
Associate Professor
Department of Radiology
University of Iowa College of Medicine
Iowa City, Iowa

WILLIAM T.C. YUH, M.D.
Assistant Professor
Department of Radiology
University of Iowa College of Medicine
Iowa City, Iowa

PREFACE

In recent years, as a response to giant strides in imaging technology, there has been a surge of interest in anatomy by radiologists. The most acute need has been in the area of the musculoskeletal system. However, most of the current books and atlases that we have consulted in our clinical practice have failed to provide necessary information and to satisfy our curiosity. Yet, detailed anatomic reviews with our anatomist colleagues resulted in a deeper understanding of our imaging studies, improved our insight into disease processes, and enhanced our ability to communicate with the referring physicians.

As work in sectional anatomy proceeded, this new excitement and enthusiasm grew and, in some instances, became contagious. Our residents demanded more instruction in clinical anatomy, and we established courses to teach sectional anatomy to fourth year medical students and to introduce sectional anatomy at the freshman level. The desire to share our new mode of providing information led us to contact Toni M. Tracy, President of Churchill Livingstone Inc., who encouraged us to prepare a detailed sectional anatomy atlas.

This atlas, *Sectional Anatomy by MRI/CT*, is intended to be used by radiologists and other clinicians interested in sectional anatomy, and by anatomists, principally as an anatomic reference for the body sectioned in all three standard planes.

There are some areas of necessary duplication within the atlas. For instance, the coronal and sagittal sections of the pelvis include the proximal thigh. Similarly, in the thigh, there are images of the adjacent pelvic region. We think this is of value, as visualization of adjacent structures beyond the traditional compartments are frequently necessary in clinical practice. We also believe that the systematic study of anatomy in multiple planes leads to a greater understanding of the spatial relationships between structures.

The book is divided into anatomic regions. These regions are then imaged in the three standard planes. The more familiar axial plane is portrayed first, followed by the coronal and sagittal planes. All images are from normal volunteers; no cadaveric studies are included. This accounts for some of the variability in muscle mass and body fat between different subjects.

Computed tomography (CT) has been used in conjunction with magnetic resonance imaging (MRI) in the abdomen and thorax. CT is used to demonstrate the axial anatomy of the upper abdomen, because respiratory motion degrades MRI quality. Images from a ciné-CT (ultra-fast) scanner have been used to augment the MRI of the thorax.

In this atlas, axial sections start proximally or cephalad and advance distally or caudally. Coronal sections start posteriorly or dorsally and advance anteriorly or ventrally, and sagittal sections, in most regions, start medially and advance laterally. Through figure labelling, the anatomic make-up of the image is identified, and the atlas uses the following abbreviations: *m.*, muscle; *mm.*, muscles; *a.*, artery, *aa.*, arteries; *v.*, vein; and *vv.*, veins.

Subjects were scanned lying in the anatomic position, i.e., the subject lying straight with the feet together and toes directed upward, arms by the side, and palms of the hands facing upward. In sections of the foot, the definition of axial and coronal is strictly based on the position of the feet of the recumbent subject in the anatomic position.

For us, the creation of this book has fulfilled a need, which started with the early days of CT and became acute with the advent of MRI. We are hopeful that *Sectional Anatomy by MRI/CT* will also fulfill this need for others.

Georges Y. El-Khoury, M.D.
Ronald A. Bergman, Ph.D.
William J. Montgomery, M.D.

ACKNOWLEDGMENTS

This atlas represents a long and tortuous, but nevertheless, enjoyable journey. We are indebted to our contributing colleagues, whose expertise greatly enhanced the quality of this effort. This atlas would not have been possible without the numerous volunteers, including medical students, residents, and faculty, who spent time in the scanner.

The technical staff has been especially patient with us. Our earliest trials were performed by Chuck Armstrong and Heidi Mueller-Berns. Much of this work, unfortunately, had to be discarded because of the rapid advances in imaging technology. The MR images in this book are mainly the work of Mary C. Connor, who worked many hours and on weekends. Her attention to detail and pride in her work took a large burden from our shoulders and made our job manageable. The authors are much indebted to Russell Bodin for preparing the sections of the spine. Our thanks are also expressed to Linda Mohr for her expert secretarial assistance, Franklin J. Sindelar and Brenda Robinson for line drawings, and Phyllis S. Bergman for generously providing editorial assistance. Kamely Dahir, Associate Managing Editor at Churchill Livingstone, has, with great care, guided us around the many pitfalls that authors encounter in preparing a manuscript for publication. Our gratitude to Toni M. Tracy, President of Churchill Livingstone, for her generous support and also for the cover design. Finally, we acknowledge the gracious and loving contributions of our families who gave us time and relief from household duties to complete this book.

Georges Y. El-Khoury, M.D.
Ronald A. Bergman, Ph.D.
William J. Montgomery, M.D.

CONTENTS

1
UPPER LIMB

Chapter 1

SHOULDER

Figure 1.1.1

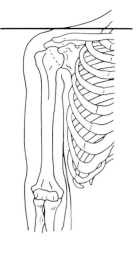

1. This section is through the superior aspect of the shoulder.

2. The trapezius is well seen. Its most superior fibers insert on the posterior aspect of the lateral third of the clavicle. Lower cervical and upper thoracic fibers insert on the acromion process and upper border of the scapular spine.

3. Levator scapulae arises from the transverse processes of the first four cervical vertebrae and inserts on the superior angle of the scapula.

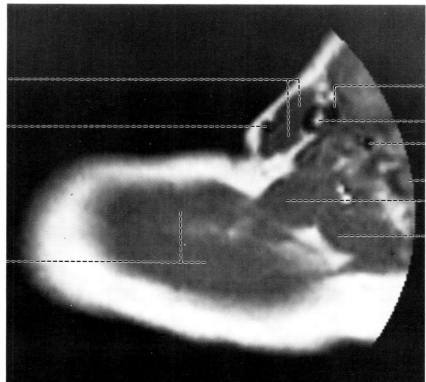

Sternocleidomastoid m.

External jugular v.

Trapezius m.

Common carotid a.

Internal jugular v.

Vertebral a.

Spinal cord

Levator scapulae m.

Splenius capitis m.

Figure 1.1.2

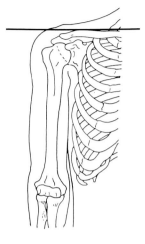

1. The portions of the trapezius inserting on the clavicle and the scapula are distinctly separated.

2. The sternocleidomastoid is seen on the anterior aspect of the neck.

3. Beneath sternocleidomastoid are the internal jugular vein and common carotid artery.

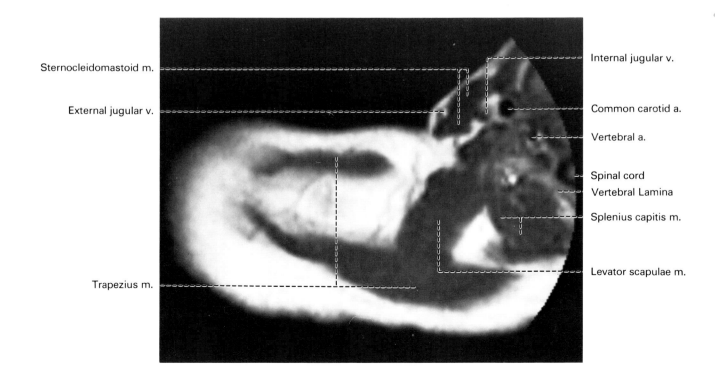

Sternocleidomastoid m.

External jugular v.

Trapezius m.

Internal jugular v.

Common carotid a.

Vertebral a.

Spinal cord
Vertebral Lamina
Splenius capitis m.

Levator scapulae m.

Figure 1.1.3

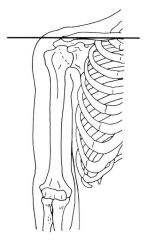

1. The supraspinatus fossa houses the supraspinatus muscle anterior to the scapular spine.

2. Note the origin of the deltoid from the scapular spine, acromion, and lateral third of the clavicle.

3. The serratus anterior, levator scapulae, and rhomboideus major converge to insert on the medial border of the scapula.

4. The acromioclavicular joint is demonstrated in this section.

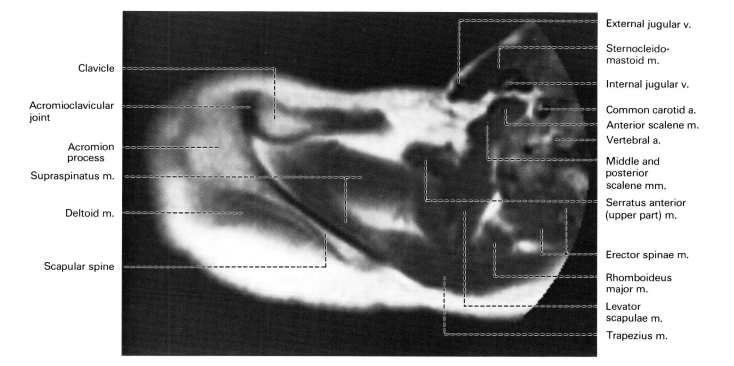

Figure 1.1.4

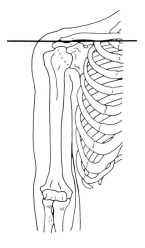

1. The supraspinatus muscle courses below the acromion process to insert on the superior aspect of the greater tuberosity.

2. The multipennate configuration of the deltoid is demonstrated in this section.

3. The infraspinatus fossa is situated inferior to the scapular spine and houses the infraspinatus muscle.

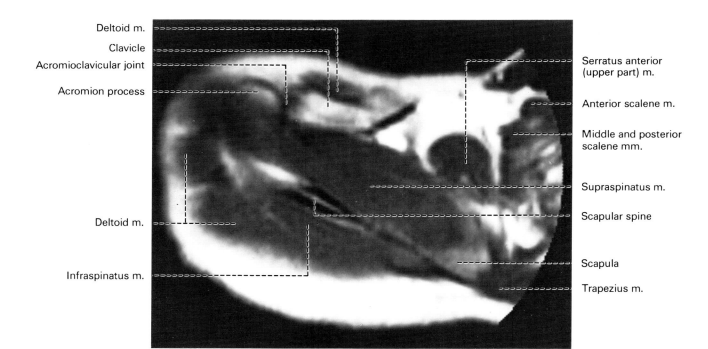

Figure 1.1.5

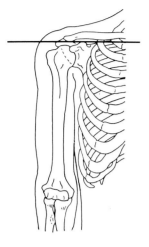

1. The anterior portion of the deltoid originates from the clavicle.

2. The supraspinatus tendon lies between the humeral head and acromion.

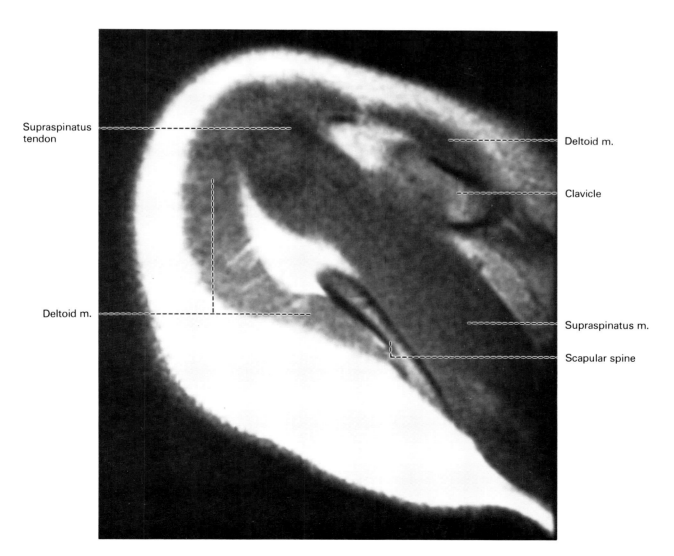

Figure 1.1.6

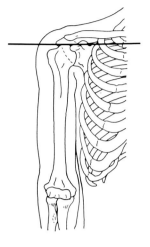

1. The infraspinatus courses laterally to insert on the greater tuberosity of the humerus. It originates from the infraspinous fossa.

2. The scapular spine separates the supraspinous and infraspinous fossae.

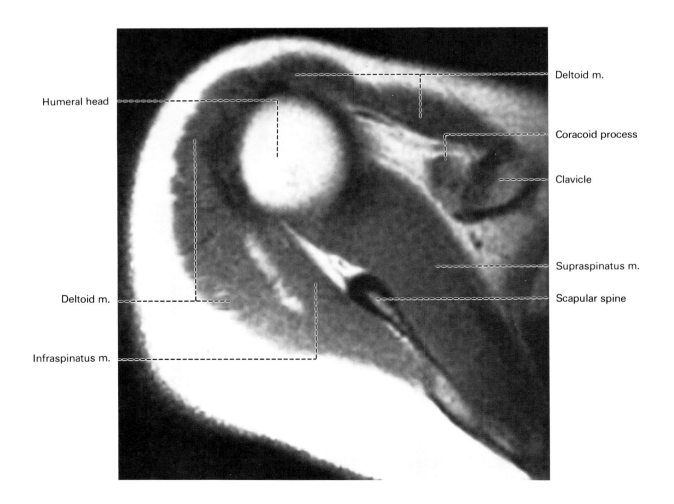

Figure 1.1.7

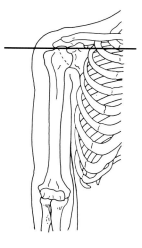

1. This section is through the coracoid process, which acts as the origin for the short head of biceps and coracobrachialis. Pectoralis minor inserts on the coracoid process also.

2. The coracoacromial and coracoclavicular ligaments attach to the coracoid process.

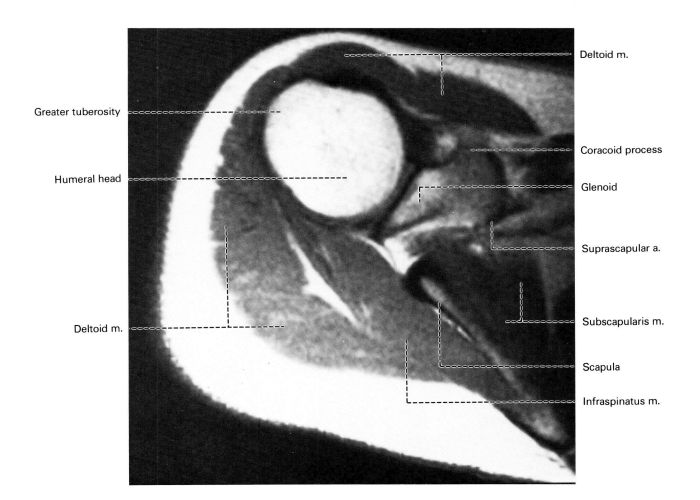

Figure 1.1.8

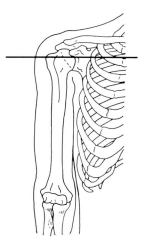

1. The glenoid labrum forms the rim of the glenoid fossa.

2. The bicipital groove is situated between the greater and lesser tuberosities. The bicipital tendon or the long head of the biceps tendon lies within the bicipital groove.

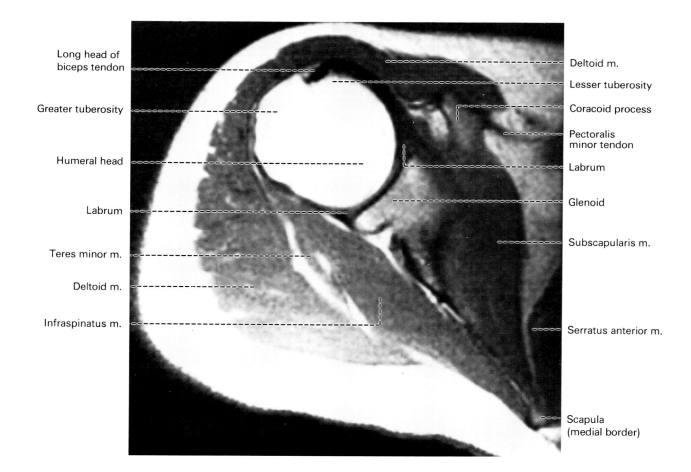

Figure 1.1.9

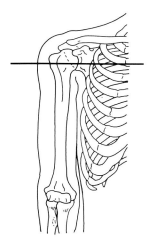

1. Note the insertion of the pectoralis minor tendon on the coracoid process.

2. The clavicular portion of pectoralis major is partially demonstrated; it originates from the medial half of the clavicle.

3. The long head of the biceps tendon can be seen within the bicipital groove.

4. Subscapularis inserts on the lesser tuberosity.

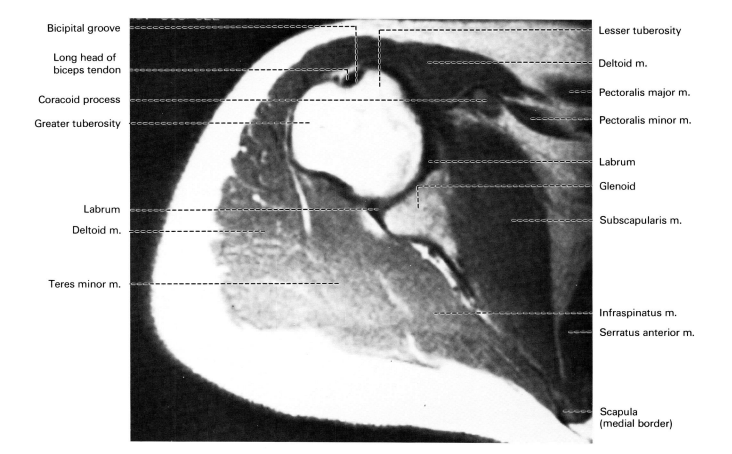

Figure 1.1.10

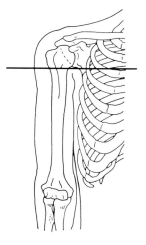

1. Note the origin of the long head of triceps tendon from the infraglenoid tuberosity.

2. The neurovascular bundle courses laterally, posterior to the clavicle and pectoralis minor.

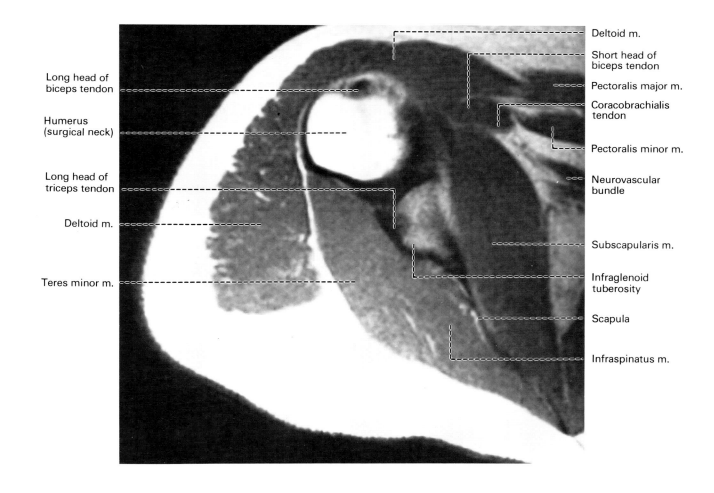

Figure 1.1.11

1. This section is directly inferior to the glenoid.

2. The long head of triceps is clearly demonstrated after it descends from its origin at the infraglenoid tuberosity.

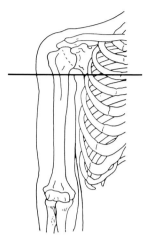

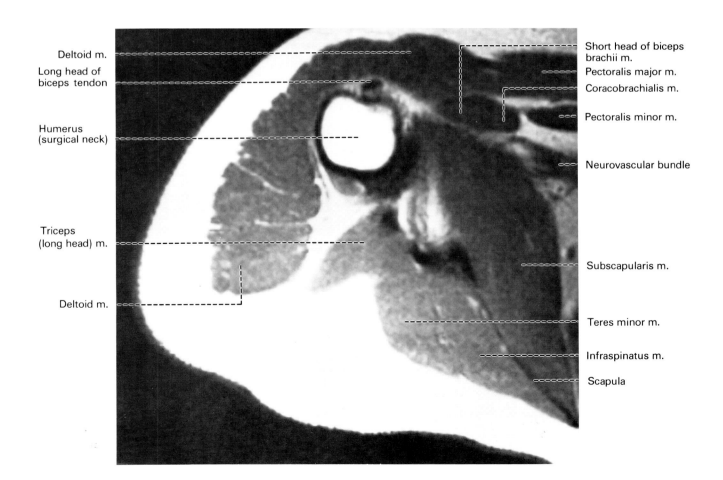

Deltoid m.

Long head of biceps tendon

Humerus (surgical neck)

Triceps (long head) m.

Deltoid m.

Short head of biceps brachii m.

Pectoralis major m.

Coracobrachialis m.

Pectoralis minor m.

Neurovascular bundle

Subscapularis m.

Teres minor m.

Infraspinatus m.

Scapula

Figure 1.1.12

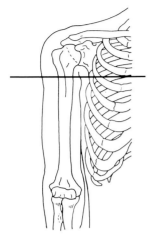

1. The long head of the triceps divides the space inferior to teres minor into the quadrangular space and triangular space.

2. The posterior humeral circumflex artery courses posteriorly through the quadrangular space.

3. Coracobrachialis and short head of biceps continue to course distally together.

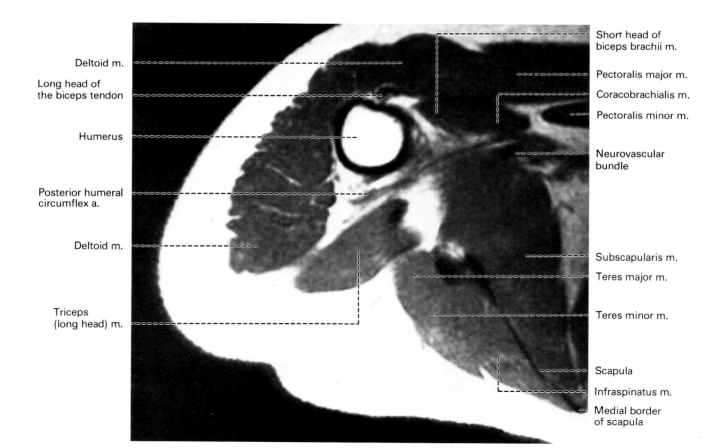

Figure 1.1.13

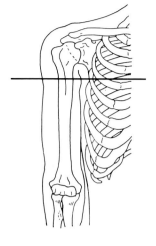

1. The lateral head of the triceps is at its origin from the posterior aspect of the humerus.

2. Teres major and latissimus dorsi merge as they course toward their insertion on the crest of the lesser tuberosity.

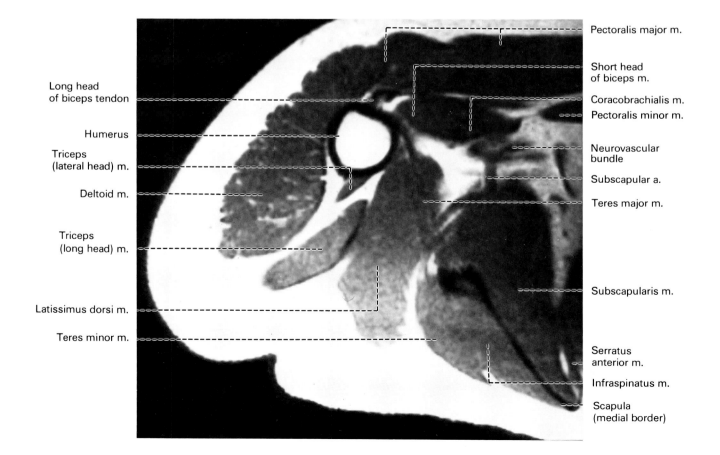

Long head of biceps tendon

Humerus

Triceps (lateral head) m.

Deltoid m.

Triceps (long head) m.

Latissimus dorsi m.

Teres minor m.

Pectoralis major m.

Short head of biceps m.

Coracobrachialis m.

Pectoralis minor m.

Neurovascular bundle

Subscapular a.

Teres major m.

Subscapularis m.

Serratus anterior m.

Infraspinatus m.

Scapula (medial border)

Figure 1.1.14

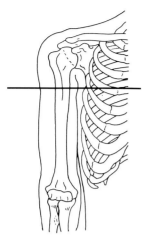

1. Pectoralis major is approaching its insertion on the crest of the greater tuberosity.

2. Teres major and latissimus dorsi are seen inserting on the crest of the lesser tuberosity.

3. Serratus anterior is demonstrated on the posterolateral aspect of the chest wall. It usually arises from the upper eight ribs.

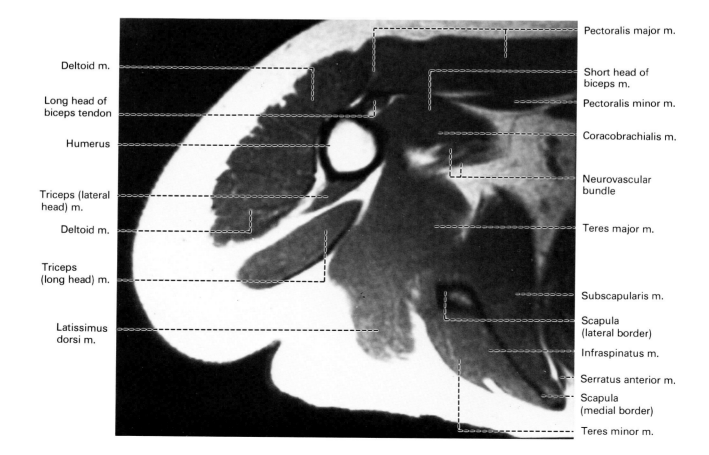

Figure 1.1.15

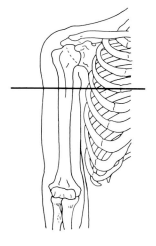

1. The neurovascular bundle courses distally along the posteromedial surface of coracobrachialis.

2. The long and short heads of biceps are seen separately before they merge into one muscle.

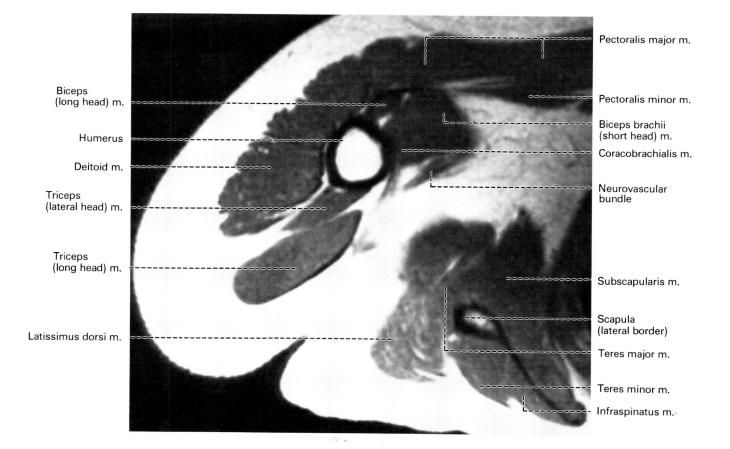

Biceps (long head) m.

Humerus

Deltoid m.

Triceps (lateral head) m.

Triceps (long head) m.

Latissimus dorsi m.

Pectoralis major m.

Pectoralis minor m.

Biceps brachii (short head) m.

Coracobrachialis m.

Neurovascular bundle

Subscapularis m.

Scapula (lateral border)

Teres major m.

Teres minor m.

Infraspinatus m.

Figure 1.1.16

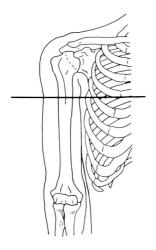

1. This section is at the inferior limit of the axilla.

2. Pectoralis major forms the anterior boundary of the axilla.

3. The lateral and long heads of triceps merge together into one muscle mass.

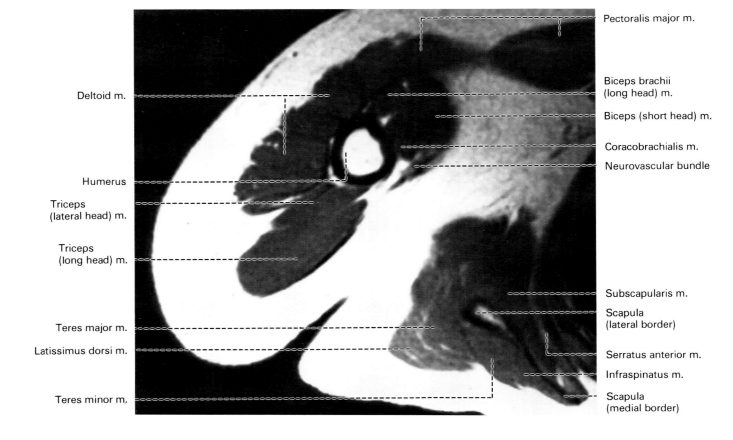

Figure 1.1.17

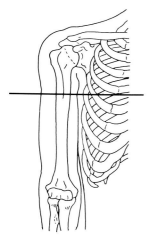

1. The radial nerve separates from the neurovascular bundle; it courses behind the humerus in the radial nerve groove accompanied by the deep (profunda) brachial artery.

2. Deltoid diminishes in size as it approaches its insertion on the deltoid tuberosity.

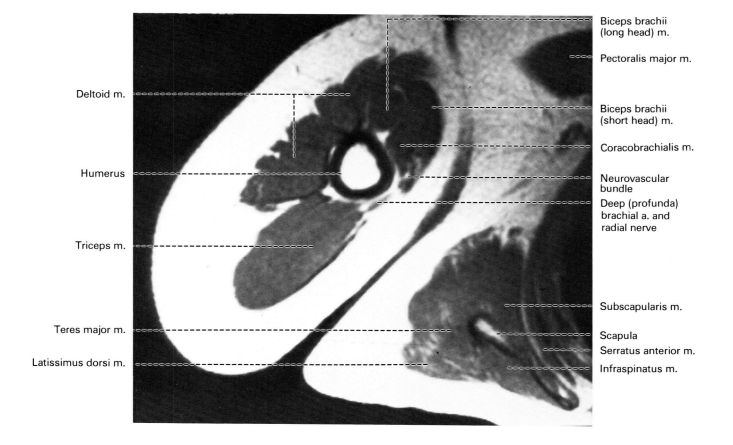

Figure 1.1.18

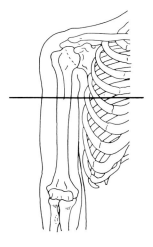

1. The neurovascular bundle continues to course distally in the medial intermuscular septum; the radial nerve and deep (profunda) brachial artery are behind the humerus.

2. Coracobrachialis is completing its insertion on the medial surface of the proximal humerus.

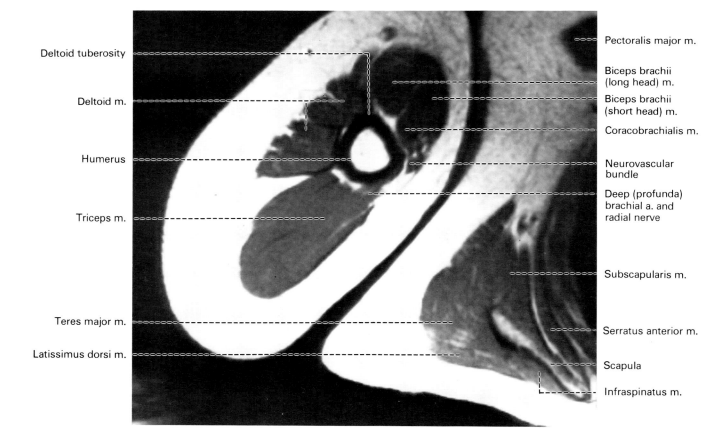

Figure 1.1.19

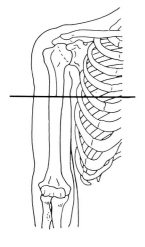

1. This section is through the lower part of the scapula close to the inferior angle.

2. The deltoid converges on the deltoid tuberosity for insertion. The tuberosity is quite prominent in this section.

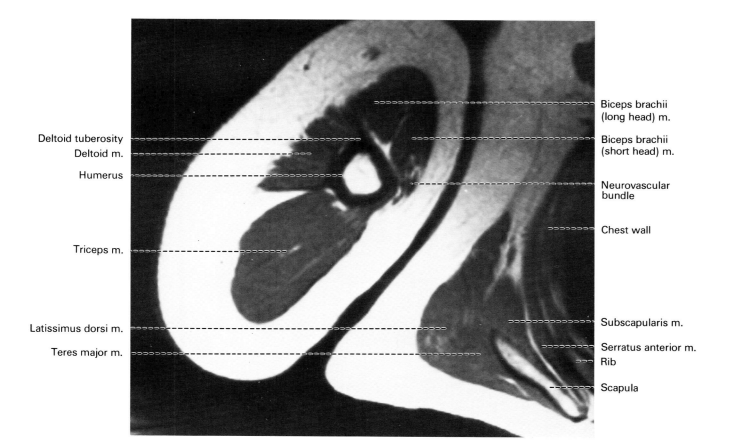

CORONAL

Figure 1.2.1

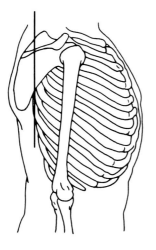

1. This posterior section cuts through the scapula, because of its oblique orientation, as it attaches to the chest wall.

2. The scapula-thoracic attachment is totally muscular.

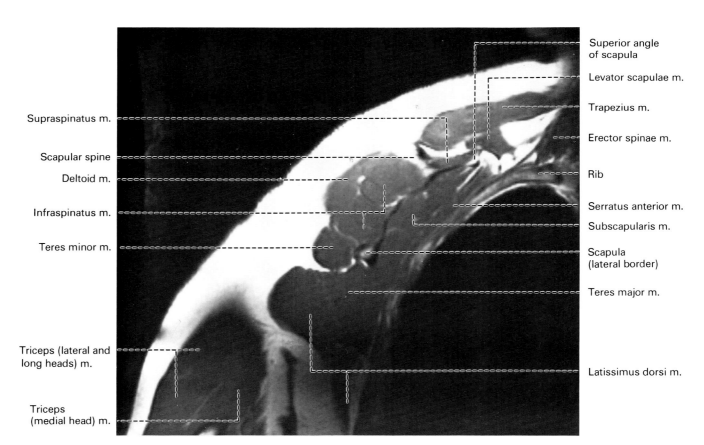

Supraspinatus m.

Scapular spine

Deltoid m.

Infraspinatus m.

Teres minor m.

Triceps (lateral and long heads) m.

Triceps (medial head) m.

Superior angle of scapula

Levator scapulae m.

Trapezius m.

Erector spinae m.

Rib

Serratus anterior m.

Subscapularis m.

Scapula (lateral border)

Teres major m.

Latissimus dorsi m.

Figure 1.2.2

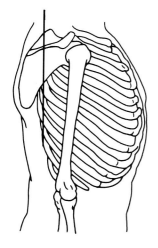

1. All rotator cuff muscles are demonstrated in this section.

2. Teres major courses laterally and anteriorly just inferior to the lateral border of the scapula.

3. The levator scapulae inserts on the superior angle of the scapula.

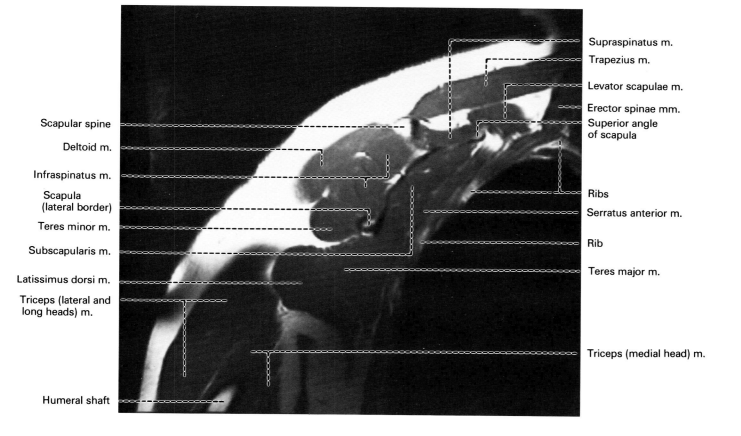

Supraspinatus m.

Trapezius m.

Levator scapulae m.

Erector spinae mm.

Superior angle of scapula

Scapular spine

Deltoid m.

Infraspinatus m.

Scapula (lateral border)

Teres minor m.

Subscapularis m.

Latissimus dorsi m.

Triceps (lateral and long heads) m.

Ribs

Serratus anterior m.

Rib

Teres major m.

Triceps (medial head) m.

Humeral shaft

Figure 1.2.3

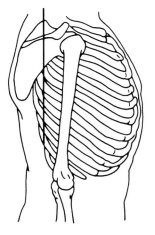

1. Note the flat middle part of serratus anterior lying between the chest wall and subscapularis muscle.

2. In this posterior section of the shoulder, teres major and latissimus dorsi can be seen as separate entities before they merge.

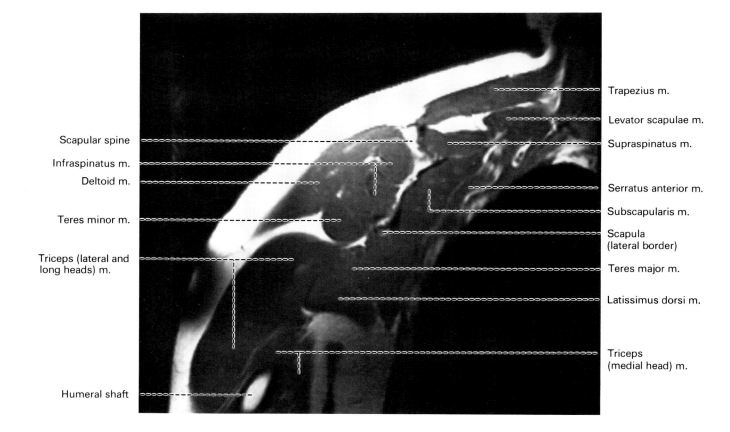

Scapular spine

Infraspinatus m.

Deltoid m.

Teres minor m.

Triceps (lateral and long heads) m.

Humeral shaft

Trapezius m.

Levator scapulae m.

Supraspinatus m.

Serratus anterior m.

Subscapularis m.

Scapula (lateral border)

Teres major m.

Latissimus dorsi m.

Triceps (medial head) m.

Figure 1.2.4

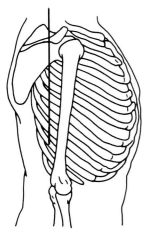

1. This section depicts most of the shoulder muscles, in particular, the rotator cuff muscles (supraspinatus, infraspinatus, teres minor, and subscapularis).

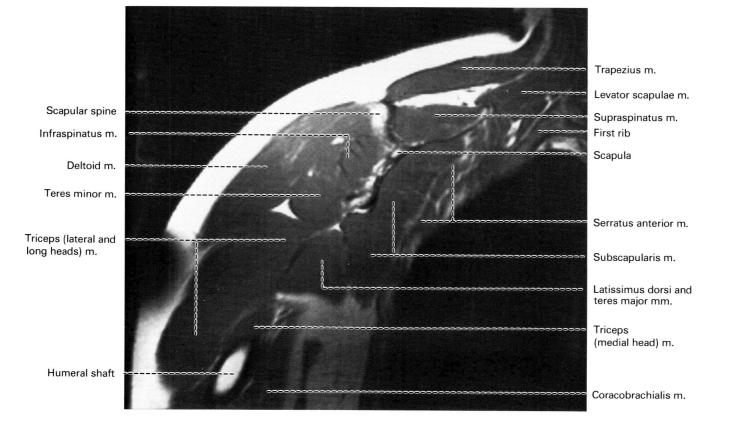

Figure 1.2.5

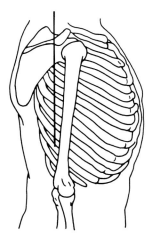

1. Note the origin of the long head of the biceps from the infraglenoid tuberosity.

2. The scapular spine separates the infraspinatus fossa from the supraspinatus fossa.

3. Note the flat middle part of the serratus anterior compared to its bulkier upper part.

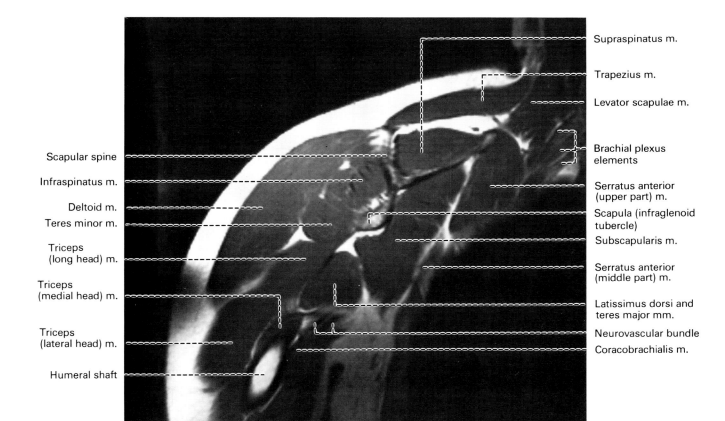

Figure 1.2.6

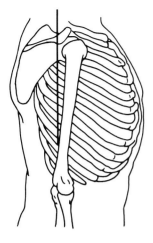

1. The long head of the triceps passes between teres minor and teres major. It separates the quadrangular space from the triangular space.

2. The long head of the triceps originates from the infraglenoid tuberosity of the scapula.

3. The posterior circumflex humeral artery and axillary nerve (not demonstrated) pass through the quadrangular space.

4. Levator scapulae and upper part of serratus anterior are clearly depicted in this section.

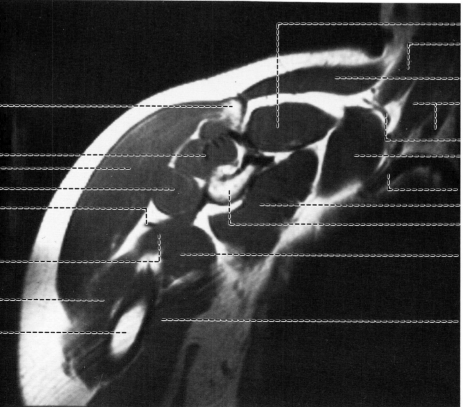

Acromion process

Infraspinatus m.
Deltoid m.

Teres minor m.

Posterior humeral circumflex a.

Triceps (long head) m.

Triceps (lateral head) m.

Humeral shaft

Supraspinatus m.

Levator scapulae m.

Trapezius m.

Scalene mm.

Transverse cervical a.

Serratus anterior (upper part) m.

Subclavian a.

Subscapularis m.

Scapular neck

Latissimus dorsi and teres major mm.

Coracobrachialis m.

Figure 1.2.7

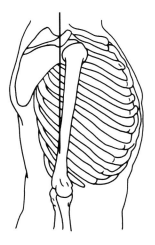

1. In the neck, the subclavian vein courses anterior to the anterior scalene muscle whereas the subclavian artery passes posterior to it.

2. Serratus anterior has an extensive fleshy origin from the upper eight ribs and inserts on the medial border of the scapula. Serratus anterior is divided into three parts; the upper and lower parts form the bulk of the muscle. The middle part is thin and may be absent.

3. The upper part of the serratus anterior is partially demonstrated in this section.

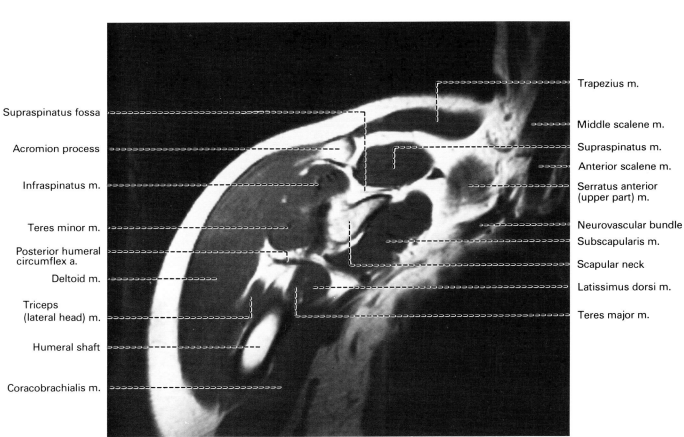

Supraspinatus fossa

Acromion process

Infraspinatus m.

Teres minor m.

Posterior humeral circumflex a.

Deltoid m.

Triceps (lateral head) m.

Humeral shaft

Coracobrachialis m.

Trapezius m.

Middle scalene m.

Supraspinatus m.

Anterior scalene m.

Serratus anterior (upper part) m.

Neurovascular bundle

Subscapularis m.

Scapular neck

Latissimus dorsi m.

Teres major m.

Figure 1.2.8

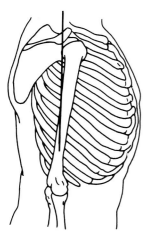

1. This section is through the posterior aspect of the glenohumeral joint.

2. The latissimus dorsi and teres major tendons are approaching their insertion on the crest of the lesser tuberosity.

3. Deltoid inserts on the deltoid tuberosity of the humerus.

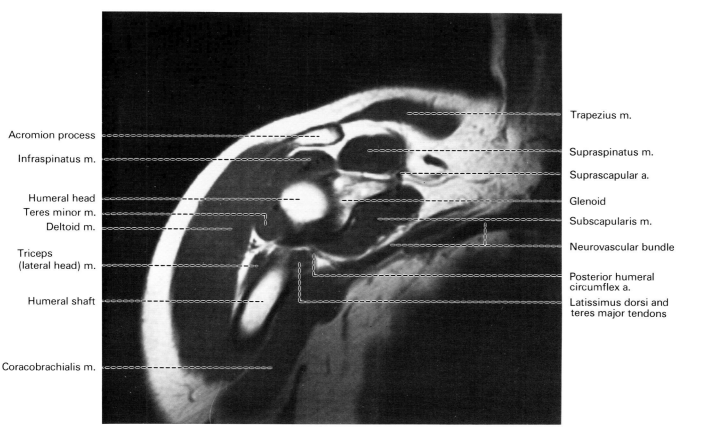

Acromion process
Infraspinatus m.
Humeral head
Teres minor m.
Deltoid m.
Triceps (lateral head) m.
Humeral shaft
Coracobrachialis m.

Trapezius m.
Supraspinatus m.
Suprascapular a.
Glenoid
Subscapularis m.
Neurovascular bundle
Posterior humeral circumflex a.
Latissimus dorsi and teres major tendons

Figure 1.2.9

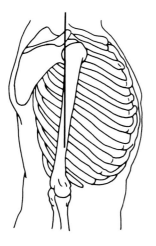

1. The occipital and upper cervical bundles of the trapezius insert on the posterior aspect of the lateral third of the clavicle.

2. Within the neurovascular bundle the axillary vein courses anterior to the artery.

3. Subscapularis inserts on the lesser tuberosity.

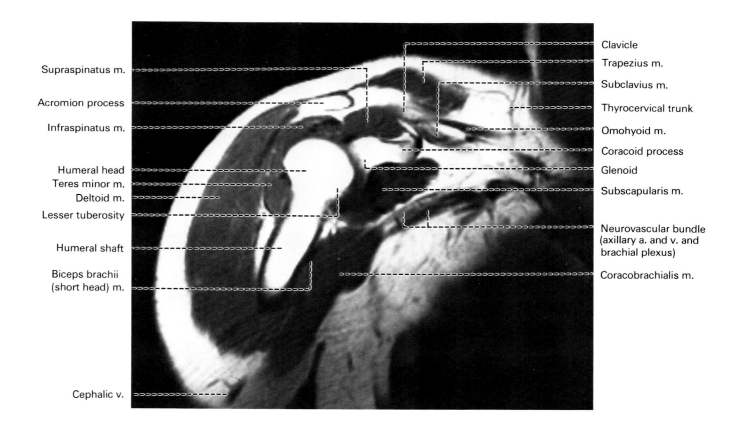

Figure 1.2.10

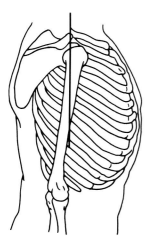

1. Subclavius is clearly depicted in this section. It is a small muscle that originates from the first rib and inserts on the inferior surface of the clavicle.

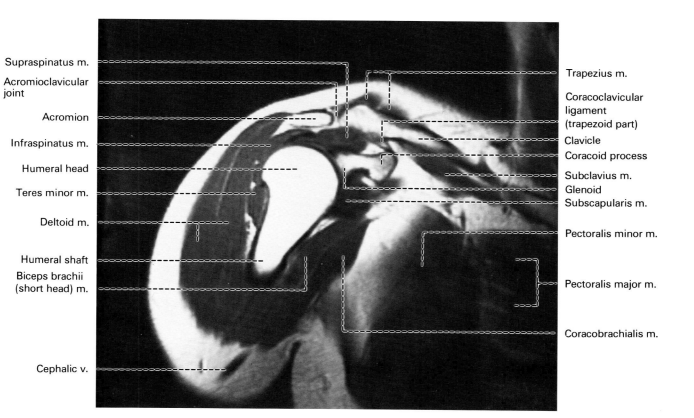

Supraspinatus m.

Acromioclavicular joint

Acromion

Infraspinatus m.

Humeral head

Teres minor m.

Deltoid m.

Humeral shaft

Biceps brachii (short head) m.

Cephalic v.

Trapezius m.

Coracoclavicular ligament (trapezoid part)

Clavicle

Coracoid process

Subclavius m.

Glenoid

Subscapularis m.

Pectoralis minor m.

Pectoralis major m.

Coracobrachialis m.

Figure 1.2.11

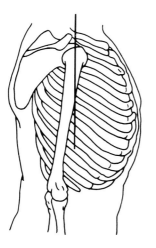

1. Note the trapezoid and conoid parts of the coracoclavicular ligament.

2. Pectoralis minor is demonstrated deep to pectoralis major.

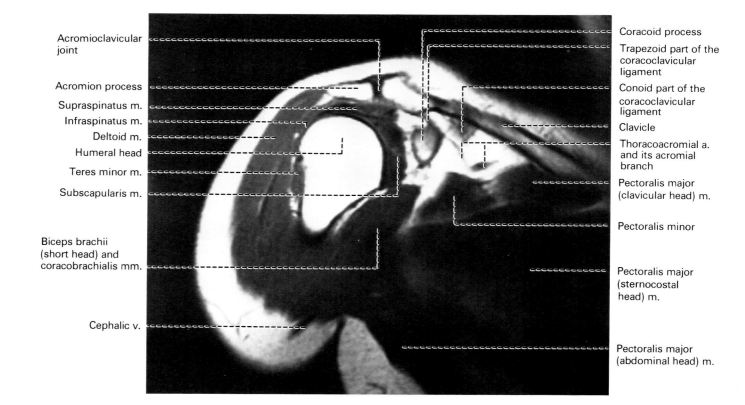

Acromioclavicular joint

Acromion process

Supraspinatus m.

Infraspinatus m.

Deltoid m.

Humeral head

Teres minor m.

Subscapularis m.

Biceps brachii (short head) and coracobrachialis mm.

Cephalic v.

Coracoid process

Trapezoid part of the coracoclavicular ligament

Conoid part of the coracoclavicular ligament

Clavicle

Thoracoacromial a. and its acromial branch

Pectoralis major (clavicular head) m.

Pectoralis minor

Pectoralis major (sternocostal head) m.

Pectoralis major (abdominal head) m.

Figure 1.2.12

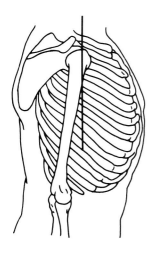

1. This section is through the tip of the coracoid process. The short head of biceps and coracobrachialis are demonstrated originating from the coracoid process.

2. The abdominal head of pectoralis major is depicted in this section.

3. All three heads of pectoralis major converge laterally and fold in a bilaminar fashion before they insert on the crest of the greater tuberosity.

4. The insertion of pectoralis major is covered by the deltoid muscle.

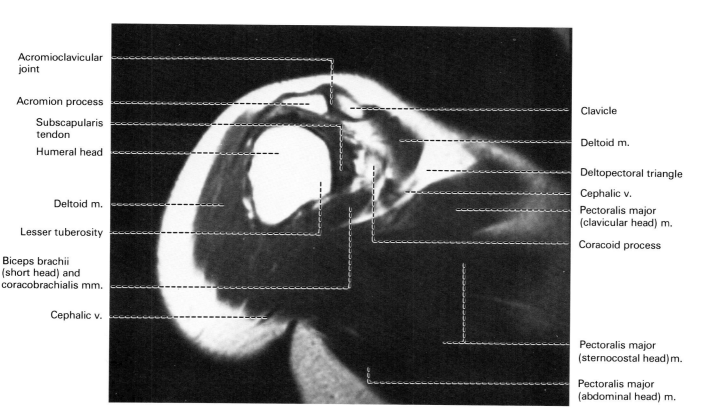

Figure 1.2.13

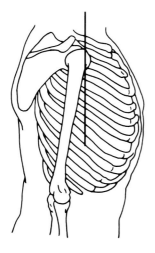

1. The tip of the coracoid process gives origin to the short head of biceps and coracobrachialis. More proximal on the coracoid process, pectoralis minor inserts (not shown on this section).

2. Note the tendon of subscapularis approaching its insertion on the lesser tuberosity.

3. The origin of deltoid from the clavicle and acromion process can be appreciated in this section.

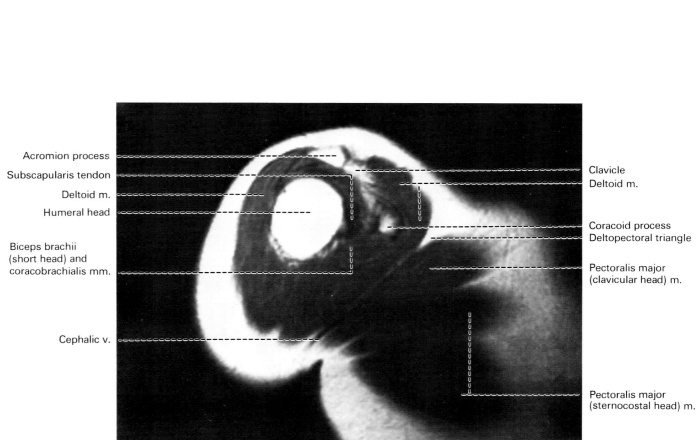

Acromion process

Subscapularis tendon

Deltoid m.

Humeral head

Biceps brachii
(short head) and
coracobrachialis mm.

Cephalic v.

Clavicle
Deltoid m.

Coracoid process
Deltopectoral triangle

Pectoralis major
(clavicular head) m.

Pectoralis major
(sternocostal head) m.

Figure 1.2.14

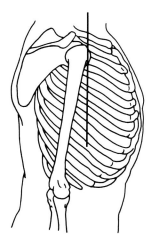

1. Pectoralis major has three heads: clavicular, sternocostal, and abdominal, with the sternocostal being the largest.

2. Note the course of the cephalic vein within the deltopectoral groove.

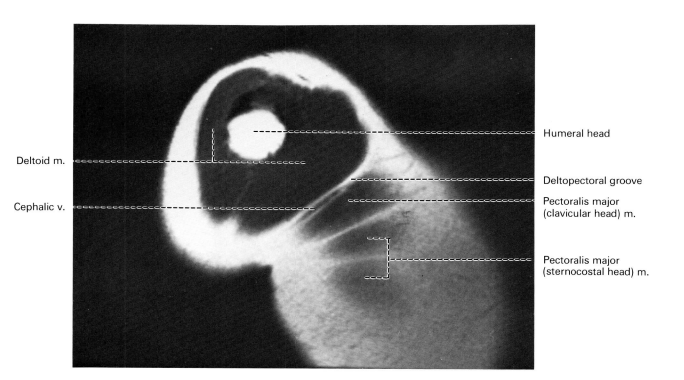

Figure 1.2.15

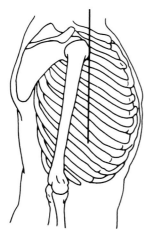

1. The deltoid originates from the lateral third of the clavicle anteriorly, from the acromion laterally, and from the spine of the scapula posteriorly. Its origin corresponds closely to the insertion of the trapezius.

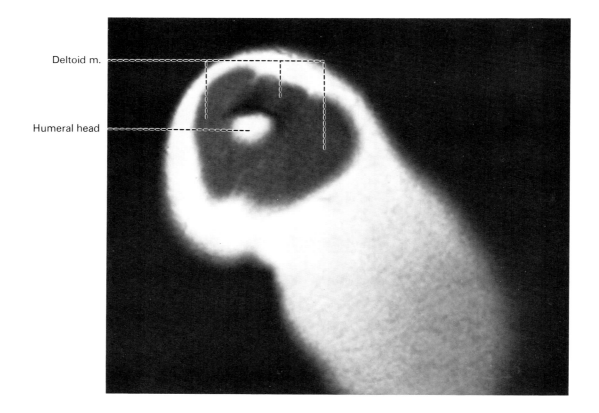

Deltoid m.

Humeral head

Figure 1.2.16

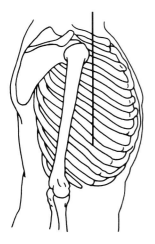

1. This is the most anterior section of the shoulder. It passes through the anterior part of deltoid, which is the most prominent muscle of the shoulder.

Deltoid m.

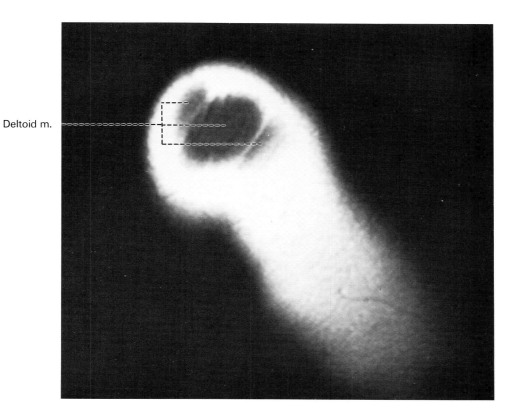

Figure 1.3.1

1. Note the size and extent of pectoralis major and latissimus dorsi muscles.

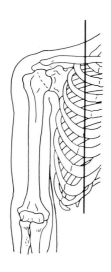

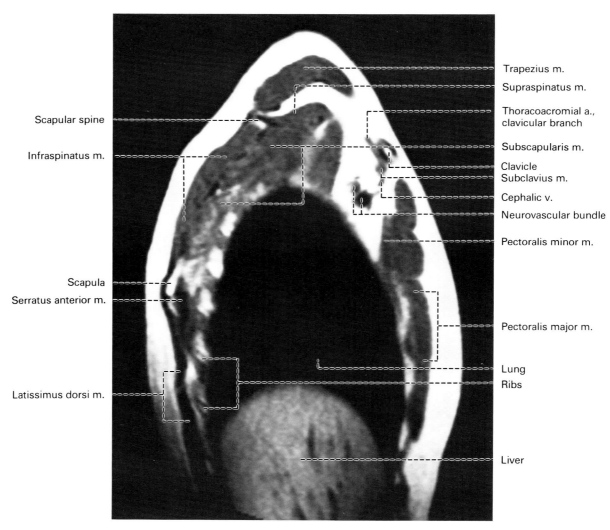

Trapezius m.

Supraspinatus m.

Thoracoacromial a., clavicular branch

Scapular spine

Subscapularis m.

Infraspinatus m.

Clavicle
Subclavius m.

Cephalic v.

Neurovascular bundle

Pectoralis minor m.

Scapula

Serratus anterior m.

Pectoralis major m.

Lung

Ribs

Latissimus dorsi m.

Liver

Figure 1.3.2

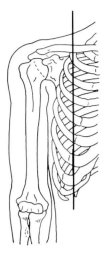

1. The scapula is heavily invested with muscular attachments.

2. Note the course of the neurovascular bundle posterior to pectoralis major.

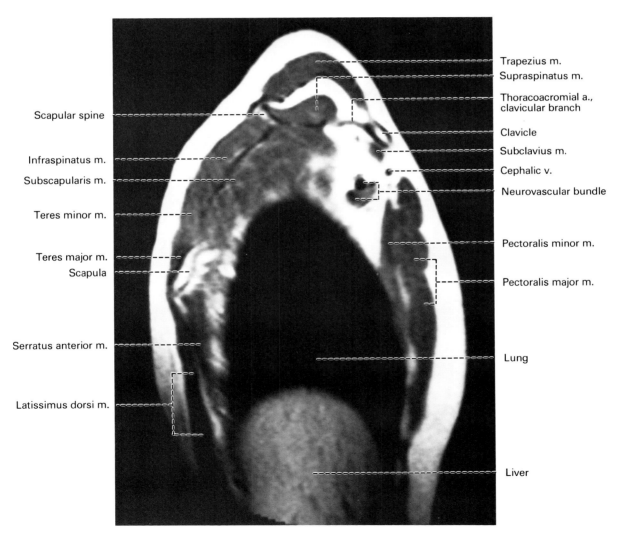

Figure 1.3.3

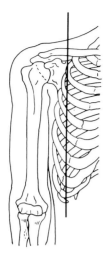

1. Note that portions of the scapula are extremely thin.

2. Note the extent of the serratus anterior muscle. It is a large flat muscle arising from the upper eight ribs and inserts on the medial border of the scapula.

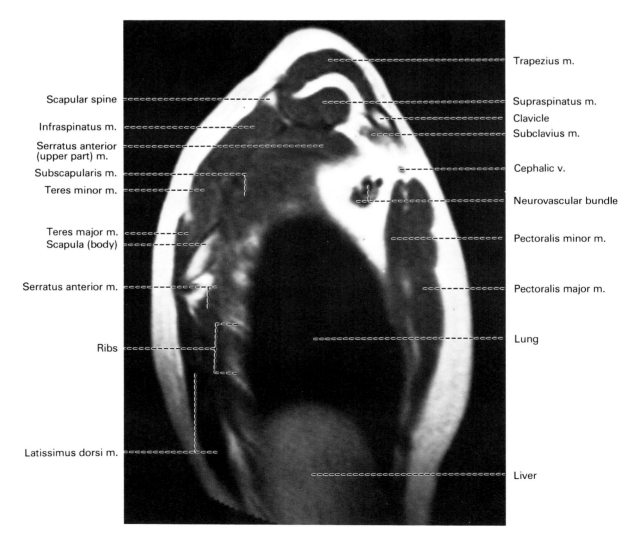

Figure 1.3.4

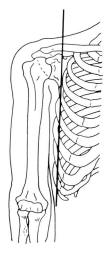

1. The cephalic vein courses in the deltopectoral groove before draining into the axillary vein.

2. The subclavian artery is renamed the axillary artery after it crosses the first rib. The axillary artery is renamed the brachial artery after it crosses teres major muscle.

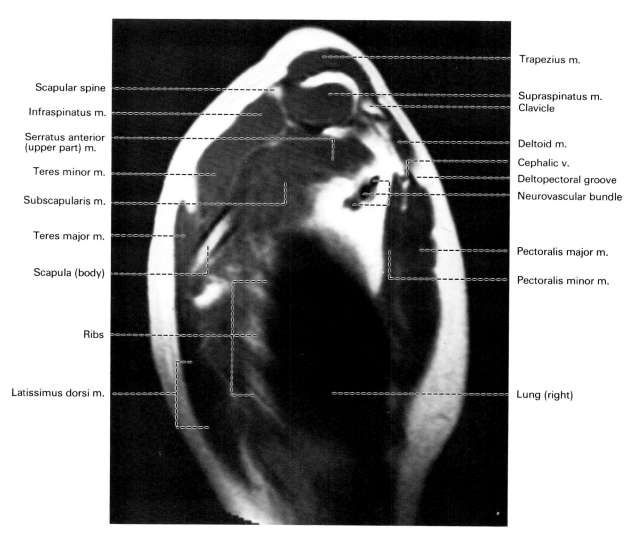

Scapular spine — Trapezius m.

Infraspinatus m. — Supraspinatus m.

Serratus anterior (upper part) m. — Clavicle

Teres minor m. — Deltoid m.

Subscapularis m. — Cephalic v.

Teres major m. — Deltopectoral groove

Scapula (body) — Neurovascular bundle

Ribs — Pectoralis major m.

Latissimus dorsi m. — Pectoralis minor m.

Lung (right)

Figure 1.3.5

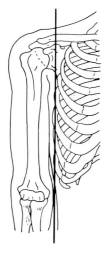

1. The origin of serratus anterior is depicted in this section. It arises from the surface of the upper eight or nine ribs and inserts on the medial border of the scapula.

2. Subscapularis occupies the entire subscapular fossa.

3. Note that the scapula is obliquely oriented on the chest wall.

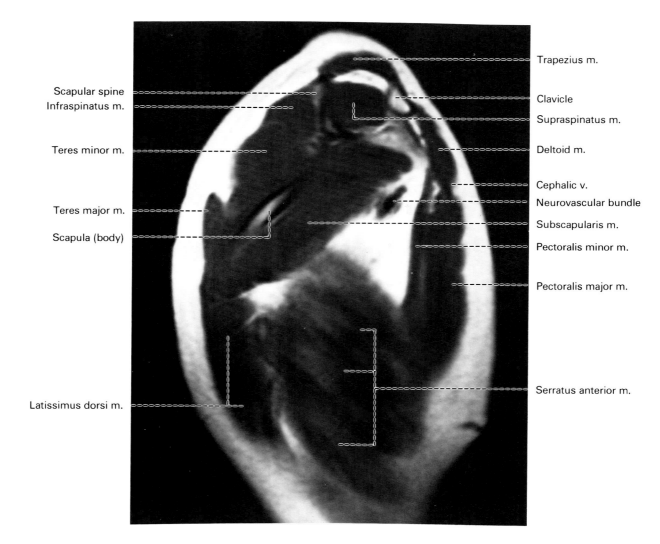

Figure 1.3.6

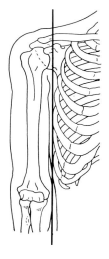

1. The trapezius is demonstrated on the superior aspect of the shoulder; it has insertions on the clavicle and scapular spine.

2. Note the insertion of pectoralis minor on the tip of the coracoid process.

3. The scapular spine is an important landmark in identifying shoulder muscles.

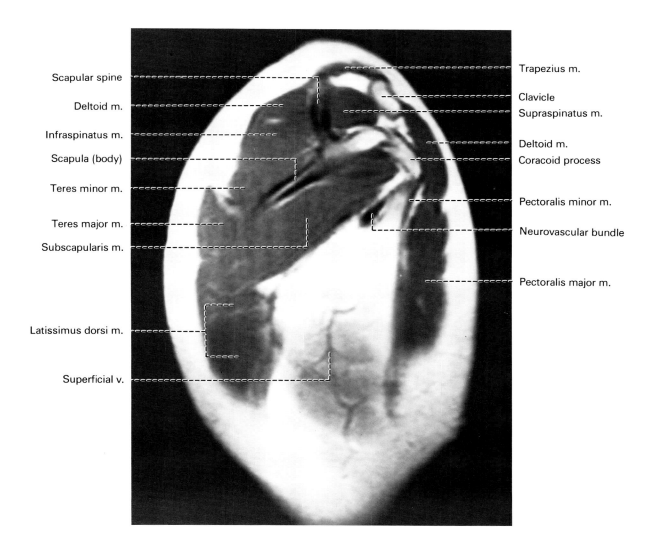

Figure 1.3.7

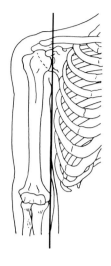

1. Anteriorly the deltoid originates from the clavicle.

2. Note the relationship of the rotator cuff muscles to the scapula from which they all originate.

3. The coracobrachialis and short head of biceps cannot be separated close to their origin from the coracoid process.

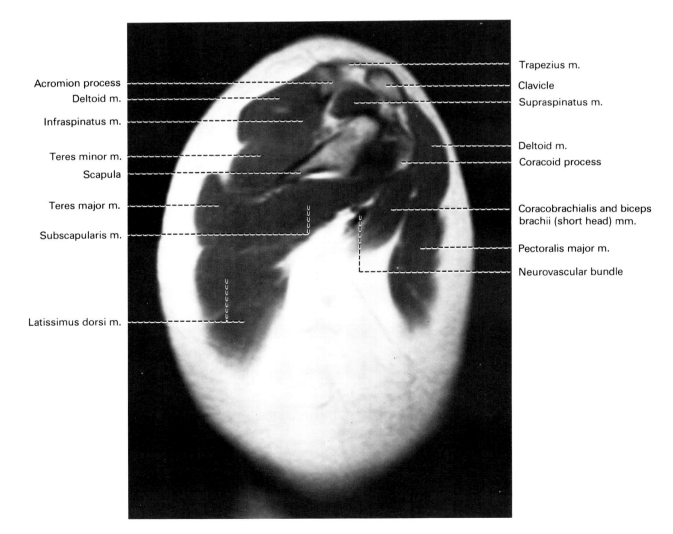

Figure 1.3.8

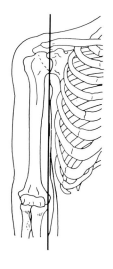

1. Subscapularis is demonstrated coursing toward its insertion on the lesser tuberosity.

2. The neurovascular bundle is seen posteromedial to the coracobrachialis.

3. The glenoid is partially demonstrated on this section.

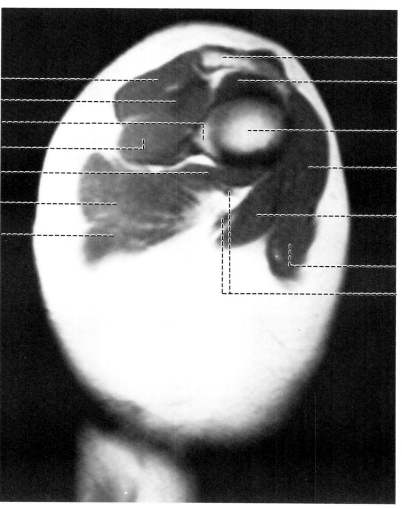

Deltoid m.

Infraspinatus m.

Glenoid

Teres minor m.

Subscapularis m.

Teres major m.

Latissimus dorsi m.

Acromion process

Supraspinatus m.

Humeral head

Deltoid m.

Coracobrachialis and biceps brachii (short head) mm.

Pectoralis major m.

Neurovascular bundle

Figure 1.3.9

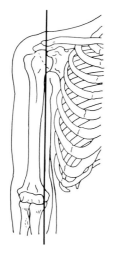

1. Teres major and latissimus dorsi have inserted on the crest of the lesser tuberosity.

2. In this section the muscle bellies of supraspinatus, infraspinatus, and teres minor are well demonstrated.

3. Coracobrachialis is seen on the medial aspect of the humeral shaft.

4. Note that a portion of the deltoid originates from the acromion process.

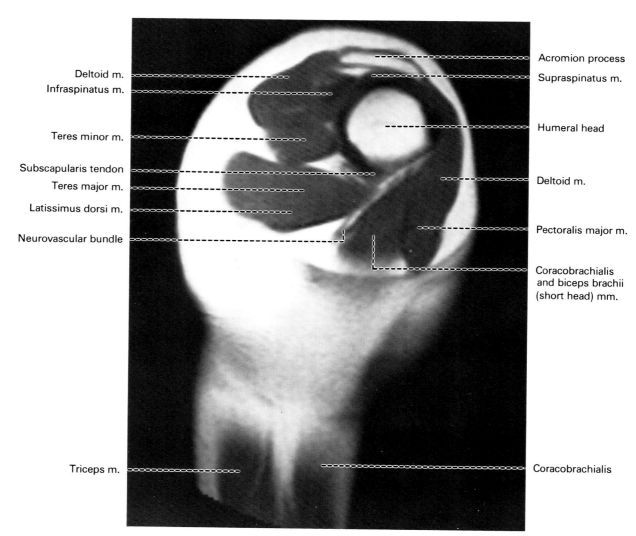

Figure 1.3.10

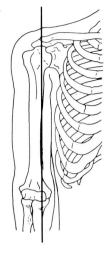

1. Note the relationship of the acromion process to the rotator cuff and the supraspinatus tendon immediately beneath the acromion.

2. Prior to its insertion, pectoralis major courses over the tendon of the long head of the biceps on the anterior aspect of the humerus.

3. Anteriorly, the deltoid muscle covers both the tendon of the long head of biceps and tendon of pectoralis major.

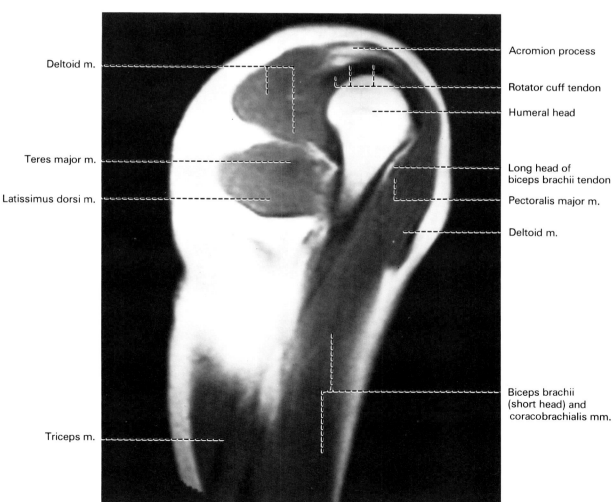

Deltoid m.

Teres major m.

Latissimus dorsi m.

Triceps m.

Acromion process

Rotator cuff tendon

Humeral head

Long head of biceps brachii tendon

Pectoralis major m.

Deltoid m.

Biceps brachii (short head) and coracobrachialis mm.

Figure 1.3.11

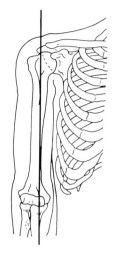

1. The posterior humeral circumflex artery is demonstrated after it exits the quadrangular space.

2. Teres major and latissimus dorsi have merged before their insertion and are difficult to separate.

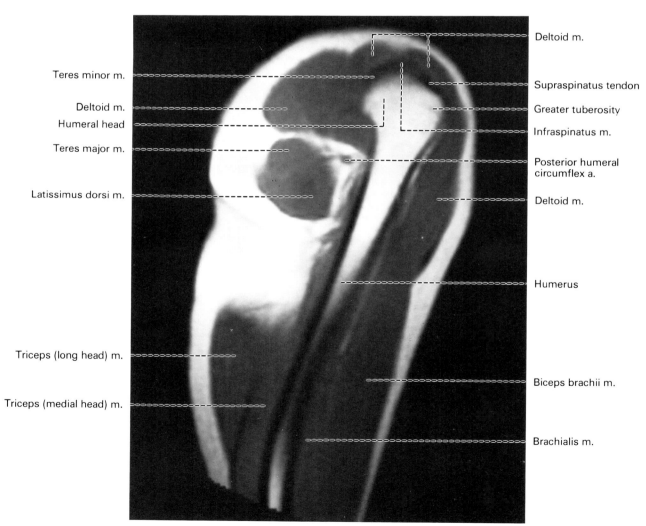

Figure 1.3.12

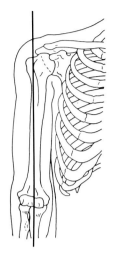

1. The long head of triceps originates from the infraglenoid tuberosity.

2. Note the insertion of supraspinatus, infraspinatus, and teres minor tendons on the greater tuberosity as they form part of the rotator cuff.

3. The deltoid surrounds the rotator cuff tendons and muscles.

4. Teres major and latissimus dorsi course together to insert on the crest of the lesser tuberosity on the crest of the greater tuberosity of the humerus.

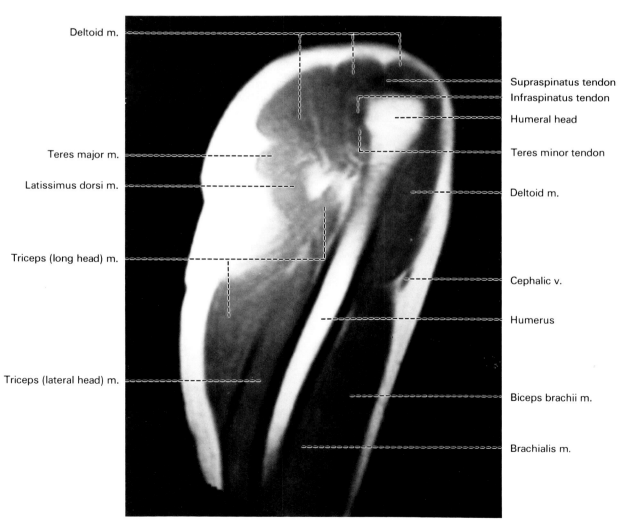

Figure 1.3.13

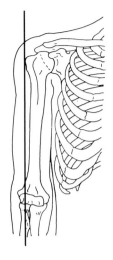

1. Note the multipennate configuration of the deltoid muscle.

2. The fascicles of the deltoid converge to insert on the deltoid tuberosity.

3. The biceps and triceps are demonstrated on the anterior and posterior aspects of the arm, respectively.

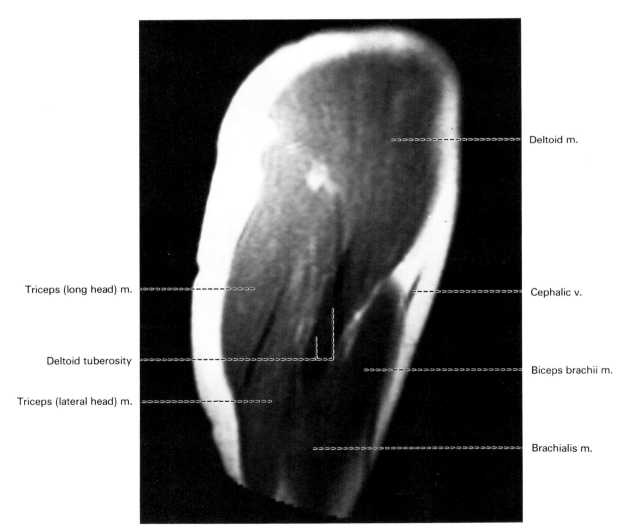

Deltoid m.

Triceps (long head) m.

Cephalic v.

Deltoid tuberosity

Biceps brachii m.

Triceps (lateral head) m.

Brachialis m.

Chapter 2

ARM

AXIAL

Figure 2.1.1

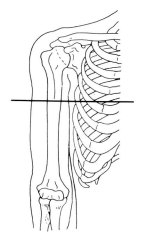

1. This section is through the proximal arm just distal to the axilla.

2. Deltoid inserts on the deltoid tuberosity.

3. Coracobrachialis inserts on the medial aspect of the proximal humerus.

4. Note the spiral course of the radial nerve behind the humerus accompanied by the deep (profunda) brachial artery.

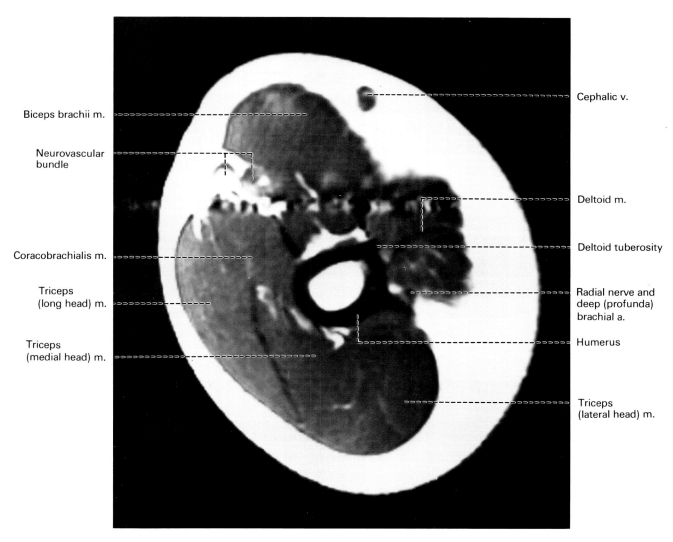

Biceps brachii m.

Neurovascular bundle

Coracobrachialis m.

Triceps (long head) m.

Triceps (medial head) m.

Cephalic v.

Deltoid m.

Deltoid tuberosity

Radial nerve and deep (profunda) brachial a.

Humerus

Triceps (lateral head) m.

Figure 2.1.2

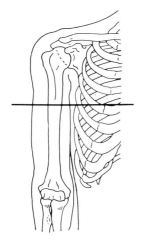

1. The cephalic vein courses proximally in the subcutaneous tissues on the anterolateral surface of the arm. It then courses medially in the deltopectoral groove prior to draining into the axillary vein.

2. Deltoid and coracobrachialis diminish in size as they complete their insertion on the humerus.

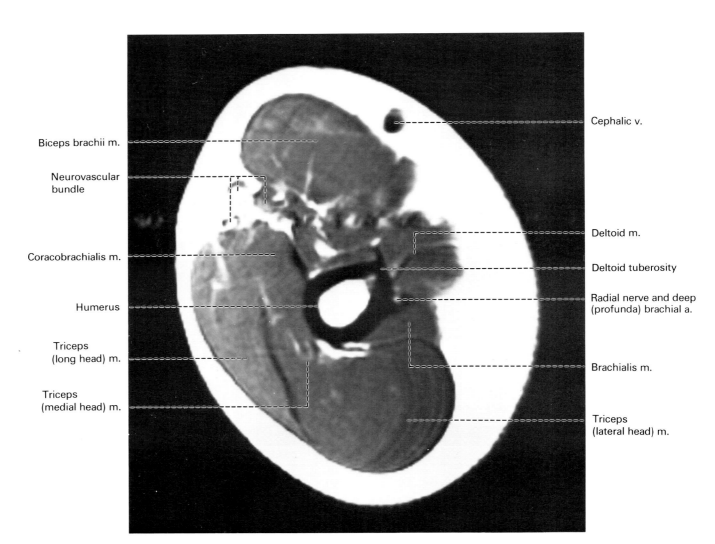

Figure 2.1.3

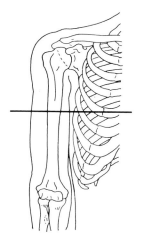

1. Note the origin of brachialis from the humerus.

2. All three heads of triceps are clearly depicted in this section.

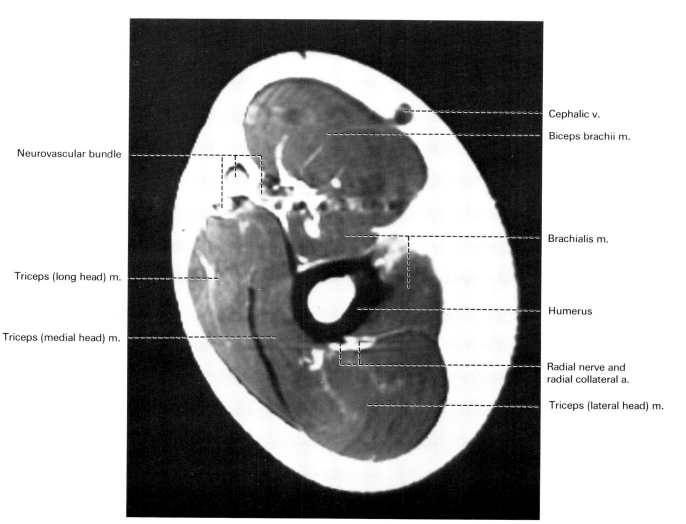

Neurovascular bundle

Triceps (long head) m.

Triceps (medial head) m.

Cephalic v.

Biceps brachii m.

Brachialis m.

Humerus

Radial nerve and radial collateral a.

Triceps (lateral head) m.

Figure 2.1.4

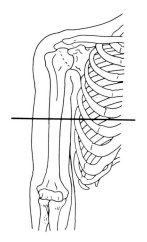

1. Brachialis continues to enlarge as sections move distally in the arm.

2. Note the location of the medial and lateral intermuscular septa.

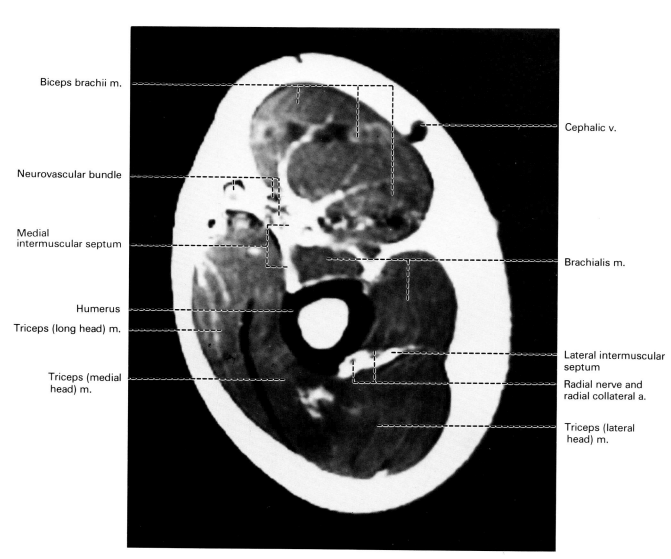

Biceps brachii m.

Neurovascular bundle

Medial intermuscular septum

Humerus

Triceps (long head) m.

Triceps (medial head) m.

Cephalic v.

Brachialis m.

Lateral intermuscular septum

Radial nerve and radial collateral a.

Triceps (lateral head) m.

Figure 2.1.5

1. The three principal muscles of the arm depicted in this section are biceps brachii, brachialis, and triceps.

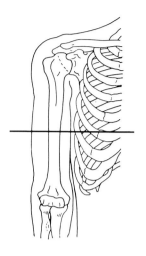

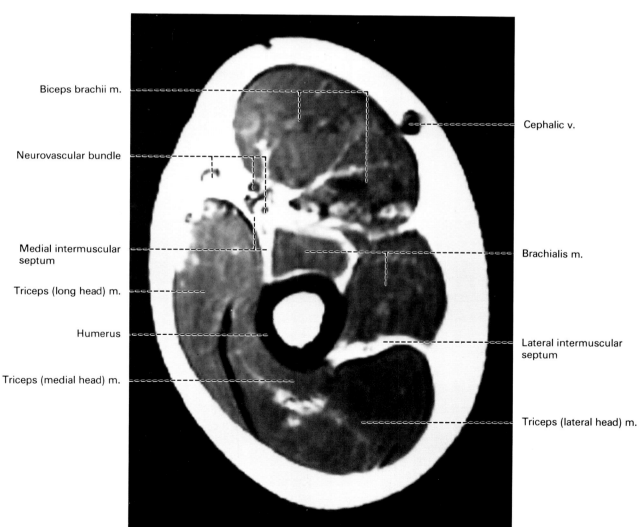

Biceps brachii m.

Neurovascular bundle

Medial intermuscular septum

Triceps (long head) m.

Humerus

Triceps (medial head) m.

Cephalic v.

Brachialis m.

Lateral intermuscular septum

Triceps (lateral head) m.

Figure 2.1.6

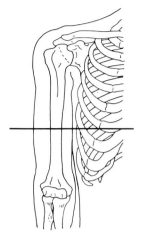

1. The radial nerve courses distally in the radial groove. It is accompanied by the radial collateral artery, a branch of the deep brachial artery.

2. At this level, the neurovascular bundle consists of the brachial artery and veins, basilic vein, and median and ulnar nerves.

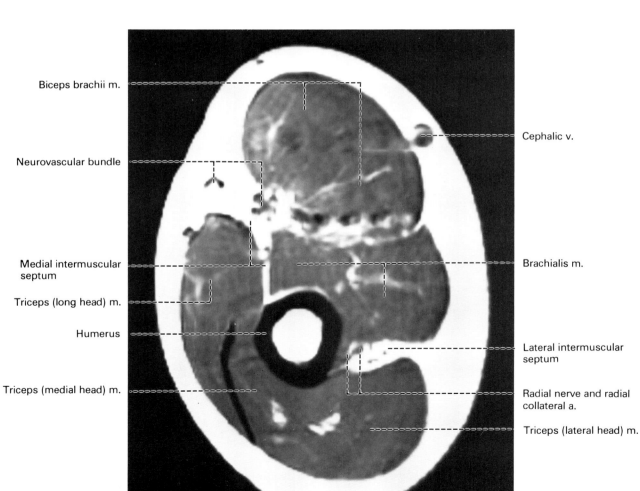

Biceps brachii m.

Cephalic v.

Neurovascular bundle

Medial intermuscular septum

Brachialis m.

Triceps (long head) m.

Humerus

Lateral intermuscular septum

Triceps (medial head) m.

Radial nerve and radial collateral a.

Triceps (lateral head) m.

Figure 2.1.7

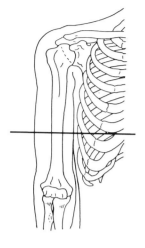

1. The section is through the insertion of the coracobrachialis on the medial aspect of the midshaft of the humerus.

2. The triceps muscle is well developed into three heads.

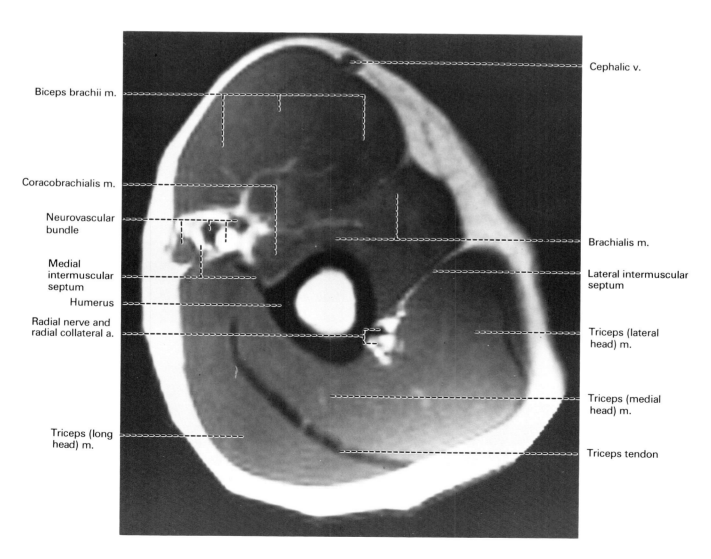

Biceps brachii m.

Coracobrachialis m.

Neurovascular bundle

Medial intermuscular septum

Humerus

Radial nerve and radial collateral a.

Triceps (long head) m.

Cephalic v.

Brachialis m.

Lateral intermuscular septum

Triceps (lateral head) m.

Triceps (medial head) m.

Triceps tendon

Figure 2.1.8

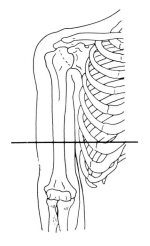

1. The brachialis muscle originates from the anterior surface of the distal half of the humerus.

2. The cephalic vein is demonstrated in the subcutaneous tissues on the anterior surface of the arm. It courses proximally to drain into the axillary vein at the deltopectoral triangle.

3. The medial and lateral intermuscular septa are clearly seen in this section.

4. A thick tendon separates the medial and long heads of triceps.

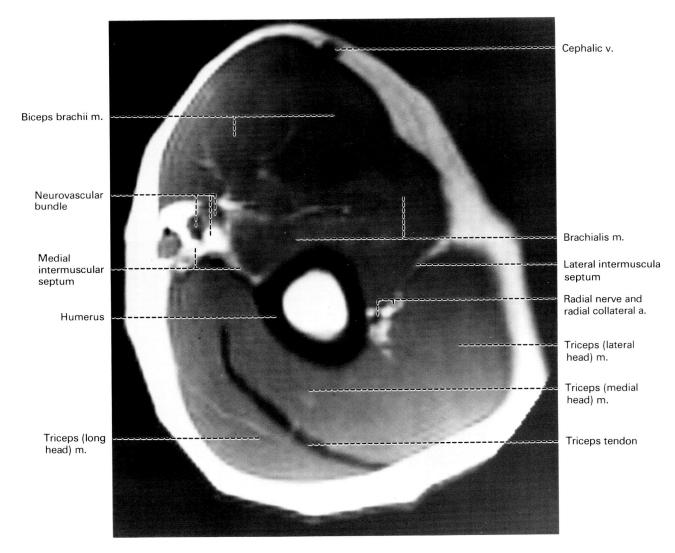

Cephalic v.

Biceps brachii m.

Neurovascular bundle

Medial intermuscular septum

Humerus

Triceps (long head) m.

Brachialis m.

Lateral intermuscula septum

Radial nerve and radial collateral a.

Triceps (lateral head) m.

Triceps (medial head) m.

Triceps tendon

Figure 2.1.9

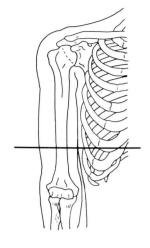

1. The ulnar nerve separates from the neurovascular bundle in this section. It has an independent course and lies posterior to the medial epicondyle at the elbow.

2. The radial nerve leaves the radial groove of the humerus and becomes anterolaterally located in the distal arm.

3. At this level, the largest muscle in the anterior compartment is biceps brachii.

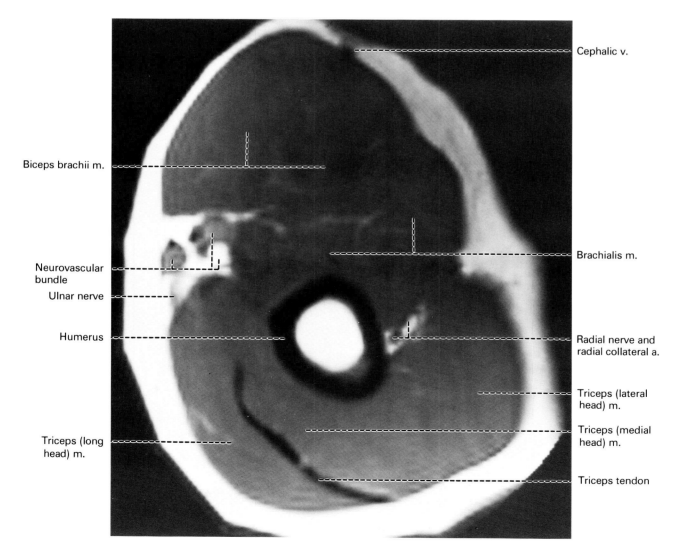

Biceps brachii m.

Neurovascular bundle

Ulnar nerve

Humerus

Triceps (long head) m.

Cephalic v.

Brachialis m.

Radial nerve and radial collateral a.

Triceps (lateral head) m.

Triceps (medial head) m.

Triceps tendon

Figure 2.1.10

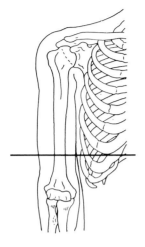

1. The distal humerus begins to flatten, and the lateral supracondylar crest appears at this level.

2. Brachioradialis originates on the proximal part of the lateral supracondylar crest.

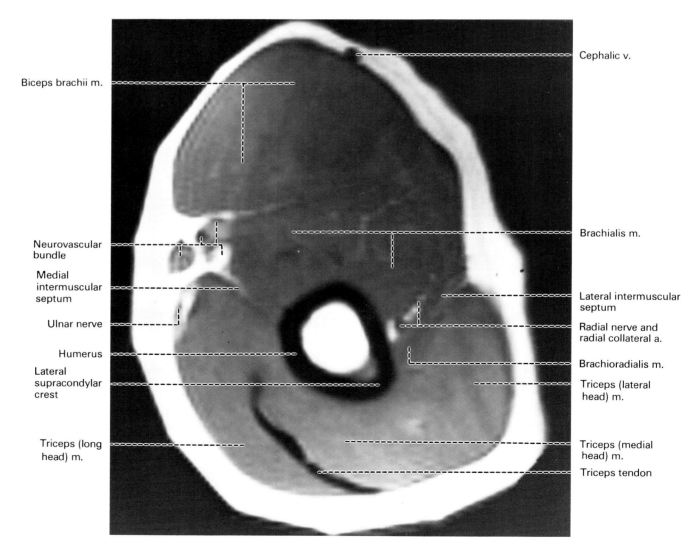

Figure 2.1.11

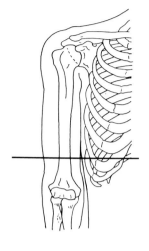

1. The ulnar nerve continues its course posterior to the neurovascular bundle on the medial surface of the triceps muscle.

2. As the radial nerve assumes a more anterior position in the distal arm, it courses between the brachioradialis and brachialis muscles.

3. The median nerve continues in the distal arm as part of the neurovascular bundle in close proximity to the brachial artery.

4. A nutrient vessel is identified in the medullary space of the humerus.

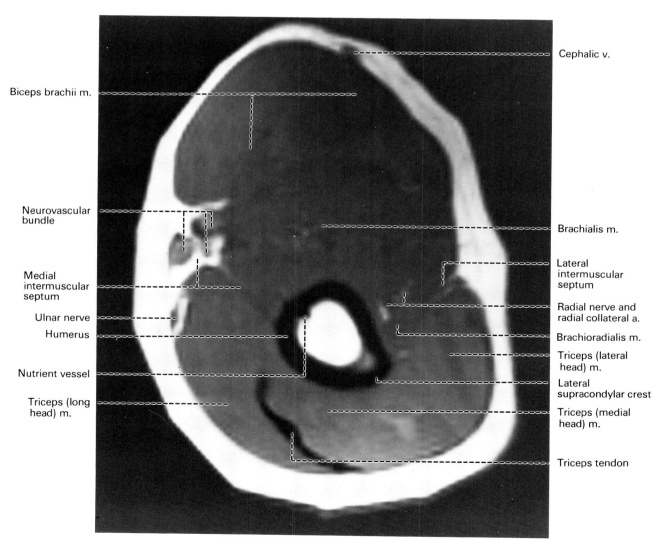

Figure 2.1.12

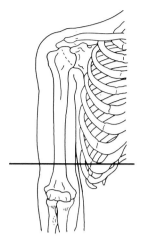

1. Extensor carpi radialis longus originates from the distal part of the lateral supracondylar crest.

2. Brachialis becomes the largest muscle of the anterior compartment in the distal arm.

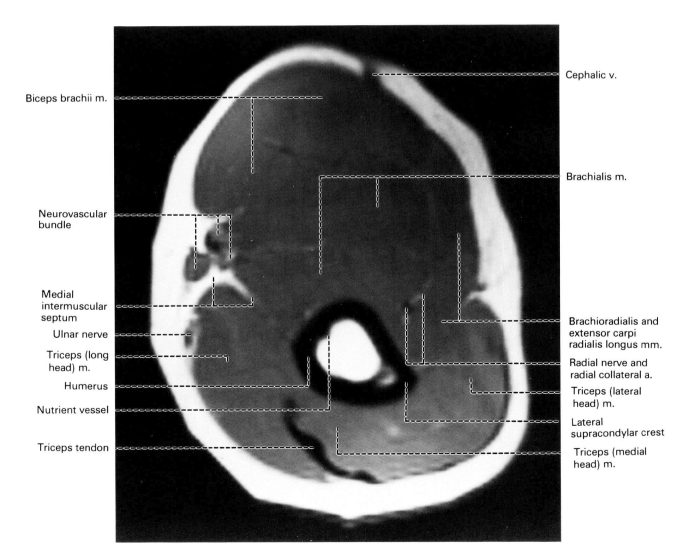

Figure 2.1.13

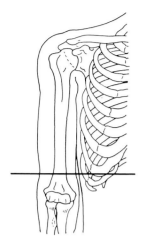

1. Biceps brachii tapers in the distal arm.

2. Both brachioradialis and extensor carpi radialis longus originate from the lateral supracondylar crest. The two muscles cannot be separated in this section.

3. The triceps tapers distally and its tendinous part becomes more prominent.

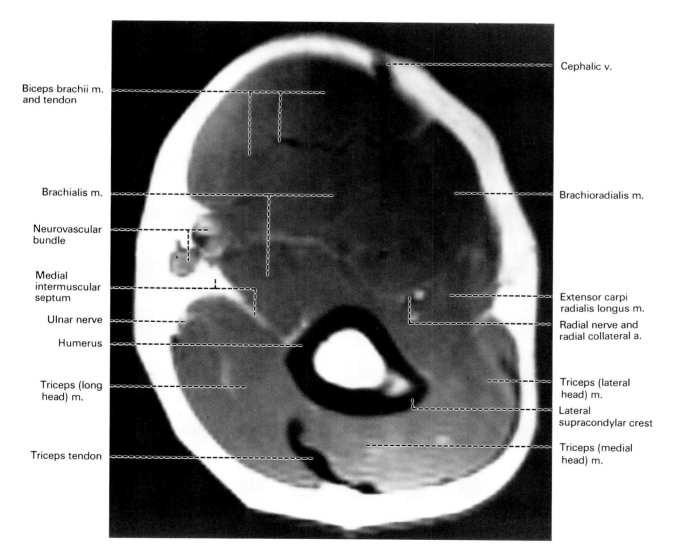

Biceps brachii m. and tendon

Brachialis m.

Neurovascular bundle

Medial intermuscular septum

Ulnar nerve

Humerus

Triceps (long head) m.

Triceps tendon

Cephalic v.

Brachioradialis m.

Extensor carpi radialis longus m.

Radial nerve and radial collateral a.

Triceps (lateral head) m.

Lateral supracondylar crest

Triceps (medial head) m.

Figure 2.1.14

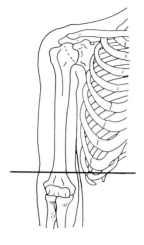

1. This section is through the supracondylar region. The continued flattening of the humerus is seen.

2. Compared to brachialis, biceps brachii appears smaller at this level.

3. In the distal arm the radial nerve courses distally in the anterior compartment between brachialis and brachioradialis.

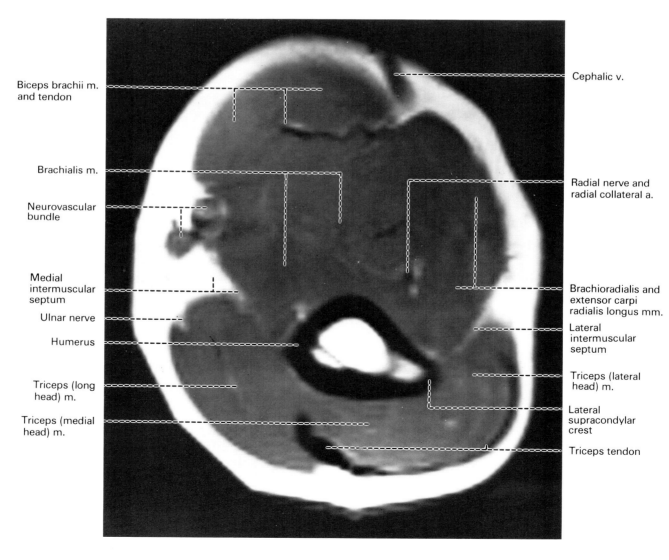

Biceps brachii m. and tendon

Brachialis m.

Neurovascular bundle

Medial intermuscular septum

Ulnar nerve

Humerus

Triceps (long head) m.

Triceps (medial head) m.

Cephalic v.

Radial nerve and radial collateral a.

Brachioradialis and extensor carpi radialis longus mm.

Lateral intermuscular septum

Triceps (lateral head) m.

Lateral supracondylar crest

Triceps tendon

CORONAL

Figure 2.2.1

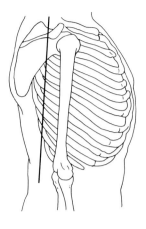

1. This section passes through the most posterior aspect of the arm.

2. The triceps (long head) is partially demonstrated.

3. Some of the shoulder muscles are depicted in this section but they are demonstrated to better advantage on the sections of the shoulder (see Ch. 1).

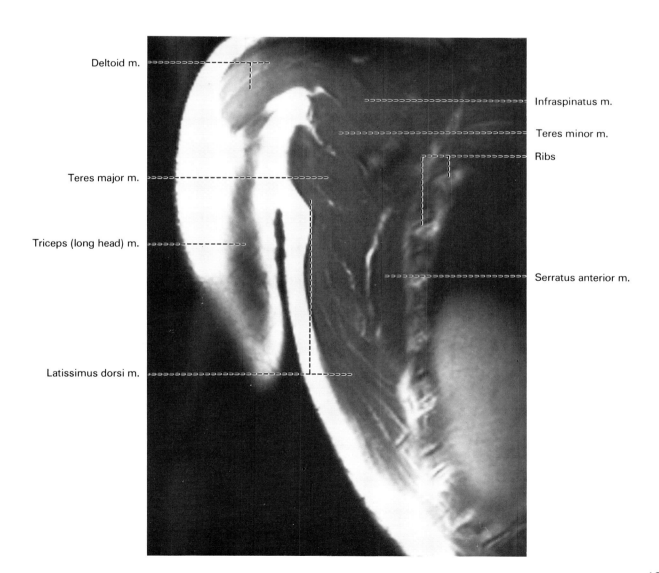

Deltoid m.

Infraspinatus m.

Teres minor m.

Ribs

Teres major m.

Triceps (long head) m.

Serratus anterior m.

Latissimus dorsi m.

Figure 2.2.2

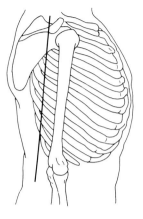

1. The long head of the triceps courses distally, posterior to teres major and latissimus dorsi and anterior to teres minor.

2. The posterior portion of the deltoid originates from the spine of the scapula.

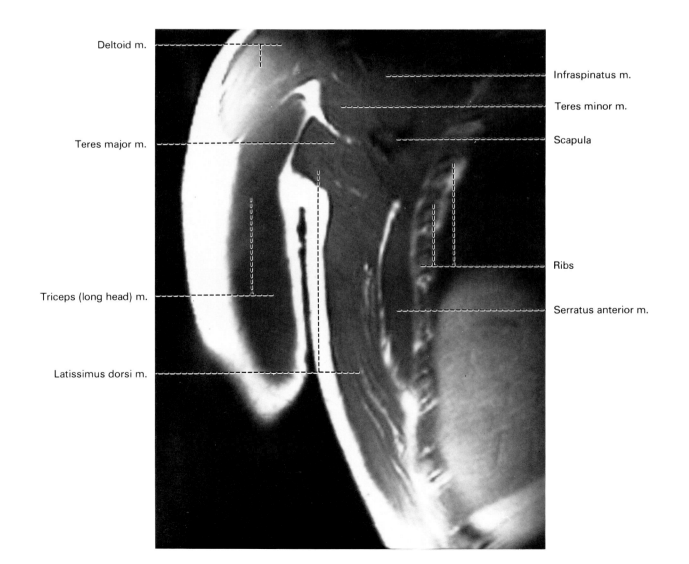

Figure 2.2.3

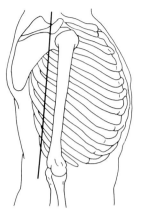

1. The only muscle of the posterior compartment of the arm is triceps.

2. Triceps is separated from the anterior compartment muscles by the medial and lateral intermuscular septa.

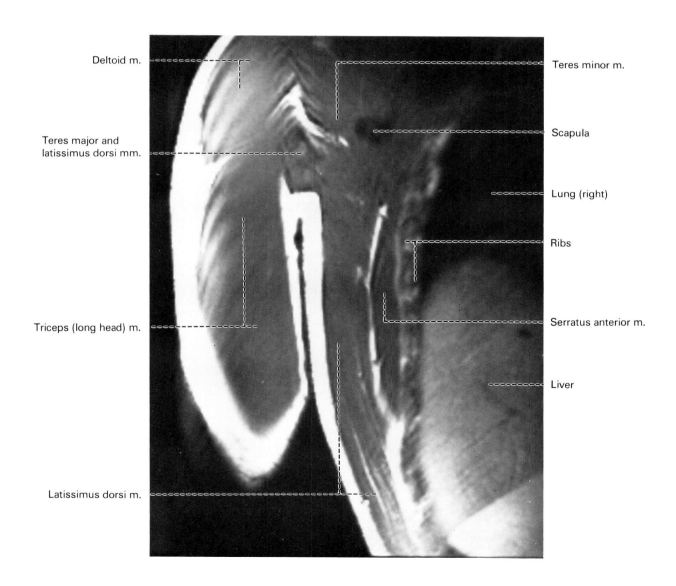

Deltoid m.

Teres major and latissimus dorsi mm.

Triceps (long head) m.

Latissimus dorsi m.

Teres minor m.

Scapula

Lung (right)

Ribs

Serratus anterior m.

Liver

Figure 2.2.4

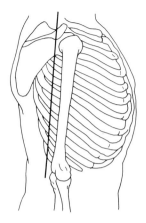

1. Note the extent of latissimus dorsi and serratus anterior muscles.

2. Latissimus dorsi originates from the lower six thoracic spinous processes, lumbar and sacral spinous processes, crest of the ilium, and lower four ribs. It inserts along with teres major on the crest of the lesser tuberosity.

3. The lateral head of the triceps is partially outlined.

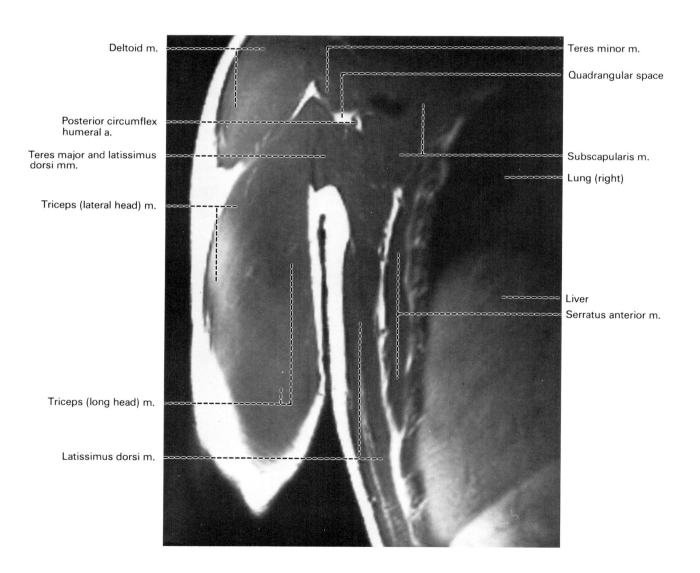

Figure 2.2.5

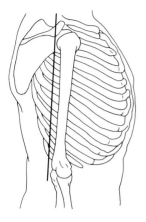

1. All three heads of triceps are demonstrated in this section.

2. The posterior circumflex humeral artery and axillary nerve exit through the quadrangular space.

3. The long and lateral heads of triceps cover the posterior surface of its medial head.

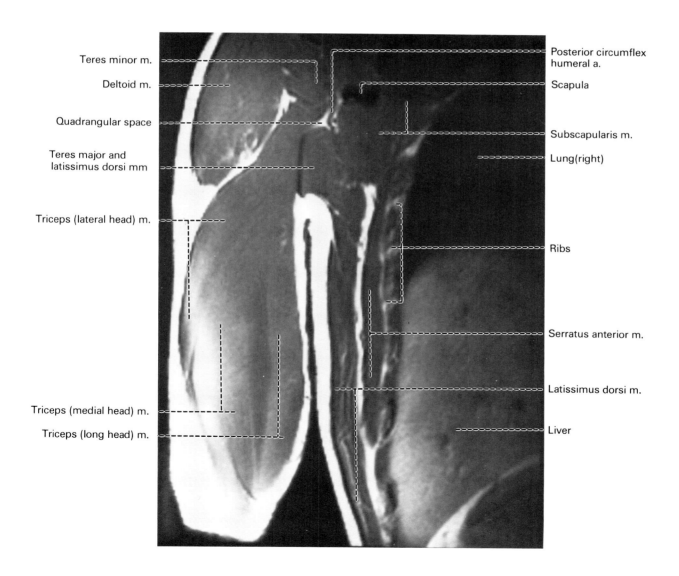

Teres minor m.
Deltoid m.
Quadrangular space
Teres major and latissimus dorsi mm
Triceps (lateral head) m.
Triceps (medial head) m.
Triceps (long head) m.

Posterior circumflex humeral a.
Scapula
Subscapularis m.
Lung(right)
Ribs
Serratus anterior m.
Latissimus dorsi m.
Liver

Figure 2.2.6

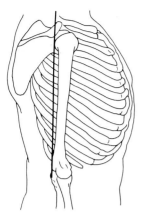

1. The course of the radial nerve and deep (profunda) brachial artery is partially outlined in this section.

2. The radial nerve and deep (profunda) brachial artery have a spiral posterior course close to the surface of the bone in the radial groove.

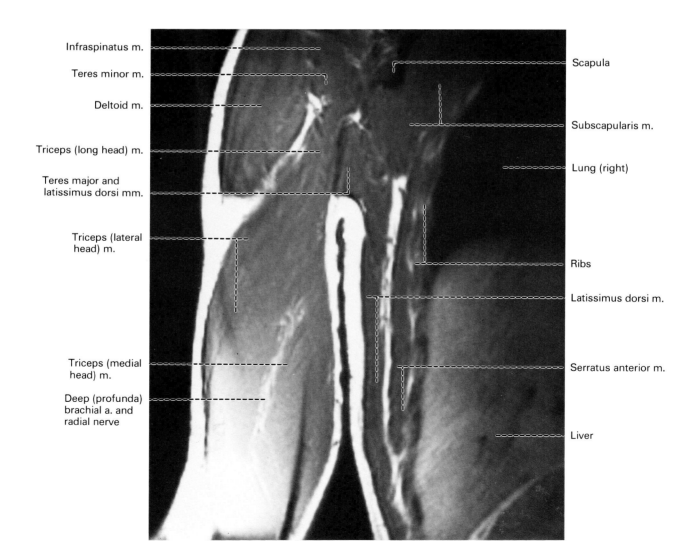

Infraspinatus m.

Teres minor m.

Deltoid m.

Triceps (long head) m.

Teres major and latissimus dorsi mm.

Triceps (lateral head) m.

Triceps (medial head) m.

Deep (profunda) brachial a. and radial nerve

Scapula

Subscapularis m.

Lung (right)

Ribs

Latissimus dorsi m.

Serratus anterior m.

Liver

Figure 2.2.7

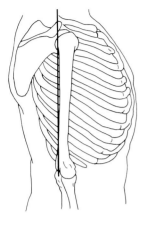

1. Note the relationship of teres minor to the long head of triceps. The long head of triceps passes between teres minor and teres major.

2. The long head of triceps originates at the infraglenoid tuberosity.

3. Note the posterior humeral circumflex artery in this section just posterior to the humeral neck.

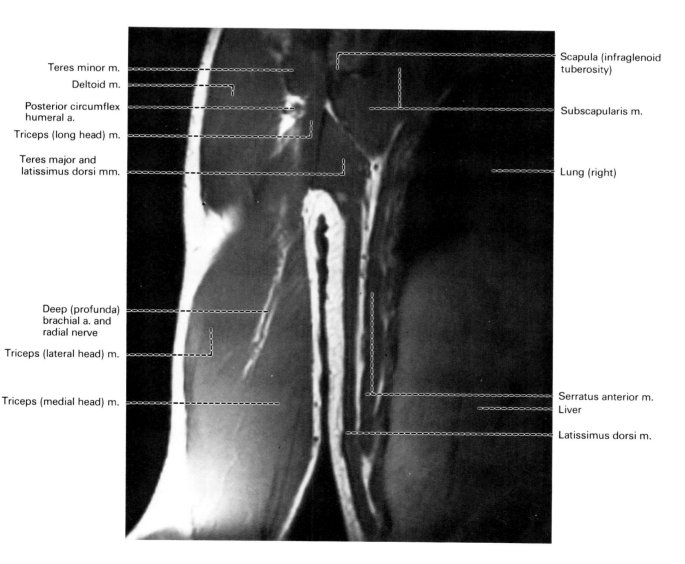

Teres minor m.

Deltoid m.

Posterior circumflex humeral a.

Triceps (long head) m.

Teres major and latissimus dorsi mm.

Deep (profunda) brachial a. and radial nerve

Triceps (lateral head) m.

Triceps (medial head) m.

Scapula (infraglenoid tuberosity)

Subscapularis m.

Lung (right)

Serratus anterior m.
Liver

Latissimus dorsi m.

Figure 2.2.8

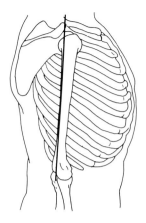

1. This section is through the posterior shaft of the humerus.

2. The origin of brachialis is partially demonstrated. It originates from the distal half of the anterior surface of the humerus.

3. Note the radial collateral artery (a terminal branch of the deep brachial) and the radial nerve posterior to the brachialis muscle.

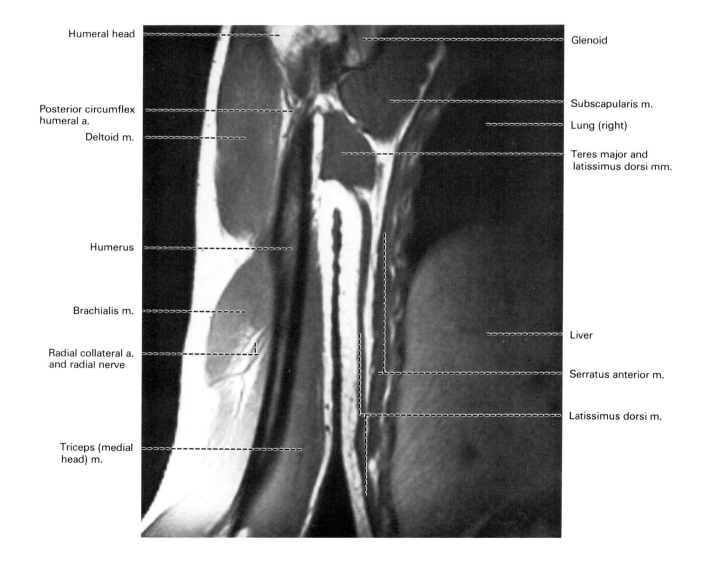

Figure 2.2.9

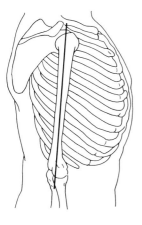

1. Note the deltoid insertion on the deltoid tuberosity.

2. Teres major and latissimus dorsi are seen approaching their insertion on the crest of the lesser tuberosity.

3. The anterior margin of latissimus dorsi is demonstrated in this section.

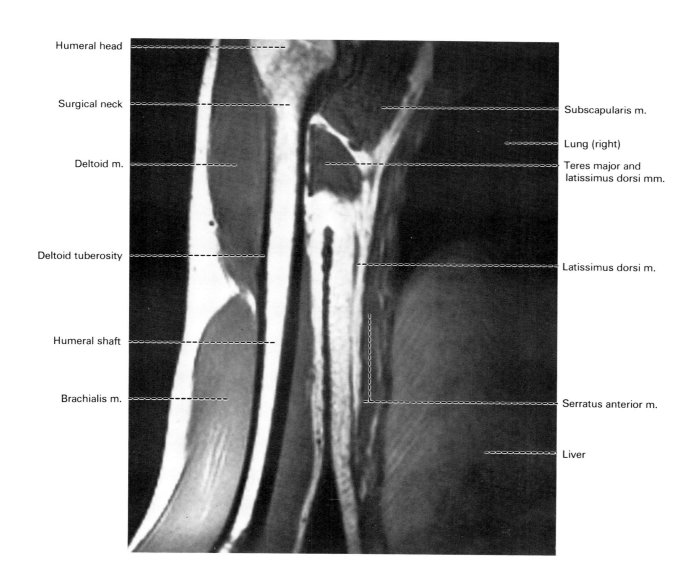

Humeral head

Surgical neck

Deltoid m.

Deltoid tuberosity

Humeral shaft

Brachialis m.

Subscapularis m.

Lung (right)

Teres major and latissimus dorsi mm.

Latissimus dorsi m.

Serratus anterior m.

Liver

Figure 2.2.10

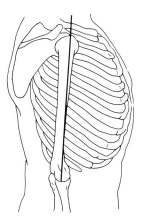

1. This section passes through the anterior shaft of the humerus.

2. Teres major and latissimus dorsi are seen inserting on the crest of the lesser tuberosity.

3. Note serratus anterior covering the lateral aspect of the rib cage. It originates from the upper eight ribs.

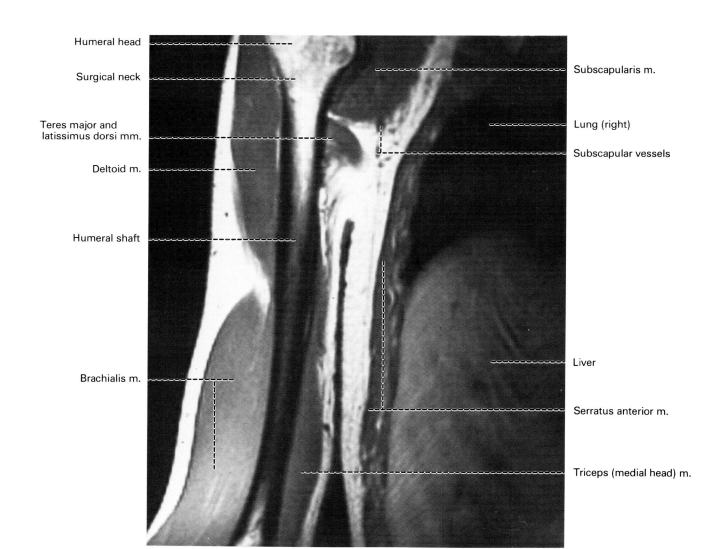

Figure 2.2.11

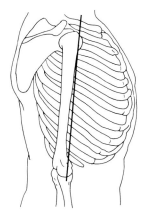

1. Note the insertion of pectoralis major on the crest of the greater tuberosity.

2. Neurovascular bundle is seen coursing distally on the anterior surface of subscapularis and medial surface of coracobrachialis.

3. The long head of the biceps tendon is demonstrated in this section. It is situated just lateral to the short head of biceps.

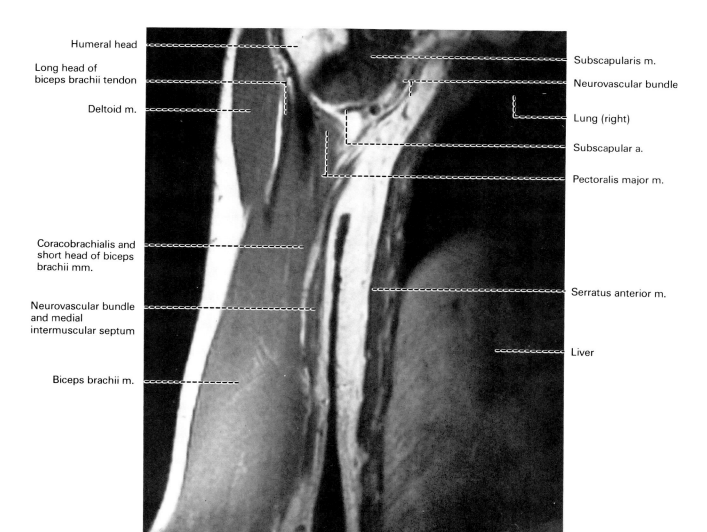

Humeral head

Long head of biceps brachii tendon

Deltoid m.

Coracobrachialis and short head of biceps brachii mm.

Neurovascular bundle and medial intermuscular septum

Biceps brachii m.

Subscapularis m.

Neurovascular bundle

Lung (right)

Subscapular a.

Pectoralis major m.

Serratus anterior m.

Liver

Figure 2.2.12

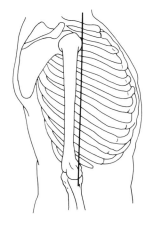

1. Note the insertion of the subscapularis muscle on the lesser tuberosity.

2. The deltoid muscle covers all the other muscle insertions at the humeral head and neck.

3. The anterior humeral circumflex artery is clearly depicted in this section as it originates from the axillary artery.

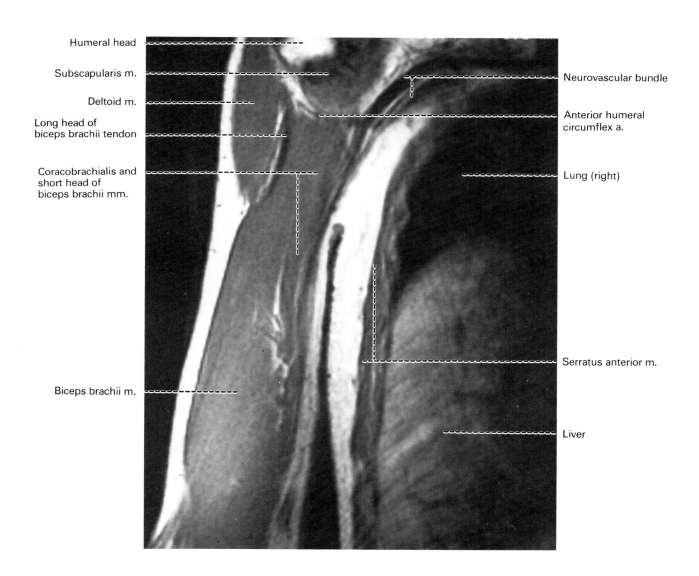

Humeral head

Subscapularis m.

Deltoid m.

Long head of biceps brachii tendon

Coracobrachialis and short head of biceps brachii mm.

Biceps brachii m.

Neurovascular bundle

Anterior humeral circumflex a.

Lung (right)

Serratus anterior m.

Liver

Figure 2.2.13

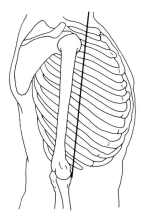

1. The axillary vein courses anterior to the axillary artery.

2. The anterior portion of the deltoid originates on the distal third of the clavicle and acromion process.

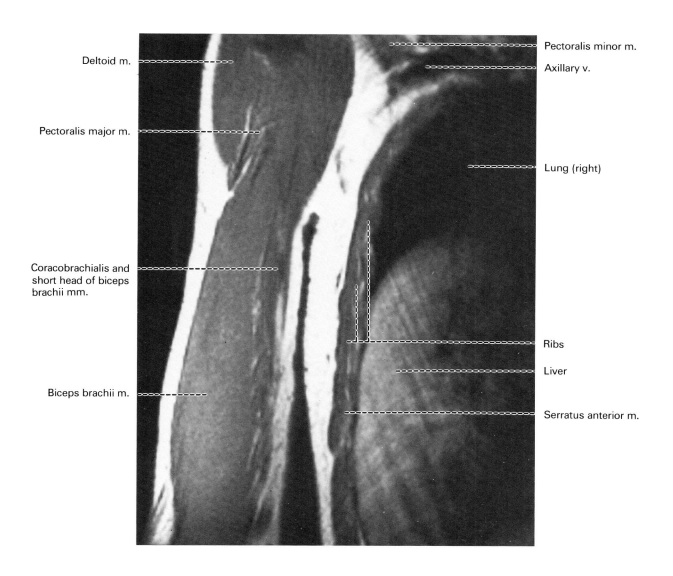

Deltoid m.

Pectoralis major m.

Coracobrachialis and short head of biceps brachii mm.

Biceps brachii m.

Pectoralis minor m.

Axillary v.

Lung (right)

Ribs

Liver

Serratus anterior m.

Figure 2.2.14

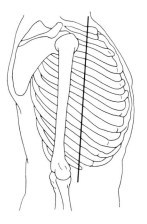

1. This section passes superficially through the anterior aspect of arm and shoulder.

2. The cephalic vein is noted in subcutaneous tissues on the anterolateral aspect of the arm prior to entering the deltopectoral groove.

3. Pectoralis minor lies anterior to the neurovascular bundle.

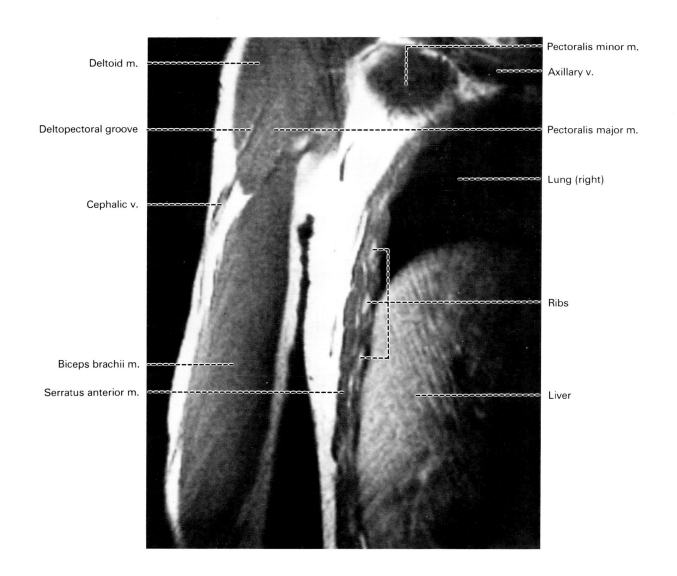

Figure 2.2.15

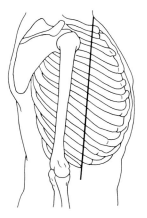

1. This section passes through the most anterior portion of biceps brachii.

2. The clavicular head of pectoralis major is demonstrated in this section.

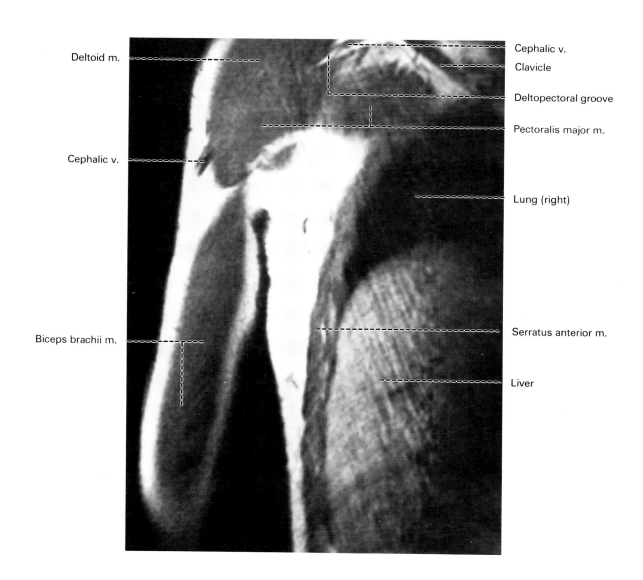

Figure 2.3.1

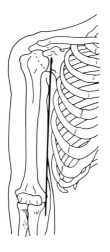

1. This is the most medial section of the arm.

2. The brachial artery and median nerve are seen coursing distally on the anterior surface of the brachialis muscle.

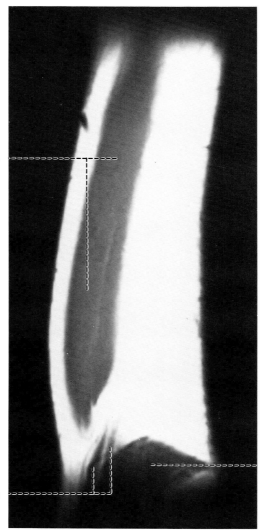

Biceps brachii m.

Superficial flexor mm.

Brachial a. and median nerve

Figure 2.3.2

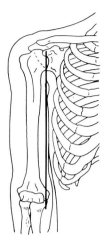

1. Note the neurovascular bundle coursing distally on the anterior surface of triceps (long head) in the proximal arm and on the anterior surface of brachialis in the distal arm.

2. Note the length of the biceps muscle. It traverses two joints, the shoulder and elbow.

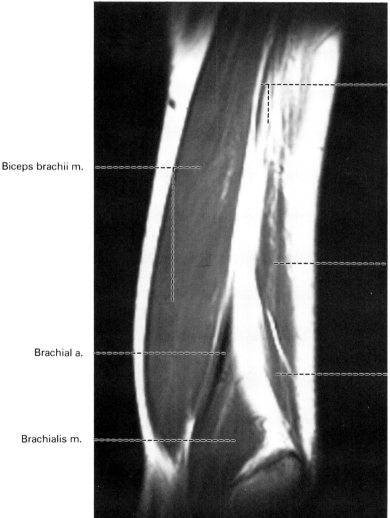

Figure 2.3.3

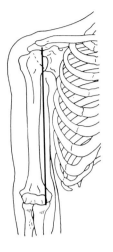

1. Note the medial intermuscular septum separating triceps from the muscles in the anterior compartment.

2. Coracobrachialis is demonstrated approaching its insertion on the shaft of the proximal humerus.

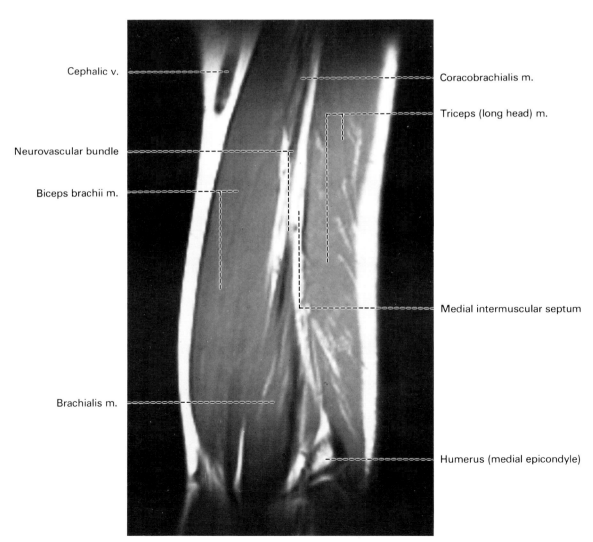

Cephalic v.

Coracobrachialis m.

Triceps (long head) m.

Neurovascular bundle

Biceps brachii m.

Medial intermuscular septum

Brachialis m.

Humerus (medial epicondyle)

Figure 2.3.4

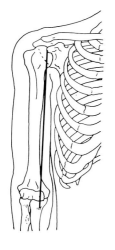

1. The olecranon fossa and posterior fat pad are well depicted in this section.

2. The coronoid fossa and anterior fat pad are also seen.

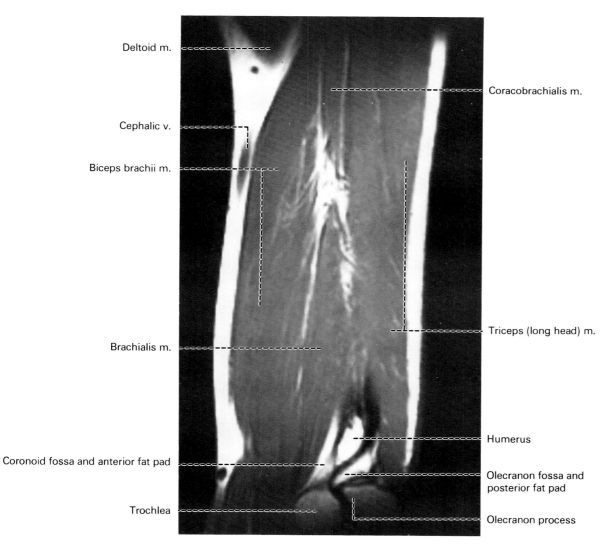

Figure 2.3.5

1. The medial head of triceps is covered by the long and lateral heads.

2. Note the origin of brachialis from the anterior surface of the humerus.

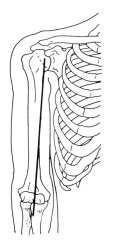

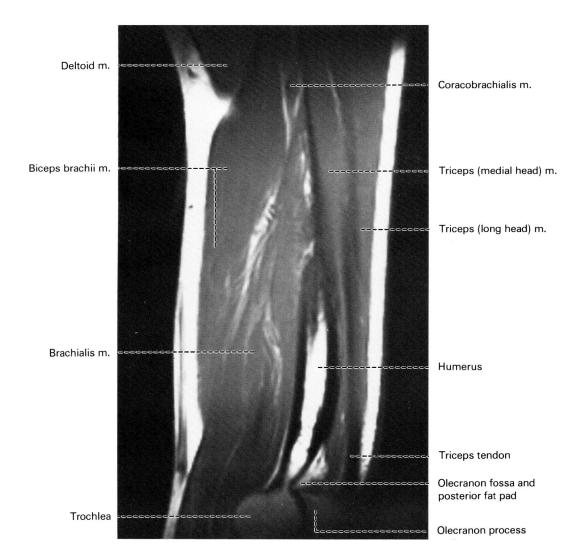

Deltoid m.

Coracobrachialis m.

Biceps brachii m.

Triceps (medial head) m.

Triceps (long head) m.

Brachialis m.

Humerus

Triceps tendon

Olecranon fossa and posterior fat pad

Trochlea

Olecranon process

Figure 2.3.6

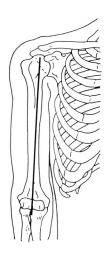

1. As the sections proceed laterally some of the extensor muscles become evident.

Deltoid m.

Triceps (lateral head) m.

Biceps brachii m.

Humerus

Brachialis m.

Triceps (medial head) m.

Brachioradialis m.

Extensor carpi radialis longus m.

Capitulum

Figure 2.3.7

1. Brachioradialis and extensor carpi radialis longus originate from the lateral supracondylar crest (ridge).

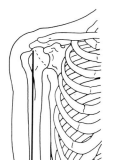

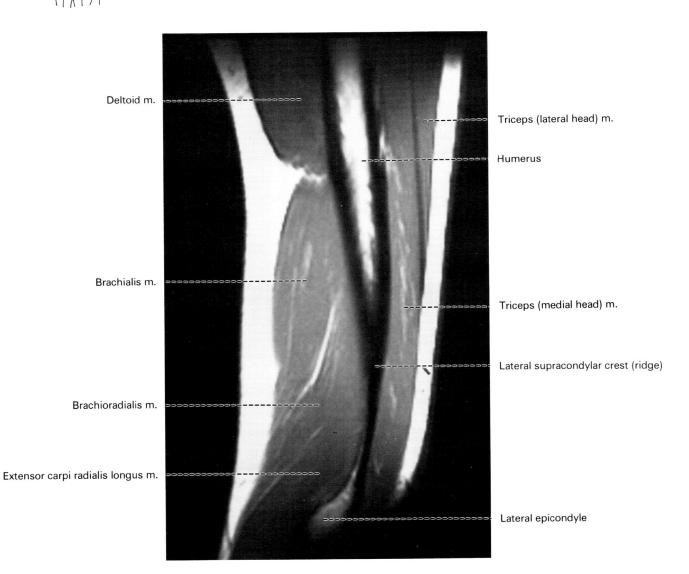

Deltoid m.

Triceps (lateral head) m.

Humerus

Brachialis m.

Triceps (medial head) m.

Lateral supracondylar crest (ridge)

Brachioradialis m.

Extensor carpi radialis longus m.

Lateral epicondyle

Figure 2.3.8

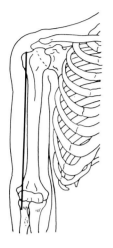

1. The radial nerve and deep (profunda) brachial artery course distally and posteriorly, adjacent to the humerus, in the radial nerve sulcus.

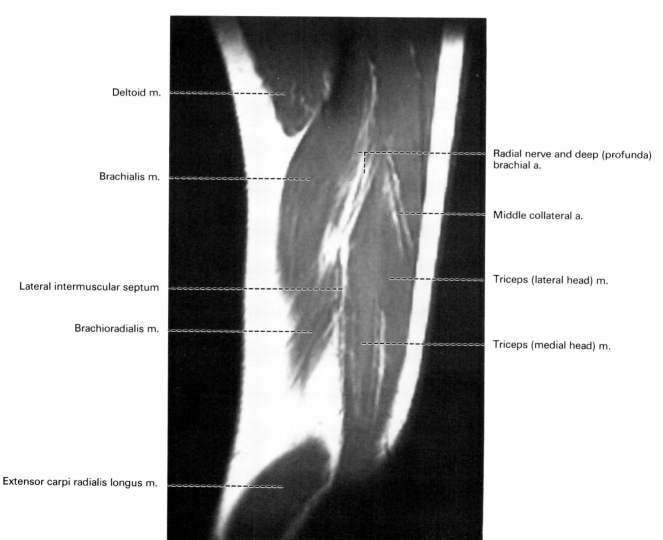

Deltoid m.

Brachialis m.

Lateral intermuscular septum

Brachioradialis m.

Extensor carpi radialis longus m.

Radial nerve and deep (profunda) brachial a.

Middle collateral a.

Triceps (lateral head) m.

Triceps (medial head) m.

Figure 2.3.9

1. In this lateral section the only prominent muscle is the lateral head of the triceps. Brachialis and deltoid are only partially demonstrated.

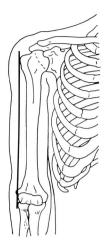

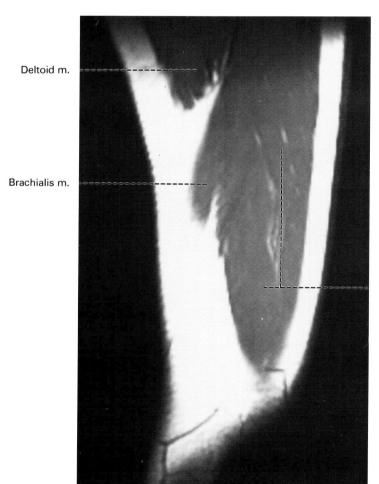

Deltoid m.

Brachialis m.

Triceps (lateral head) m.

Figure 2.3.10

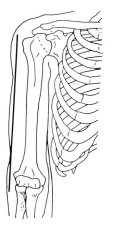

1. The lateral head of the triceps originates from the posterior and lateral surfaces of the humerus, superior and lateral to the radial (nerve) groove.

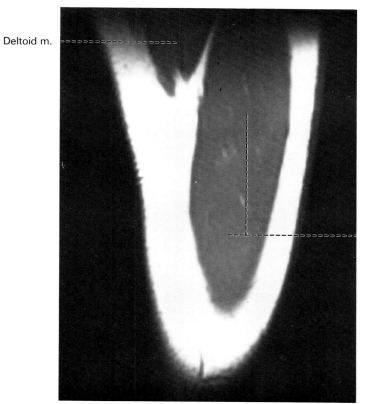

Deltoid m.

Triceps (lateral head) m.

Figure 2.3.11

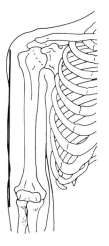

1. This is the most lateral section of the arm. Only the lateral aspect of triceps and deltoid is seen in this section.

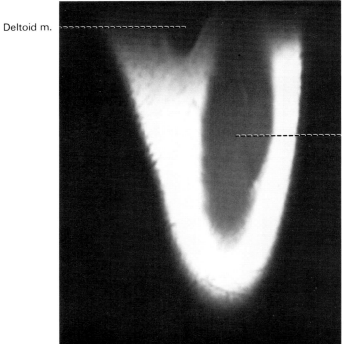

Deltoid m.

Triceps (lateral head) m.

Chapter 3

ELBOW

Figure 3.1.1

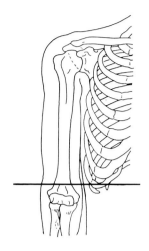

1. This section passes through the lateral epicondyle.

2. Extensor carpi radialis brevis originates from the lateral epicondyle.

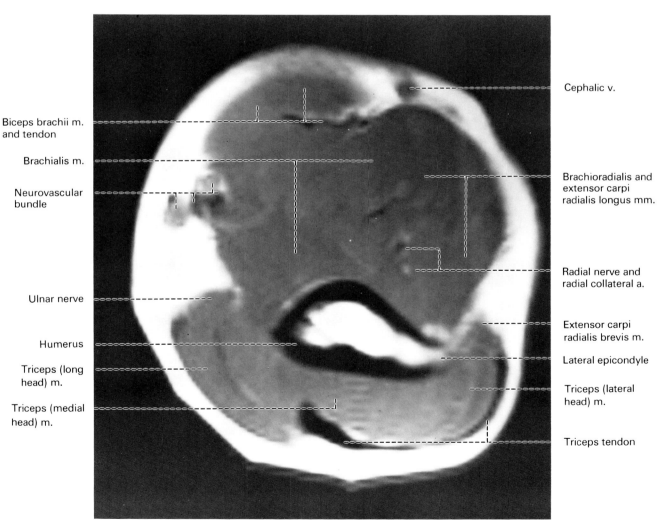

Biceps brachii m. and tendon

Brachialis m.

Neurovascular bundle

Ulnar nerve

Humerus

Triceps (long head) m.

Triceps (medial head) m.

Cephalic v.

Brachioradialis and extensor carpi radialis longus mm.

Radial nerve and radial collateral a.

Extensor carpi radialis brevis m.

Lateral epicondyle

Triceps (lateral head) m.

Triceps tendon

Figure 3.1.2

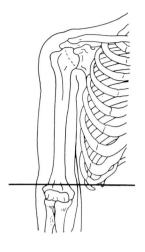

1. At this level biceps brachii is almost completely tendinous.

2. The brachialis tendon appears at this level.

3. The humerus completes its flattening and curves anteriorly (better demonstrated on the sagittal section) in this section.

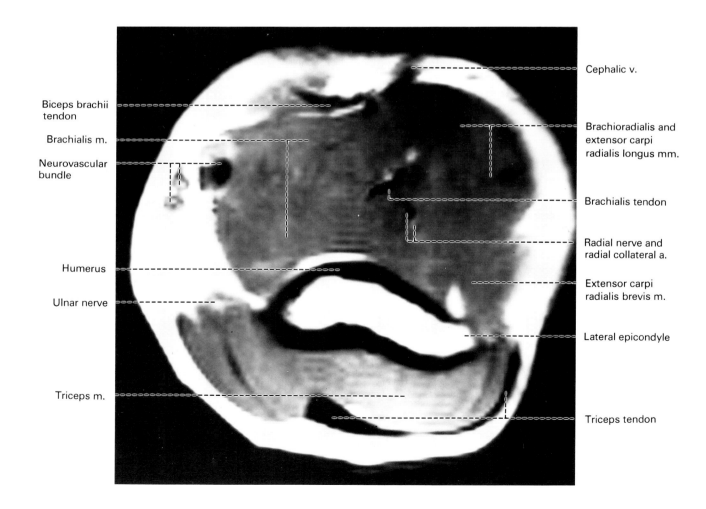

Biceps brachii tendon
Brachialis m.
Neurovascular bundle
Humerus
Ulnar nerve
Triceps m.

Cephalic v.
Brachioradialis and extensor carpi radialis longus mm.
Brachialis tendon
Radial nerve and radial collateral a.
Extensor carpi radialis brevis m.
Lateral epicondyle
Triceps tendon

Figure 3.1.3

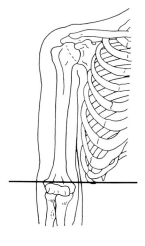

1. The olecranon fossa and posterior fat pad are seen in this section.

2. Note the location of the ulnar nerve. At the elbow its course is posterior to the medial epicondyle.

3. At the elbow, the brachial artery and median nerve move from a medial to an anterior position.

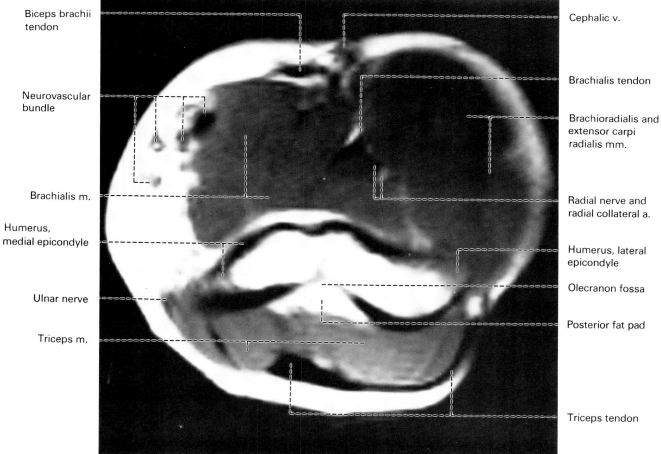

Biceps brachii tendon

Neurovascular bundle

Brachialis m.

Humerus, medial epicondyle

Ulnar nerve

Triceps m.

Cephalic v.

Brachialis tendon

Brachioradialis and extensor carpi radialis mm.

Radial nerve and radial collateral a.

Humerus, lateral epicondyle

Olecranon fossa

Posterior fat pad

Triceps tendon

Figure 3.1.4

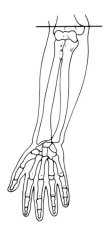

1. Anconeus originates with the common extensor tendon from the lateral epicondyle and inserts on the posterolateral aspect of the proximal ulna.

2. Note the thick tendon of biceps.

3. The radial nerve is covered by brachioradialis.

4. The lateral and medial epicondyles act as the origin of common extensor and common flexor tendons, respectively.

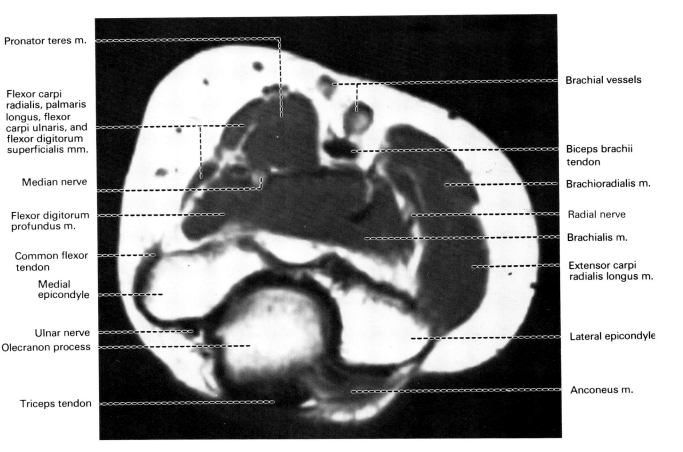

Figure 3.1.5

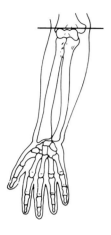

1. This section passes through the trochlea and capitulum.

2. Note the insertion of the bicipital aponeurosis on the anterior surface of pronator teres.

3. The median nerve is covered by pronator teres.

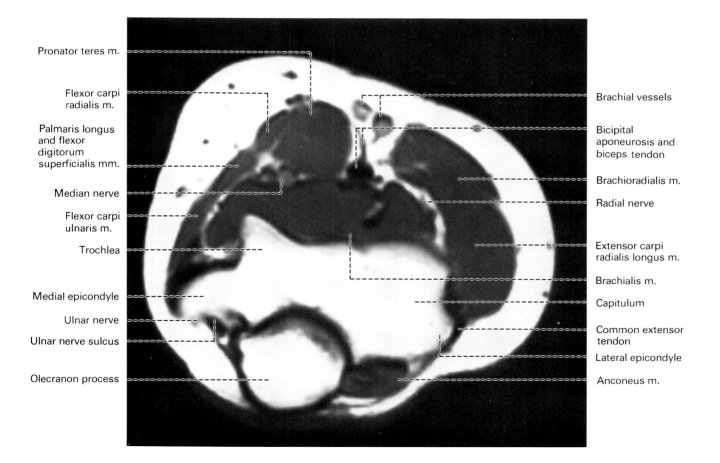

Pronator teres m.

Flexor carpi radialis m.

Palmaris longus and flexor digitorum superficialis mm.

Median nerve

Flexor carpi ulnaris m.

Trochlea

Medial epicondyle

Ulnar nerve

Ulnar nerve sulcus

Olecranon process

Brachial vessels

Bicipital aponeurosis and biceps tendon

Brachioradialis m.

Radial nerve

Extensor carpi radialis longus m.

Brachialis m.

Capitulum

Common extensor tendon

Lateral epicondyle

Anconeus m.

Figure 3.1.6

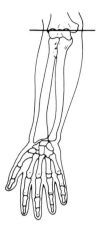

1. Brachialis diminishes in size as it approaches its insertion on the coronoid process.

2. Note the common extensor tendon posterior to extensor carpi radialis longus.

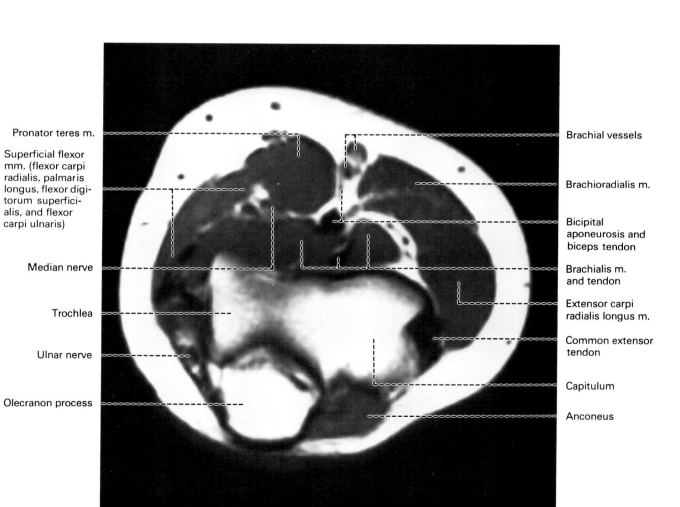

Pronator teres m.

Superficial flexor mm. (flexor carpi radialis, palmaris longus, flexor digitorum superficialis, and flexor carpi ulnaris)

Median nerve

Trochlea

Ulnar nerve

Olecranon process

Brachial vessels

Brachioradialis m.

Bicipital aponeurosis and biceps tendon

Brachialis m. and tendon

Extensor carpi radialis longus m.

Common extensor tendon

Capitulum

Anconeus

Figure 3.1.7

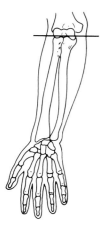

1. Flexor carpi ulnaris has two heads: a humeral head originating as part of the common flexor tendon and an ulnar head originating from the medial border of the olecranon and proximal ulna posteriorly.

2. The radial head is partially outlined in this section and is seen articulating with the radial notch of the ulna.

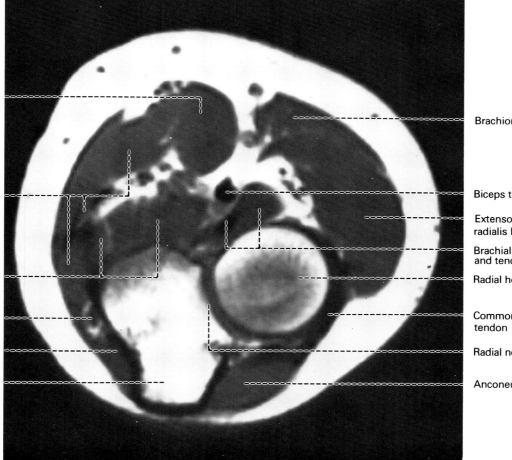

Pronator teres m.

Superficial flexor mm. flexor carpi radialis, palmaris longus, flexor digitorum superficialis, and flexor carpi ulnaris)

Flexor digitorum profundus m.

Ulnar nerve

Flexor carpi ulnaris (ulnar head) m.

Ulna

Brachioradialis m.

Biceps tendon

Extensor carpi radialis longus m.

Brachialis m. and tendon

Radial head

Common extensor tendon

Radial notch

Anconeus m.

Figure 3.1.8

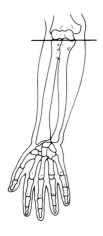

1. In this section brachialis has become totally tendinous.

2. Distal to the elbow, the ulnar nerve courses in the anterior compartment of the forearm.

3. Flexor digitorum profundus originates along with flexor carpi ulnaris from the posterior border of the ulna and also from the anterior and medial surfaces of the proximal ulna.

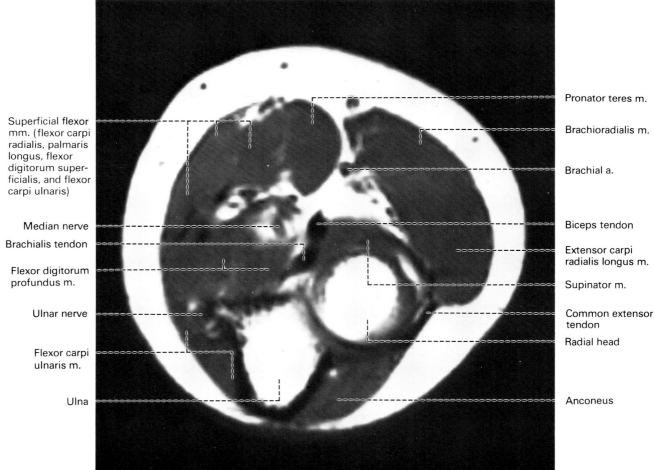

Superficial flexor mm. (flexor carpi radialis, palmaris longus, flexor digitorum superficialis, and flexor carpi ulnaris)

Median nerve

Brachialis tendon

Flexor digitorum profundus m.

Ulnar nerve

Flexor carpi ulnaris m.

Ulna

Pronator teres m.

Brachioradialis m.

Brachial a.

Biceps tendon

Extensor carpi radialis longus m.

Supinator m.

Common extensor tendon

Radial head

Anconeus

Figure 3.1.9

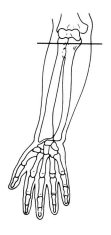

1. The supinator muscle originates from the lateral epicondyle, radial collateral ligament, annular ligament, and supinator crest and fossa of the ulna. It courses distally and laterally and wraps around the proximal radius and inserts on its lateral surface.

2. The brachialis tendon is seen inserting on the coronoid process.

3. On the extensor side of the forearm, the major muscle mass is formed by brachioradialis and extensor carpi radialis longus, which are difficult to separate in this section.

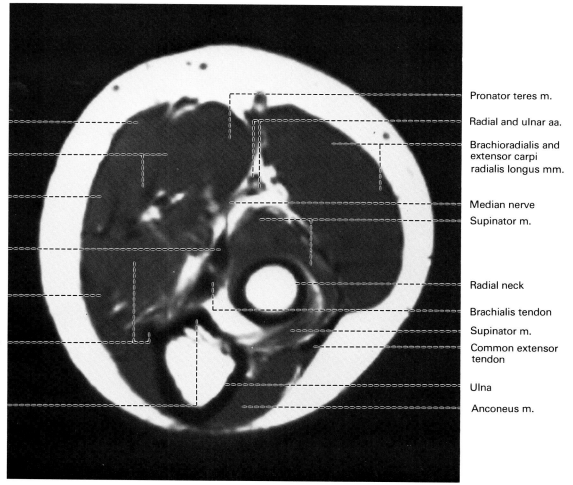

Flexor carpi radialis m.

Flexor digitorum superficialis m.

Palmaris longus m.

Biceps tendon

Flexor carpi ulnaris m.

Flexor digitorum profundus m.

Coronoid process

Pronator teres m.

Radial and ulnar aa.

Brachioradialis and extensor carpi radialis longus mm.

Median nerve
Supinator m.

Radial neck

Brachialis tendon

Supinator m.
Common extensor tendon

Ulna

Anconeus m.

Figure 3.1.10

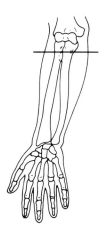

1. The brachialis tendon is completing its insertion on the coronoid process.

2. The brachial artery has already divided into the radial and ulnar arteries.

3. Individual flexor muscles can be identified in this section.

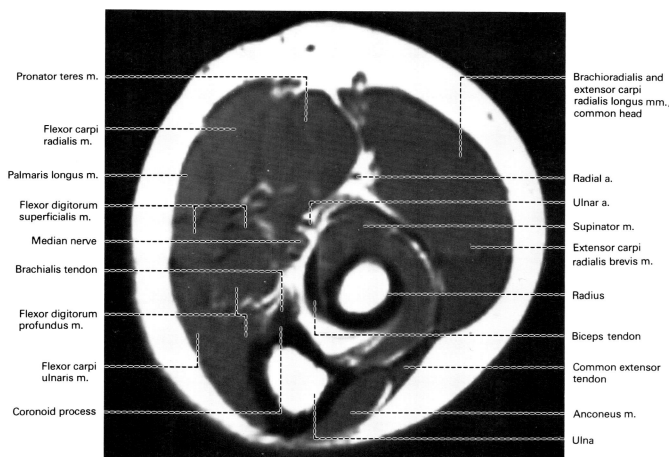

Pronator teres m.

Flexor carpi radialis m.

Palmaris longus m.

Flexor digitorum superficialis m.

Median nerve

Brachialis tendon

Flexor digitorum profundus m.

Flexor carpi ulnaris m.

Coronoid process

Brachioradialis and extensor carpi radialis longus mm., common head

Radial a.

Ulnar a.

Supinator m.

Extensor carpi radialis brevis m.

Radius

Biceps tendon

Common extensor tendon

Anconeus m.

Ulna

Figure 3.1.11

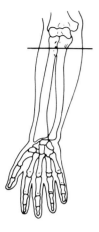

1. The biceps tendon is completing its insertion on the radial tuberosity.

2. Individual extensor muscles can be identified in this section.

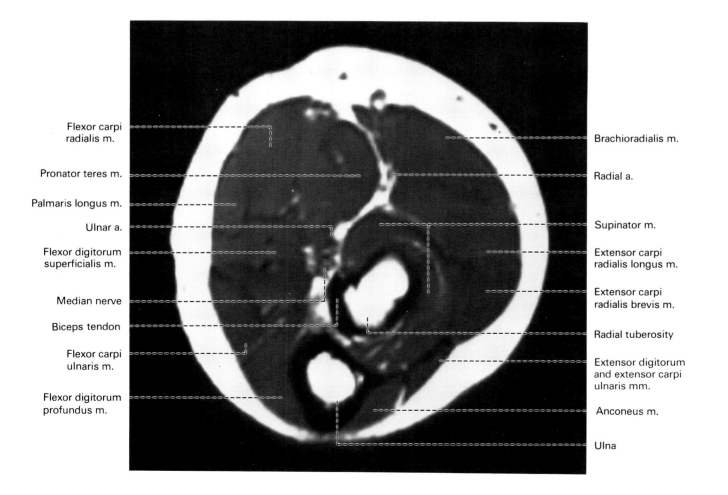

Flexor carpi radialis m.

Pronator teres m.

Palmaris longus m.

Ulnar a.

Flexor digitorum superficialis m.

Median nerve

Biceps tendon

Flexor carpi ulnaris m.

Flexor digitorum profundus m.

Brachioradialis m.

Radial a.

Supinator m.

Extensor carpi radialis longus m.

Extensor carpi radialis brevis m.

Radial tuberosity

Extensor digitorum and extensor carpi ulnaris mm.

Anconeus m.

Ulna

Figure 3.1.12

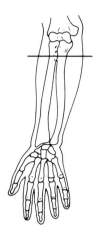

1. Note the complex course of the supinator muscle.

2. The radial tuberosity has a thin cortex compared to the radial shaft.

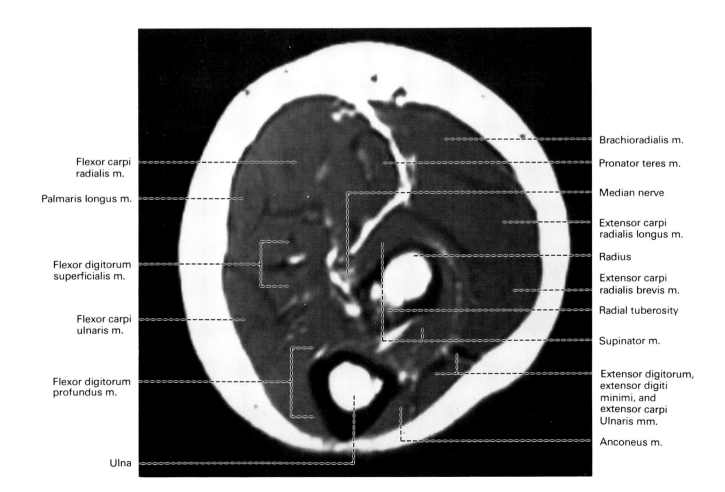

Flexor carpi radialis m.

Palmaris longus m.

Flexor digitorum superficialis m.

Flexor carpi ulnaris m.

Flexor digitorum profundus m.

Ulna

Brachioradialis m.

Pronator teres m.

Median nerve

Extensor carpi radialis longus m.

Radius

Extensor carpi radialis brevis m.

Radial tuberosity

Supinator m.

Extensor digitorum, extensor digiti minimi, and extensor carpi Ulnaris mm.

Anconeus m.

Figure 3.1.13

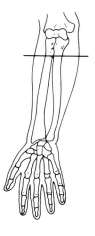

1. Pronator teres is covered by flexor carpi radialis and brachioradialis as it approaches its insertion on the radius.

2. The ulnar nerve travels in the forearm between flexor digitorum profundus and flexor carpi ulnaris.

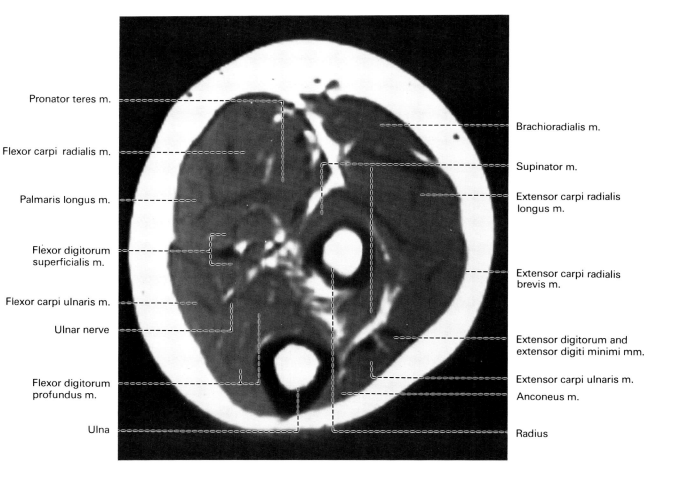

Pronator teres m.

Flexor carpi radialis m.

Palmaris longus m.

Flexor digitorum superficialis m.

Flexor carpi ulnaris m.

Ulnar nerve

Flexor digitorum profundus m.

Ulna

Brachioradialis m.

Supinator m.

Extensor carpi radialis longus m.

Extensor carpi radialis brevis m.

Extensor digitorum and extensor digiti minimi mm.

Extensor carpi ulnaris m.

Anconeus m.

Radius

Figure 3.2.1

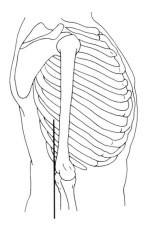

1. This section is through the posterior aspect of the elbow. It passes through the tip of the olecranon process.

2. Note the insertion of triceps onto the olecranon process.

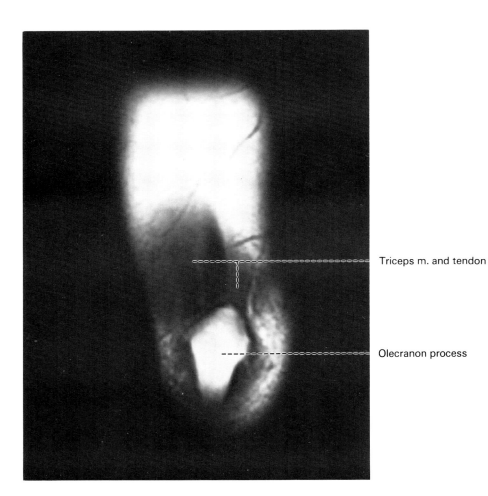

Triceps m. and tendon

Olecranon process

Figure 3.2.2

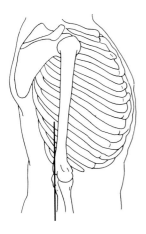

1. Note the course of the ulnar nerve posterior to the medial epicondyle.

2. Triceps approaches its insertion on the olecranon process.

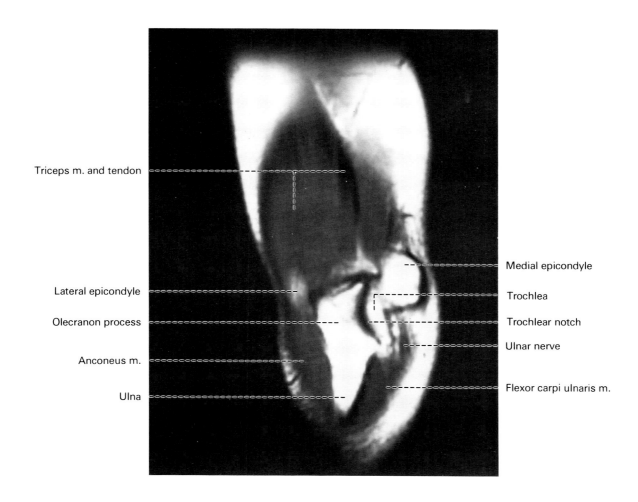

Triceps m. and tendon

Lateral epicondyle

Olecranon process

Anconeus m.

Ulna

Medial epicondyle

Trochlea

Trochlear notch

Ulnar nerve

Flexor carpi ulnaris m.

Figure 3.2.3

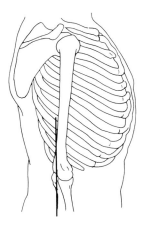

1. Triceps is the only muscle on the dorsum of the distal arm.

2. The olecranon fossa houses the olecranon process in full extension.

3. The medial epicondyle is the origin for all the superficial flexors.

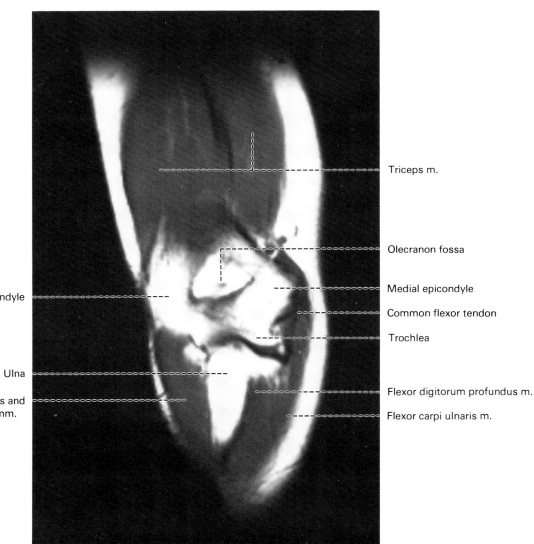

Figure 3.2.4

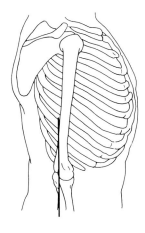

1. A large portion of flexor digitorum profundus lies deep to flexor carpi ulnaris.

2. Note the origin of brachioradialis and extensor carpi radialis longus from the lateral supracondylar crest (ridge).

3. Note the origin of extensor carpi ulnaris brevis and extensor digitorum from the lateral epicondyle.

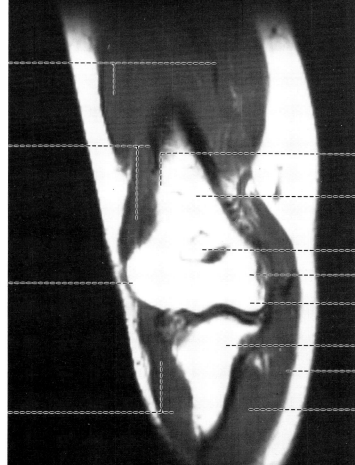

Triceps m.

Brachioradialis and extensor carpi radialis longus mm.

Lateral epicondyle

Extensor carpi ulnaris and extensor digitorum mm.

Lateral supracondylar crest (ridge)

Humerus

Olecranon fossa

Medial epicondyle

Trochlea

Ulna

Flexor carpi ulnaris m.

Flexor digitorum profundus m.

Figure 3.2.5

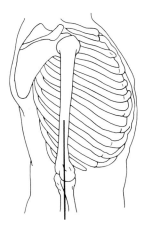

1. Brachioradialis and extensor carpi radialis longus originate from the lateral supracondylar crest (ridge).

2. Extensor carpi radialis brevis, extensor digitorum, and extensor digiti minimi originate from the lateral epicondyle.

3. Flexor digitorum profundus has a broad origin from the medial and anterior surfaces of the ulna.

4. Note the coronoid fossa; it houses the coronoid process in full flexion of the elbow.

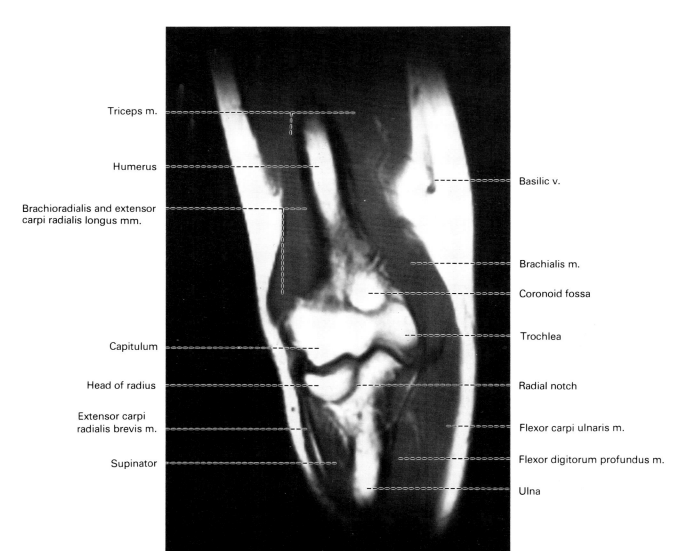

Figure 3.2.6

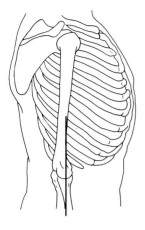

1. The radiocapitular articulation is clearly depicted in this section.

2. Brachialis courses distally toward its insertion on the coronoid process.

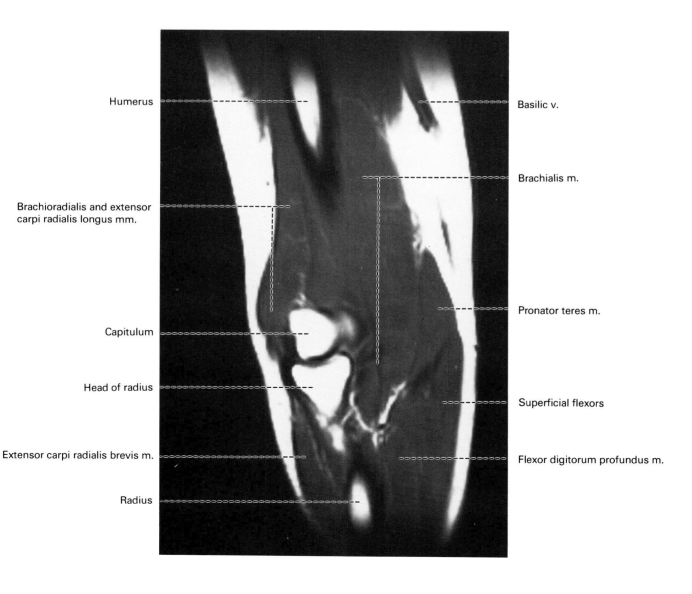

Humerus

Basilic v.

Brachialis m.

Brachioradialis and extensor carpi radialis longus mm.

Pronator teres m.

Capitulum

Head of radius

Superficial flexors

Extensor carpi radialis brevis m.

Flexor digitorum profundus m.

Radius

Figure 3.2.7

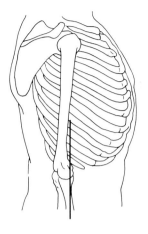

1. In this section pronator teres is clearly separated from the rest of the superficial flexors.

2. Note the origin of flexor pollicis longus from the anterior surface of the radius.

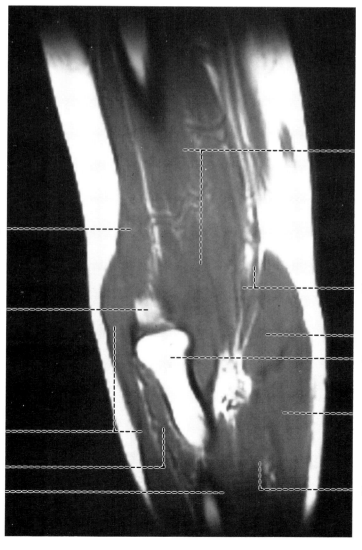

Brachioradialis m.

Capitulum

Extensor carpi radialis brevis m.

Supinator m.

Flexor pollicis longus m.

Brachialis m.

Brachial a. and median nerve

Pronator teres m.

Head of radius

Superficial flexor mm.
(flexor carpi radialis, palmaris longus, flexor carpi ulnaris, and flexor digitorum superficialis)

Flexor digitorum profundus m.

Figure 3.2.8

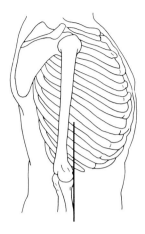

1. This section is through the floor of the cubital fossa, which is formed by brachialis and supinator.

2. Brachialis lies deep to the biceps. It originates on the anterior surface of the distal half of the humerus.

3. The cubital fossa contains the biceps tendon, brachial artery, and median nerve.

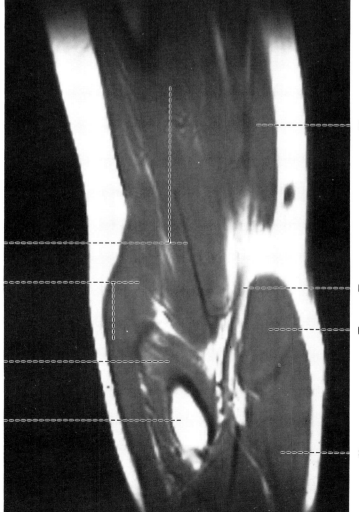

Biceps brachii m.

Brachioradialis m.

Supinator m.

Radius

Brachialis m.

Brachial a.

Pronator teres m.

Superficial flexor mm.

Figure 3.2.9

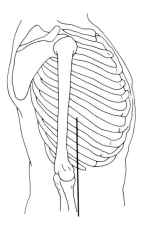

1. This section depicts the cubital fossa, a triangular space bounded laterally by brachioradialis and medially by pronator teres.

2. The brachial artery and median nerve course through the cubital fossa as they pass from arm to forearm.

3. Note the biceps tendon; it inserts on the radial tuberosity.

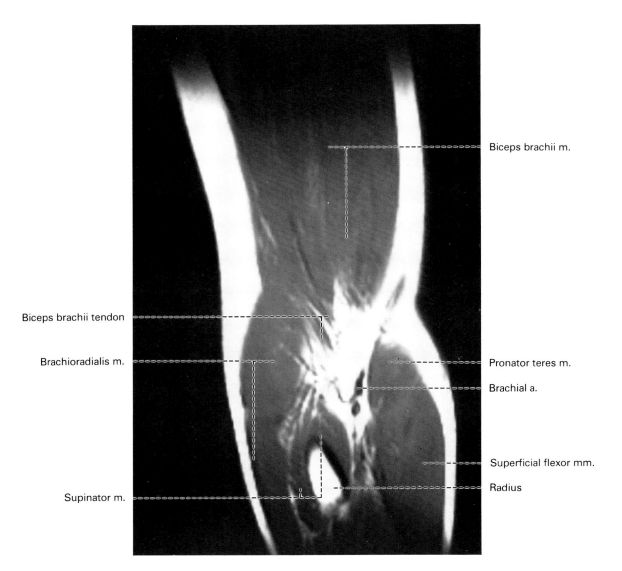

Figure 3.2.10

1. Note the supinator muscle inserting on the anterolateral aspect of the proximal radius.

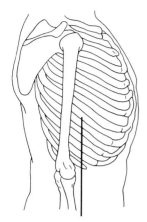

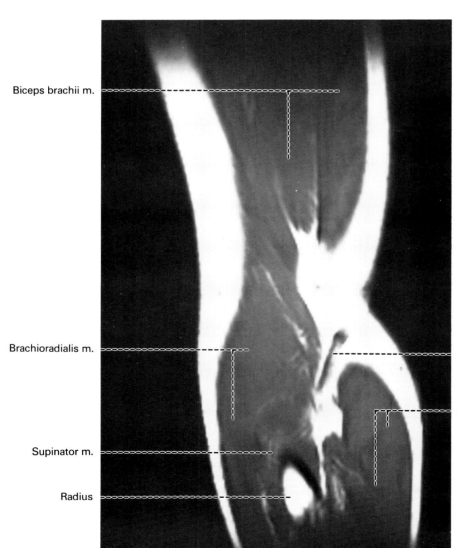

Biceps brachii m.

Brachioradialis m.

Brachial a.

Supinator m.

Superficial flexor mm.
(flexor carpi radialis, palmaris longus, flexor carpi ulnaris, and flexor digitorum superficialis)

Radius

Figure 3.2.11

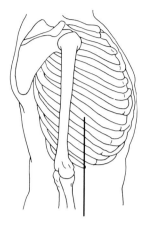

1. This section is through the anterior portion of the cubital fossa.

2. The most anterior muscles in the forearm are the superficial flexors (pronator teres, flexor carpi radialis, palmaris longus, flexor carpi ulnaris, and flexor digitorum superficialis) and brachioradialis.

3. In the arm, biceps is the most anterior muscle.

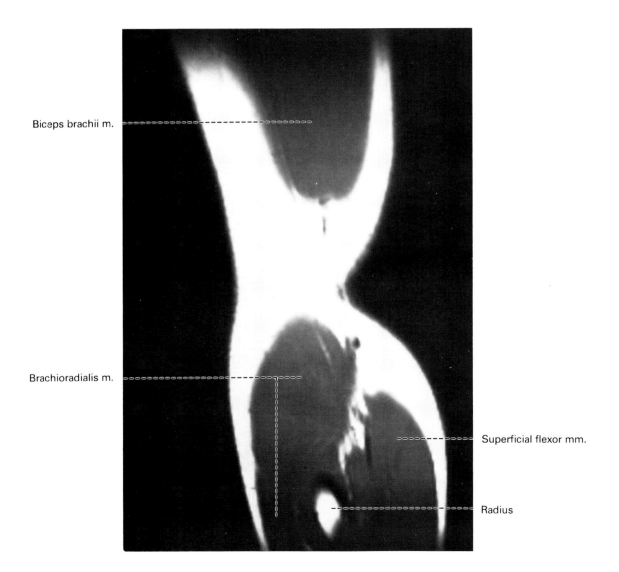

SAGITTAL

Figure 3.3.1

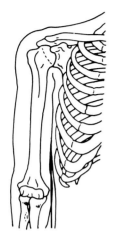

1. This is the most medial section of the elbow. It passes through the medial epicondyle, which serves as the origin of the common flexor tendon.

2. Note the course of the ulnar nerve in the arm. In the elbow, the ulnar nerve passes behind the medial epicondyle.

3. The basilic vein is clearly demonstrated in this section.

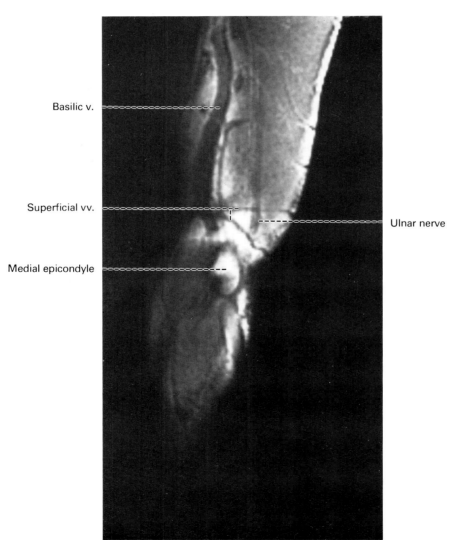

Basilic v.

Superficial vv.

Ulnar nerve

Medial epicondyle

Figure 3.3.2

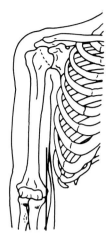

1. The most medial muscle in the elbow and forearm is flexor carpi ulnaris.

2. Pronator teres, flexor carpi radialis, palmaris longus, and flexor digitorum superficialis appear as a single muscle mass beyond their origin and are difficult to separate.

3. The ulnar nerve lies immediately posterior to the medial epicondyle.

4. The neurovascular bundle of the arm is seen in the medial intermuscular septum. The muscle mass posterior to the medial and lateral intermuscular septa is triceps.

5. The medial and long heads of the triceps muscle are included in this section.

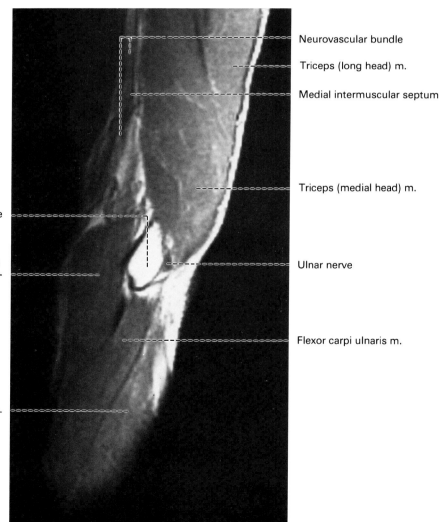

Neurovascular bundle

Triceps (long head) m.

Medial intermuscular septum

Triceps (medial head) m.

Medial epicondyle

Superficial flexor mm. (pronator teres, flexor carpi radialis, palmaris longus, and flexor digitorum superficialis)

Ulnar nerve

Flexor carpi ulnaris m.

Flexor digitorum profundus m.

Figure 3.3.3

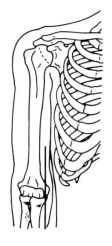

1. This section is through the medial aspect of the trochlear fossa, which articulates with the trochlea.

2. The olecranon and coronoid processes are demonstrated.

3. The triceps tendon inserts on the olecranon.

4. Brachialis is seen crossing the elbow to reach its insertion in the proximal forearm.

5. Flexor digitorum profundus originates from the posteromedial aspect of the ulna.

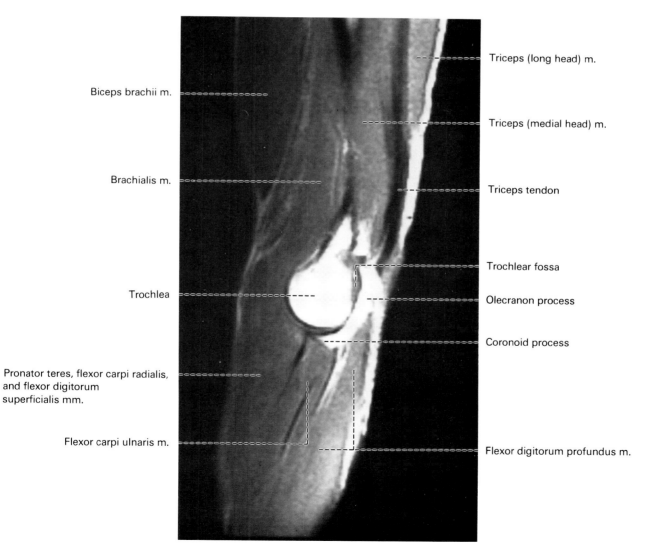

Figure 3.3.4

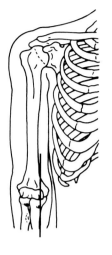

1. The olecranon and coronoid fossae house the olecranon and coronoid processes, respectively. They also contain some fat.

2. The superficial flexors are seen as one mass, and individual muscles are difficult to separate.

3. Note the insertion of the triceps tendon onto the olecranon process.

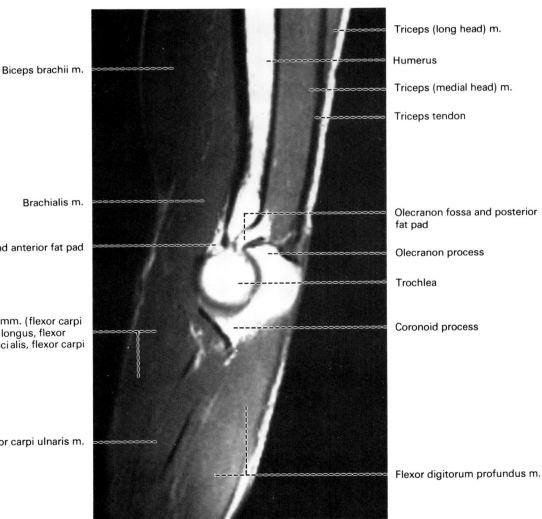

Biceps brachii m.

Brachialis m.

Coronoid fossa and anterior fat pad

Superficial flexor mm. (flexor carpi radialis, palmaris longus, flexor digitorum superficialis, flexor carpi ulnaris)

Flexor carpi ulnaris m.

Triceps (long head) m.

Humerus

Triceps (medial head) m.

Triceps tendon

Olecranon fossa and posterior fat pad

Olecranon process

Trochlea

Coronoid process

Flexor digitorum profundus m.

Figure 3.3.5

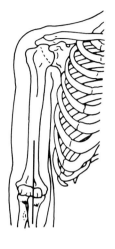

1. Note the muscular insertion of brachialis onto the tuberosity of the ulna (part of the coronoid process).

2. The trochlea and capitulum are normally anterior to the long axis of the humerus.

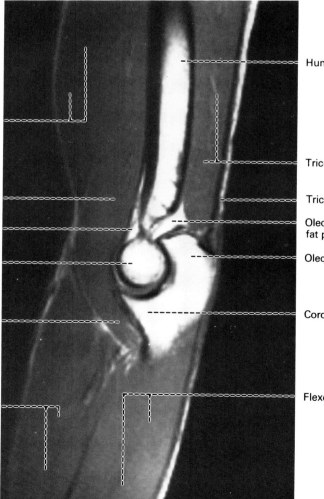

Biceps brachii m.

Brachialis m.

Coronoid fossa and anterior fat pad

Trochlea

Brachialis m.

Superficial flexor mm. (flexor carpi radialis, palmaris longus, flexor digitorum superficialis, and flexor carpi ulnaris)

Humerus

Triceps (medial head) m.

Triceps tendon

Olecranon fossa and posterior fat pad

Olecranon process

Coronoid process

Flexor digitorum profundus m.

Figure 3.3.6

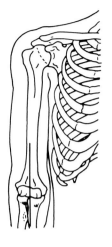

1. The brachial artery and median nerve are demonstrated on the anterior surface of the brachialis muscle.

2. The bicipital aponeurosis is seen in the anterior aspect of the cubital fossa.

3. The deep and superficial flexors are demonstrated in this section.

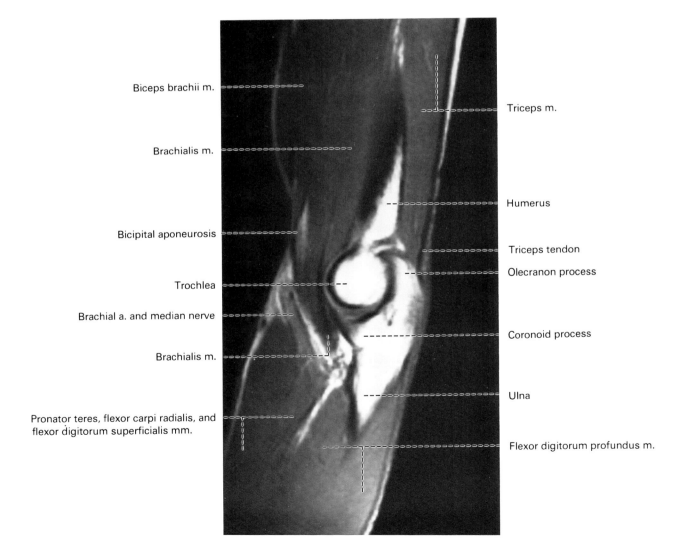

Figure 3.3.7

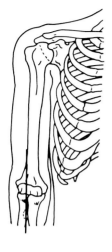

1. This section is through the medial aspect of the radial head and capitulum.

2. This section passes lateral to the humeral shaft where the lateral intermuscular septum is demonstrated. It separates triceps (posteriorly) from brachialis and biceps (anteriorly).

3. Note the biceps tendon coming to its insertion on the radial tuberosity.

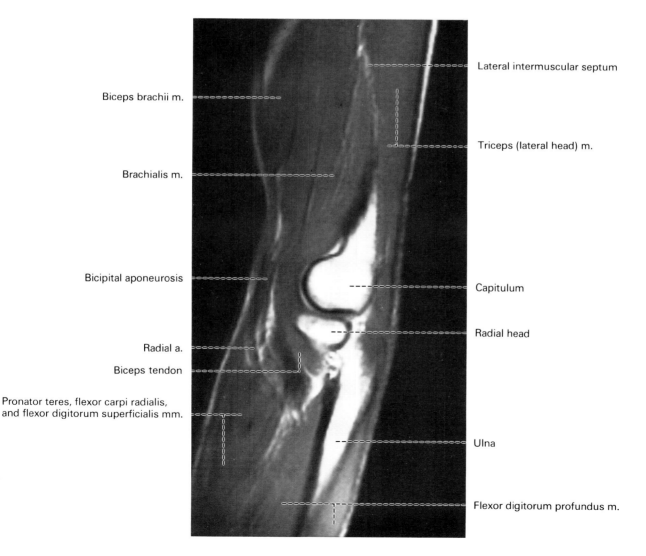

Figure 3.3.8

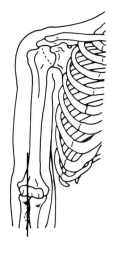

1. Anconeus is seen posterior to the elbow joint. It arises from the lateral epicondyle and inserts on the lateral aspect of the olecranon.

2. Supinator is demonstrated in this section. It is seen wrapping around the radius where it inserts on its lateral surface.

3. Brachioradialis is seen anterior to the supinator.

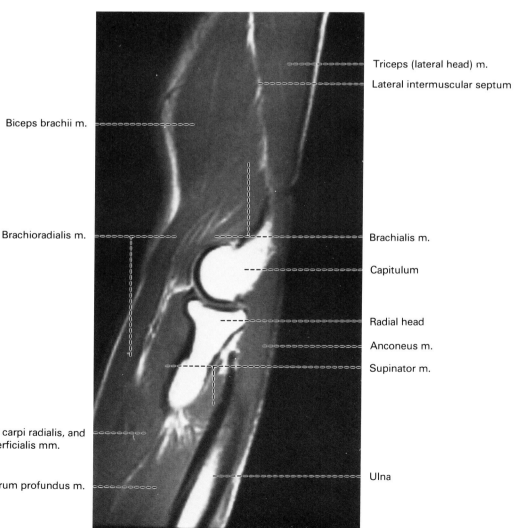

Figure 3.3.9

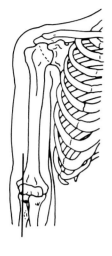

1. This section is through the lateral epicondyle. It is the origin for the common extensor tendon.

2. Extensor carpi radialis longus is seen at its origin from the lateral supracondylar crest. Brachioradialis also originates from the same crest.

3. Extensor carpi ulnaris is seen in this section; it originates from the lateral epicondyle.

4. Note the relationship of supinator to the proximal radius.

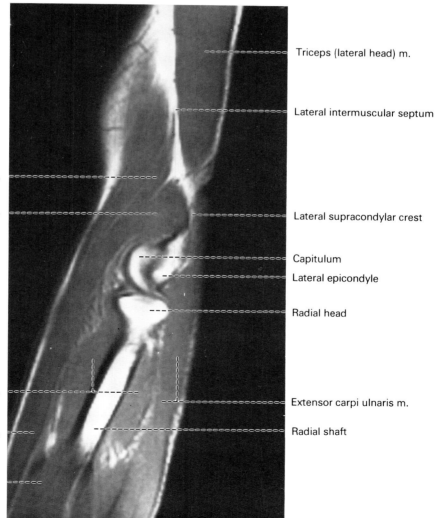

Figure 3.3.10

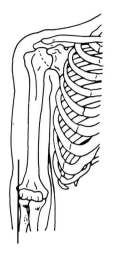

1. The common extensor tendon is demonstrated in this section.

2. Extensor digitorum is seen covering supinator and abductor pollicis longus.

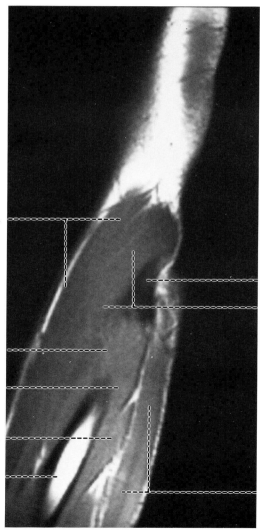

Brachioradialis m.

Common extensor tendon

Extensor carpi radialis longus m.

Extensor carpi radialis brevis m.

Supinator m.

Abductor pollicis longus m.

Radius

Extensor digitorum m.

Figure 3.3.11

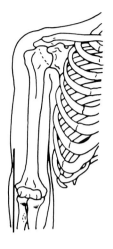

1. The most prominent muscles in the anterolateral aspect of the forearm are brachioradialis, extensor carpi radialis longus, and brevis.

2. Extensor digitorum and abductor pollicis longus beneath it are demonstrated on the posterolateral aspect of the forearm.

Extensor carpi radialis longus m.

Extensor carpi radialis brevis m.

Extensor digitorum m.

Abductor pollicis longus m.

Radius

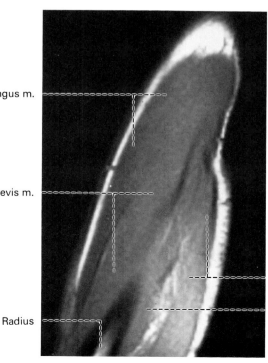

Figure 3.3.12

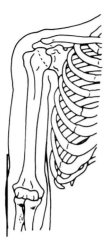

1. This section passes through the most lateral aspect of the proximal forearm.

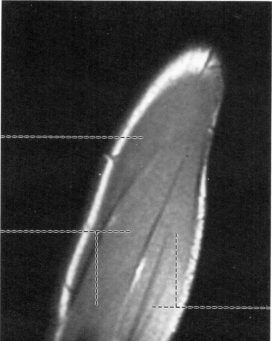

Extensor carpi radialis longus m.

Extensor carpi radialis brevis m.

Extensor digitorum m.

Chapter 4

FOREARM

Figure 4.1.1

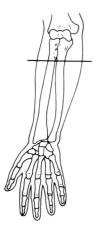

1. The brachioradialis muscle is diminishing in size and becoming partially tendinous as the sections approach the midforearm.

2. Note that the posteromedial cortex of the ulna is just underneath the subcutaneous fat.

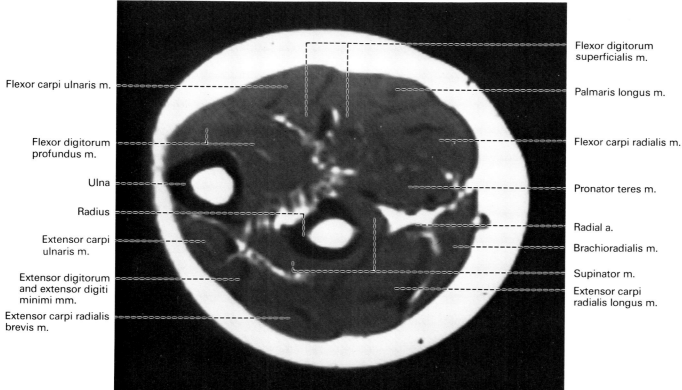

Flexor carpi ulnaris m.

Flexor digitorum profundus m.

Ulna

Radius

Extensor carpi ulnaris m.

Extensor digitorum and extensor digiti minimi mm.

Extensor carpi radialis brevis m.

Flexor digitorum superficialis m.

Palmaris longus m.

Flexor carpi radialis m.

Pronator teres m.

Radial a.

Brachioradialis m.

Supinator m.

Extensor carpi radialis longus m.

Figure 4.1.2

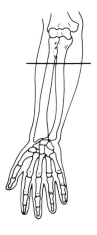

1. The interosseous membrane is distinctly seen in this section. It acts as an origin for several muscles in the forearm.

2. A small part of flexor digitorum profundus originates from the interosseous membrane.

3. The median nerve courses between flexor digitorum superficialis and flexor digitorum profundus.

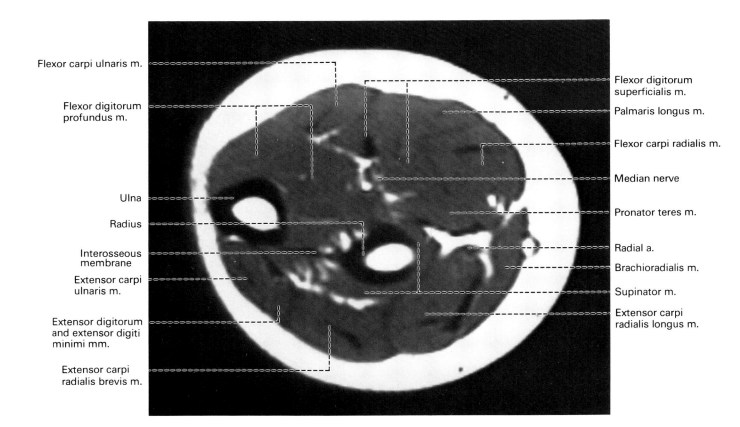

Flexor carpi ulnaris m.

Flexor digitorum profundus m.

Ulna

Radius

Interosseous membrane

Extensor carpi ulnaris m.

Extensor digitorum and extensor digiti minimi mm.

Extensor carpi radialis brevis m.

Flexor digitorum superficialis m.

Palmaris longus m.

Flexor carpi radialis m.

Median nerve

Pronator teres m.

Radial a.

Brachioradialis m.

Supinator m.

Extensor carpi radialis longus m.

Figure 4.1.3

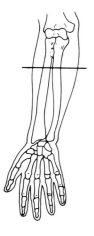

1. The pronator teres starts to insert on the anterolateral aspect of the midshaft of the radius.

2. Extensor pollicis longus is seen originating from the posterior surface of the interosseous membrane. It also originates in part from the posterolateral aspect of the ulna.

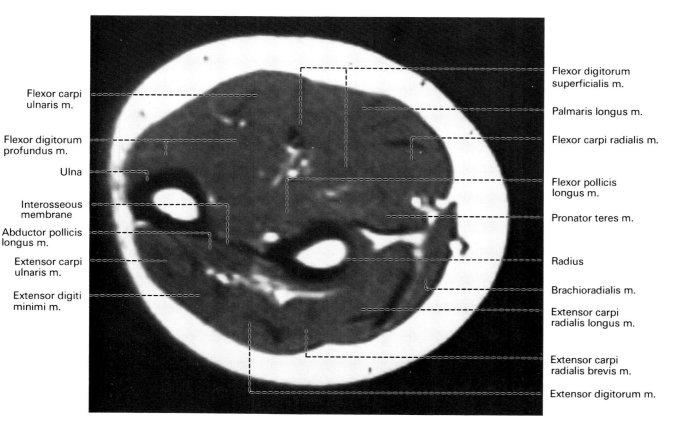

Flexor carpi ulnaris m.

Flexor digitorum profundus m.

Ulna

Interosseous membrane

Abductor pollicis longus m.

Extensor carpi ulnaris m.

Extensor digiti minimi m.

Flexor digitorum superficialis m.

Palmaris longus m.

Flexor carpi radialis m.

Flexor pollicis longus m.

Pronator teres m.

Radius

Brachioradialis m.

Extensor carpi radialis longus m.

Extensor carpi radialis brevis m.

Extensor digitorum m.

Figure 4.1.4

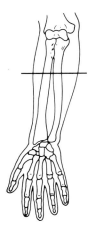

1. Note the origin of flexor pollicis longus from the anterior surface of the radius at its middle third.

2. Abductor pollicis longus originates on the posterior surface of the radius at its middle third and from the adjacent interosseous membrane.

3. The individual extensor muscles are clearly demonstrated in this section. They occupy the posterior and lateral aspects of the forearm at this level.

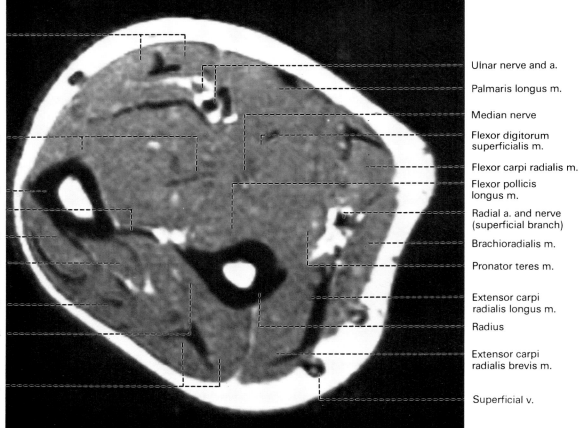

Flexor carpi ulnaris m.

Flexor digitorum profundus m.

Ulna

Interosseous membrane

Extensor carpi ulnaris m.

Extensor pollicis longus m.

Extensor digiti minimi m.

Abductor pollicis longus m.

Extensor digitorum m.

Ulnar nerve and a.

Palmaris longus m.

Median nerve

Flexor digitorum superficialis m.

Flexor carpi radialis m.

Flexor pollicis longus m.

Radial a. and nerve (superficial branch)

Brachioradialis m.

Pronator teres m.

Extensor carpi radialis longus m.

Radius

Extensor carpi radialis brevis m.

Superficial v.

Figure 4.1.5

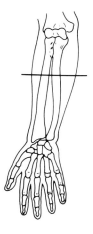

1. Many of the forearm muscles at this level have thick tendinous components.

2. Note that neither the radius nor ulna are circular in cross section.

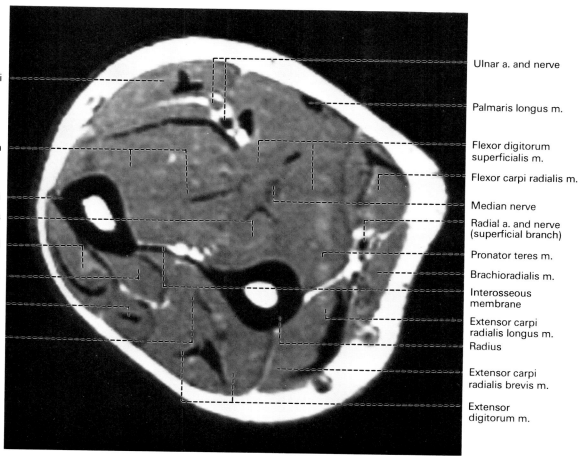

Flexor carpi ulnaris m.

Flexor digitorum profundus m.

Ulna

Flexor pollicis longus m.

Extensor carpi ulnaris m.

Extensor pollicis longus m.

Extensor digiti minimi m.

Abductor pollicis longus m.

Ulnar a. and nerve

Palmaris longus m.

Flexor digitorum superficialis m.

Flexor carpi radialis m.

Median nerve

Radial a. and nerve (superficial branch)

Pronator teres m.

Brachioradialis m.

Interosseous membrane

Extensor carpi radialis longus m.

Radius

Extensor carpi radialis brevis m.

Extensor digitorum m.

Figure 4.1.6

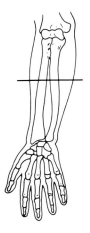

1. In this section, note that extensor pollicis longus, extensor pollicis brevis, and abductor pollicis longus are all covered by other extensor muscles.

2. The interosseous membrane is distinctly seen.

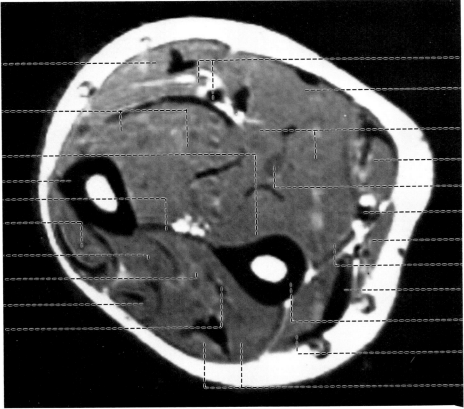

Flexor carpi ulnaris m.

Flexor digitorum profundus m.

Flexor pollicis longus m.

Ulna

Interosseous membrane

Extensor carpi ulnaris m.

Extensor pollicis longus m.

Extensor pollicis brevis m.

Extensor digiti minimi m.

Abductor pollicis longus m.

Ulnar a. and nerve

Palmaris longus m.

Flexor digitorum superficialis m.

Flexor carpi radialis m.

Median nerve

Radial a. and nerve (superficial branch)

Brachioradialis m.

Pronator teres m.

Extensor carpi radialis longus m.

Radius

Extensor carpi radialis brevis m.

Extensor digitorum m.

Figure 4.1.7

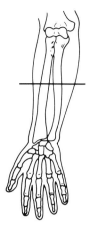

1. In this part of the forearm the median nerve travels between flexor digitorum superficialis and flexor pollicis longus.

2. The ulnar nerve continues to travel underneath flexor carpi ulnaris.

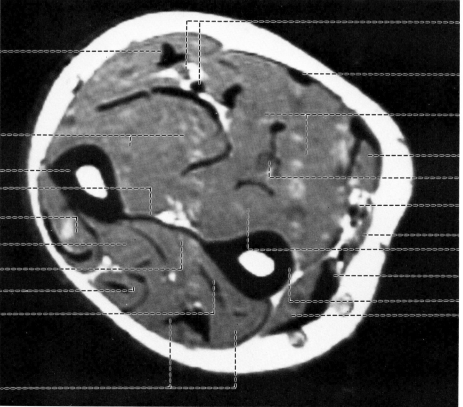

Flexor carpi ulnaris m.

Flexor digitorum profundus m.

Ulna

Interosseous membrane

Extensor carpi ulnaris m.

Extensor pollicis longus m.

Extensor pollicis brevis m.

Extensor digiti minimi m.

Abductor pollicis longus m.

Extensor digitorum m.

Ulnar a. and nerve

Palmaris longus m.

Flexor digitorum superficialis m.

Flexor carpi radialis m.

Median nerve

Radial a. and nerve (superficial branch)

Brachioradialis m.

Flexor pollicis longus m.

Extensor carpi radialis longus m.

Radius

Extensor carpi radialis brevis m.

Figure 4.1.8

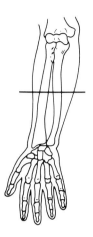

1. Brachioradialis has become completely tendinous at this level.

2. Abductor pollicis longus and extensor pollicis brevis are migrating laterally to cross over extensor carpi radialis longus and brevis in lower sections.

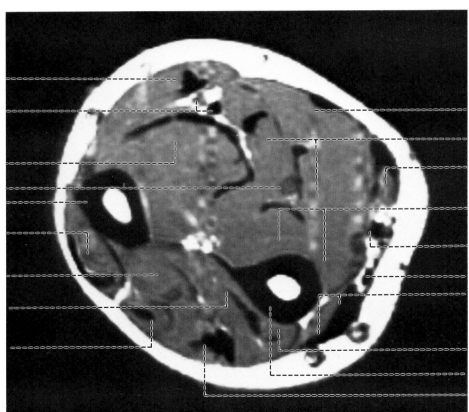

Flexor carpi ulnaris m.

Ulnar a. and nerve

Flexor digitorum profundus m.

Median nerve

Ulna

Extensor carpi ulnaris m.

Extensor pollicis longus m.

Extensor pollicis brevis m.

Extensor digiti minimi m.

Palmaris longus m.

Flexor digitorum superficialis m.

Flexor carpi radialis m.

Flexor pollicis longus m.

Radial a. and nerve (superficial branch)

Brachioradialis tendon

Extensor carpi radialis longus and brevis tendons

Abductor pollicis longus m.

Radius

Extensor digitorum m.

Figure 4.1.9

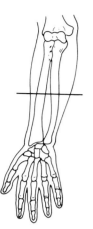

1. Flexor carpi radialis, brachioradialis, and extensor carpi radialis longus and brevis are all almost entirely tendinous in this section.

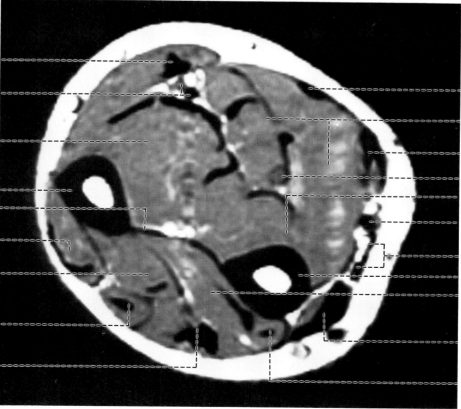

Flexor carpi ulnaris m.

Ulnar a. and nerve

Flexor digitorum profundus m.

Ulna

Interosseous membrane

Extensor carpi ulnaris m.

Extensor pollicis longus m.

Extensor digiti minimi m.

Extensor digitorum m.

Palmaris longus m.

Flexor digitorum superficialis m.

Flexor carpi radialis tendon

Median nerve

Flexor pollicis longus m.

Radial a. and nerve (superficial branch)

Brachioradialis tendon

Radius

Extensor pollicis brevis m.

Extensor carpi radialis longus and brevis tendons

Abductor pollicis longus m.

Figure 4.1.10

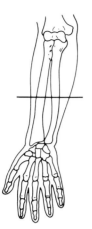

1. Abductor pollicis longus and extensor pollicis brevis continue their migration laterally.

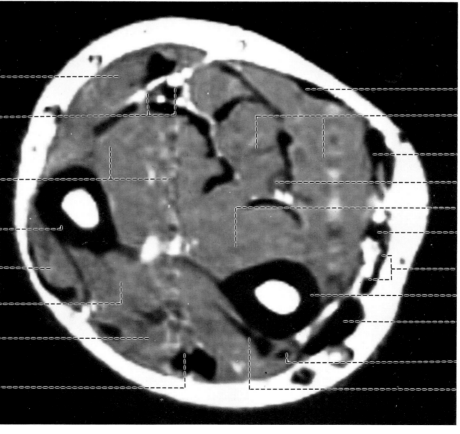

Flexor carpi ulnaris m.

Ulnar a. and nerve

Flexor digitorum profundus m.

Ulna

Extensor carpi ulnaris m.

Extensor pollicis longus m.

Extensor digiti minimi m.

Extensor digitorum m.

Palmaris longus m.

Flexor digitorum superficialis m.

Flexor carpi radialis tendon

Median nerve

Flexor pollicis longus m.

Radial a. and nerve (superficial branch)

Brachioradialis tendon

Radius

Extensor carpi radialis longus and brevis tendons

Abductor pollicis longus m.

Extensor pollicis brevis m.

Figure 4.1.11

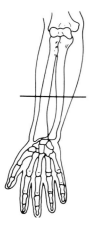

1. Extensor indicis originates on the posterior surface of the distal third of the ulna.

2. The entire muscle mass of the forearm is diminished in distal sections as the tendons of individual muscles become more prominent.

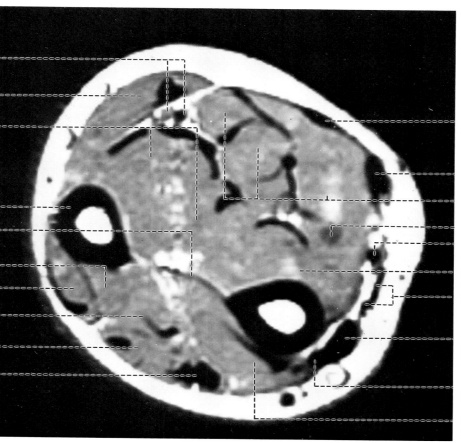

Ulnar a. and nerve

Flexor carpi ulnaris m.

Flexor digitorum profundus m.

Ulna

Interosseous membrane

Extensor indicis m.

Extensor carpi ulnaris m.

Extensor pollicis longus m.

Extensor digiti minimi m.

Extensor digitorum tendons

Palmaris longus tendon

Flexor carpi radialis tendon

Flexor digitorum superficialis m.

Median nerve

Radial a. and nerve (superficial branch)

Flexor pollicis longus m.

Brachioradialis tendon

Extensor carpi radialis longus and brevis tendons

Abductor pollicis longus m.

Extensor pollicis brevis m.

Figure 4.1.12

1. In this section, the radial artery has become superficial.

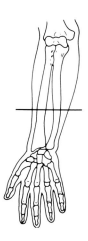

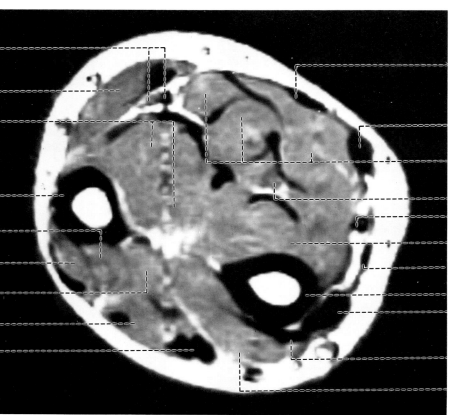

Ulnar a. and nerve

Flexor carpi
ulnaris m.

Flexor digitorum
profundus m.

Ulna

Extensor indicis m.

Extensor carpi
ulnaris m.

Extensor pollicis
longus m.

Extensor digiti
minimi m.

Extensor digitorum
tendons

Palmaris longus
tendon

Flexor carpi
radialis tendon

Flexor digitorum
superficialis m.

Median nerve

Radial a. and nerve
(superficial branch)

Flexor pollicis longus m.

Brachioradialis
tendon

Radius

Extensor carpi
radialis longus and
brevis tendons

Abductor pollicis
longus tendon

Extensor pollicis
brevis m.

Figure 4.1.13

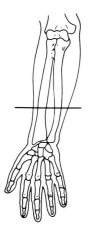

1. Abductor pollicis longus and extensor pollicis brevis are crossing over extensor carpi radialis longus and brevis tendons.

2. Extensor pollicis longus starts to migrate laterally before it also crosses over extensor carpi radialis longus and brevis tendons in more distal sections.

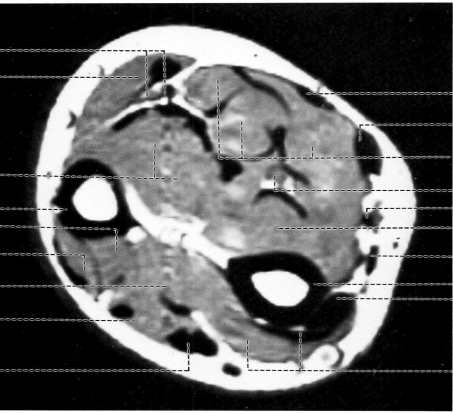

Ulnar a. and nerve

Flexor carpi ulnaris m.

Flexor digitorum profundus m.

Ulna

Extensor indicis m.

Extensor carpi ulnaris m.

Extensor pollicis longus m.

Extensor digiti minimi m.

Extensor digitorum tendons

Palmaris longus tendon

Flexor carpi radialis tendon

Flexor digitorum superficialis m.

Median nerve

Radial a.

Flexor pollicis longus m.

Brachioradialis tendon

Radius

Extensor carpi radialis longus and brevis tendons

Abductor pollicis longus tendon and extensor pollicis brevis m.

Figure 4.1.14

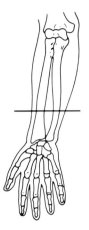

1. The ulnar artery and nerve continue to be clearly demonstrated between flexor carpi ulnaris and flexor digitorum profundus.

2. The median nerve proceeds in its course toward the wrist between flexor digitorum superficialis and flexor pollicis longus.

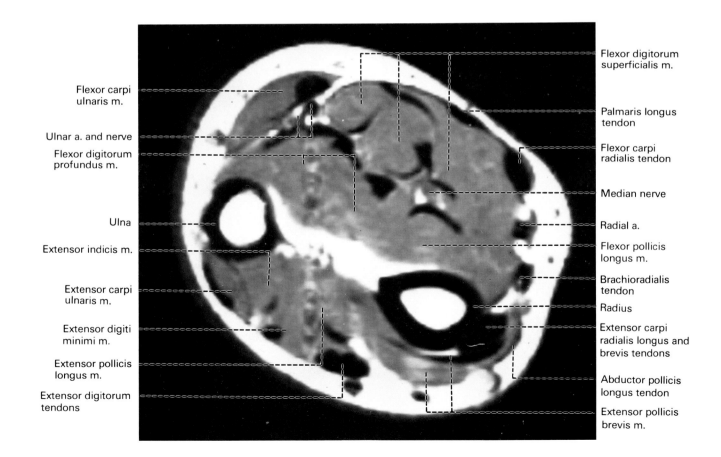

Flexor carpi ulnaris m.

Ulnar a. and nerve

Flexor digitorum profundus m.

Ulna

Extensor indicis m.

Extensor carpi ulnaris m.

Extensor digiti minimi m.

Extensor pollicis longus m.

Extensor digitorum tendons

Flexor digitorum superficialis m.

Palmaris longus tendon

Flexor carpi radialis tendon

Median nerve

Radial a.

Flexor pollicis longus m.

Brachioradialis tendon

Radius

Extensor carpi radialis longus and brevis tendons

Abductor pollicis longus tendon

Extensor pollicis brevis m.

Figure 4.1.15

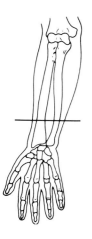

1. Abductor pollicis longus has completed its crossing over extensor carpi radialis longus and brevis tendons.

2. The diameter of the radius increases as the section approaches the wrist.

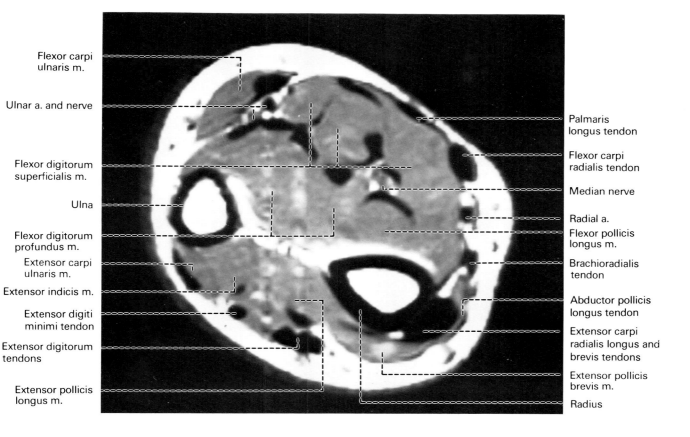

Flexor carpi ulnaris m.

Ulnar a. and nerve

Flexor digitorum superficialis m.

Ulna

Flexor digitorum profundus m.

Extensor carpi ulnaris m.

Extensor indicis m.

Extensor digiti minimi tendon

Extensor digitorum tendons

Extensor pollicis longus m.

Palmaris longus tendon

Flexor carpi radialis tendon

Median nerve

Radial a.

Flexor pollicis longus m.

Brachioradialis tendon

Abductor pollicis longus tendon

Extensor carpi radialis longus and brevis tendons

Extensor pollicis brevis m.

Radius

Figure 4.1.16

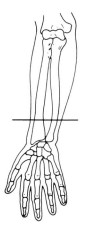

1. This section passes through the proximal portion of pronator quadratus. It originates from the anterior surface of the distal one-fourth of the ulna and runs transversely to insert on the anterior surface of the radius.

2. The radial artery runs superficially in the subcutaneous tissues adjacent to the extensor carpi radialis tendon.

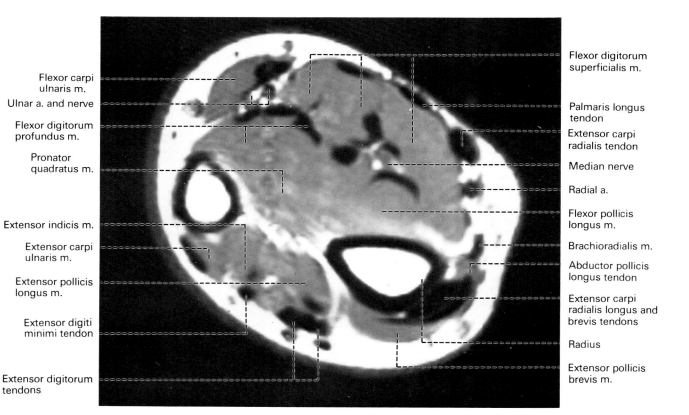

Flexor carpi ulnaris m.

Ulnar a. and nerve

Flexor digitorum profundus m.

Pronator quadratus m.

Extensor indicis m.

Extensor carpi ulnaris m.

Extensor pollicis longus m.

Extensor digiti minimi tendon

Extensor digitorum tendons

Flexor digitorum superficialis m.

Palmaris longus tendon

Extensor carpi radialis tendon

Median nerve

Radial a.

Flexor pollicis longus m.

Brachioradialis m.

Abductor pollicis longus tendon

Extensor carpi radialis longus and brevis tendons

Radius

Extensor pollicis brevis m.

Figure 4.1.17

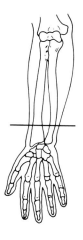

1. Pronator quadratus is seen linking the anterior surface of the radius to the ulna.

2. The radius continues to enlarge in diameter.

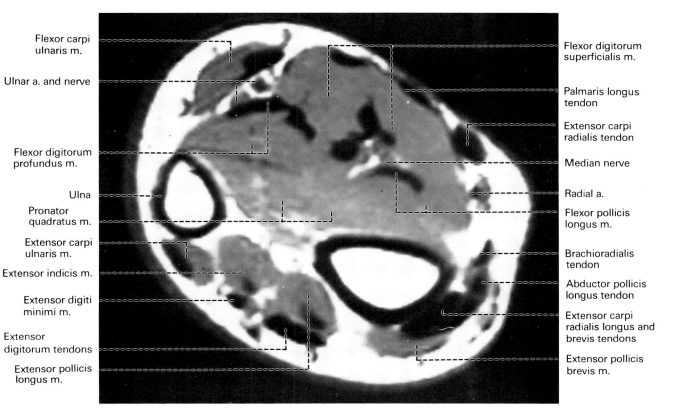

Flexor carpi ulnaris m.

Ulnar a. and nerve

Flexor digitorum profundus m.

Ulna

Pronator quadratus m.

Extensor carpi ulnaris m.

Extensor indicis m.

Extensor digiti minimi m.

Extensor digitorum tendons

Extensor pollicis longus m.

Flexor digitorum superficialis m.

Palmaris longus tendon

Extensor carpi radialis tendon

Median nerve

Radial a.

Flexor pollicis longus m.

Brachioradialis tendon

Abductor pollicis longus tendon

Extensor carpi radialis longus and brevis tendons

Extensor pollicis brevis m.

Figure 4.1.18

1. The tendons of extensor digitorum, flexor digitorum superficialis, and flexor digitorum profundus are each dividing into smaller tendons.

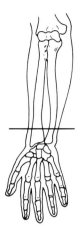

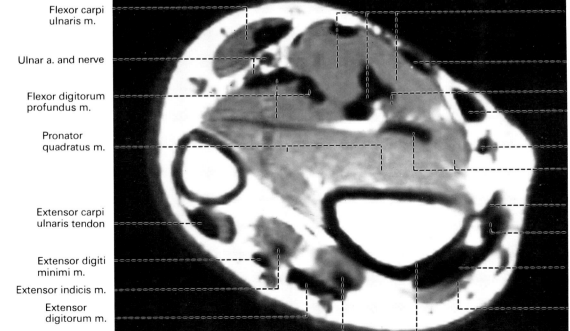

Flexor carpi ulnaris m.

Ulnar a. and nerve

Flexor digitorum profundus m.

Pronator quadratus m.

Extensor carpi ulnaris tendon

Extensor digiti minimi m.

Extensor indicis m.

Extensor digitorum m.

Extensor pollicis longus tendons

Flexor digitorum superficialis m.

Palmaris longus tendon

Median nerve

Flexor carpi radialis tendon

Radial a.

Flexor pollicis longus m.

Brachioradialis tendon

Abductor pollicis longus tendon

Extensor carpi radialis longus and brevis tendons

Extensor pollicis brevis m.

Radius

Figure 4.1.19

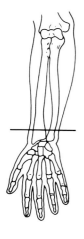

1. The extensor pollicis brevis tendon has crossed the extensor carpi radialis longus and brevis tendons.

2. All the extensor muscles have become tendinous.

3. The relative positions of the extensor tendons will be maintained until the radiocarpal joint is crossed.

4. In this section the brachioradialis tendon completes its insertion onto the lateral aspect of the distal radius.

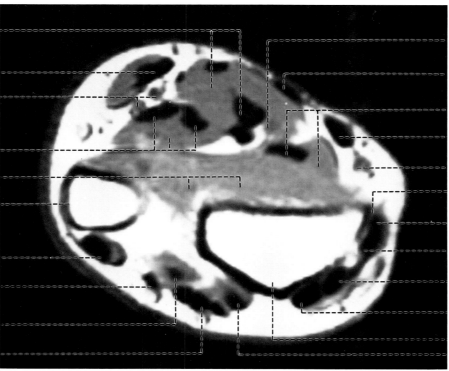

Flexor digitorum superficialis m.

Extensor carpi ulnaris tendon

Ulnar a. and nerve

Flexor digitorum profundus m.

Pronator quadratus m.

Ulna

Extensor carpi ulnaris tendon

Extensor digiti minimi tendon

Extensor indicis tendon

Extensor digitorum tendons

Median nerve

Palmaris longus tendon

Flexor pollicis longus m.

Flexor carpi radialis tendon

Radial a.

Brachioradialis tendon

Abductor pollicis longus tendon

Extensor pollicis brevis tendon

Extensor carpi radialis longus tendon

Extensor carpi radialis brevis tendon

Radius

Extensor pollicis longus m.

Figure 4.2.1

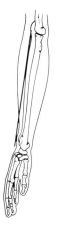

1. This section is through the posterior aspect of the forearm.

2. The posterior cortex of the ulna lies superficially under the skin.

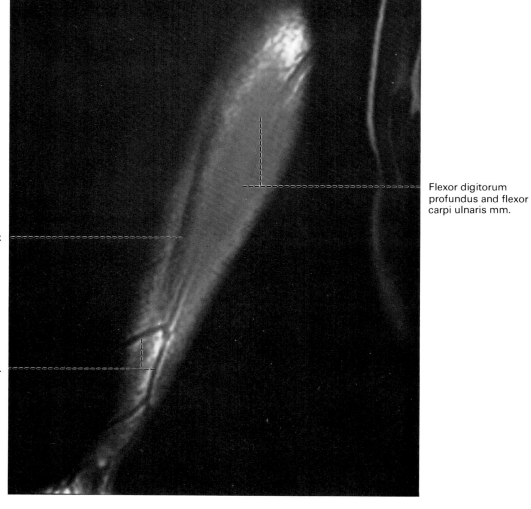

Flexor digitorum profundus and flexor carpi ulnaris mm.

Posterior cortex of ulna

Superficial v v.

Figure 4.2.2

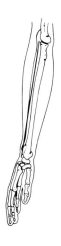

1. Extensor carpi ulnaris originates from the posterior aspect of the ulna.

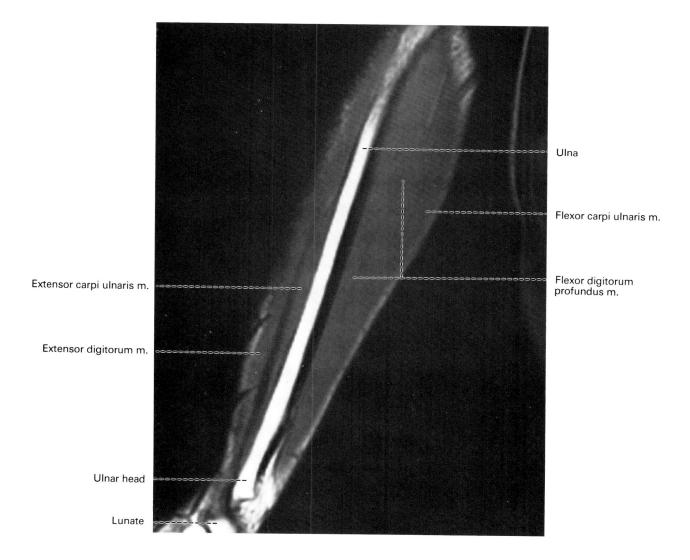

Figure 4.2.3

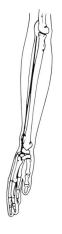

1. Flexor digitorum profundus originates in part on the posteromedial surface of the ulna.

2. Note the relationship of extensor digitorum to extensor pollicis longus. Extensor digitorum covers extensor pollicis longus.

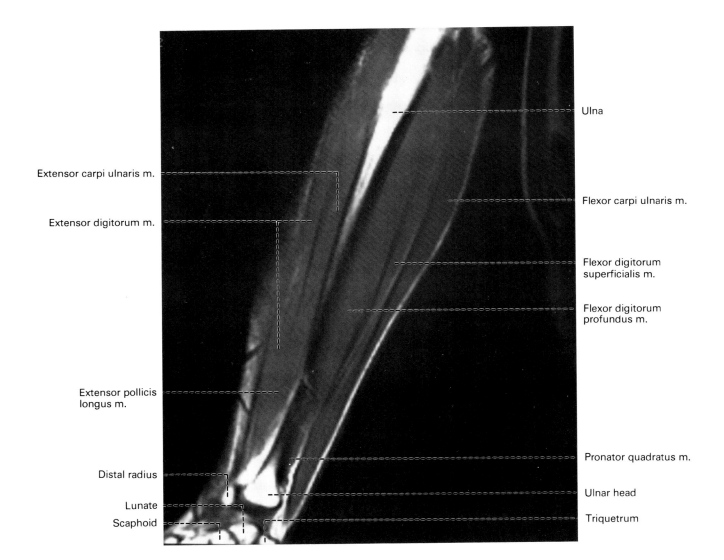

Extensor carpi ulnaris m.

Extensor digitorum m.

Extensor pollicis longus m.

Distal radius

Lunate

Scaphoid

Ulna

Flexor carpi ulnaris m.

Flexor digitorum superficialis m.

Flexor digitorum profundus m.

Pronator quadratus m.

Ulnar head

Triquetrum

Figure 4.2.4

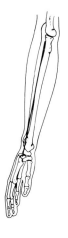

1. Extensor pollicis longus originates from the interosseous membrane and ulna.

2. Flexor carpi ulnaris lies medial to flexor digitorum superficialis and profundus.

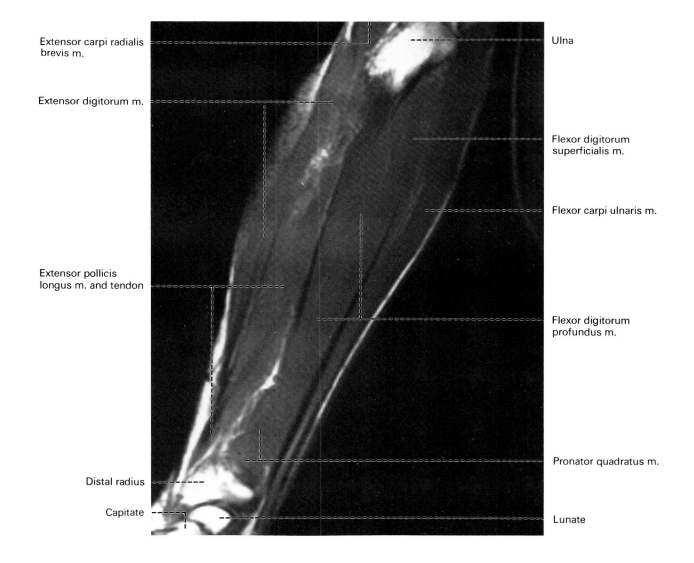

Extensor carpi radialis brevis m.

Extensor digitorum m.

Extensor pollicis longus m. and tendon

Distal radius

Capitate

Ulna

Flexor digitorum superficialis m.

Flexor carpi ulnaris m.

Flexor digitorum profundus m.

Pronator quadratus m.

Lunate

Figure 4.2.5

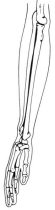

1. Pronator quadratus is partially demonstrated as it bridges the anterior surface of the distal radius and ulna.

2. Abductor pollicis longus and extensor pollicis brevis originate in part from the posterior surface of the radius.

3. Anterior to the ulna, flexor digitorum profundus is demonstrated. The anterior surface of the ulna is the origin of flexor digitorum profundus.

4. The tendon of flexor carpi ulnaris inserts on the pisiform.

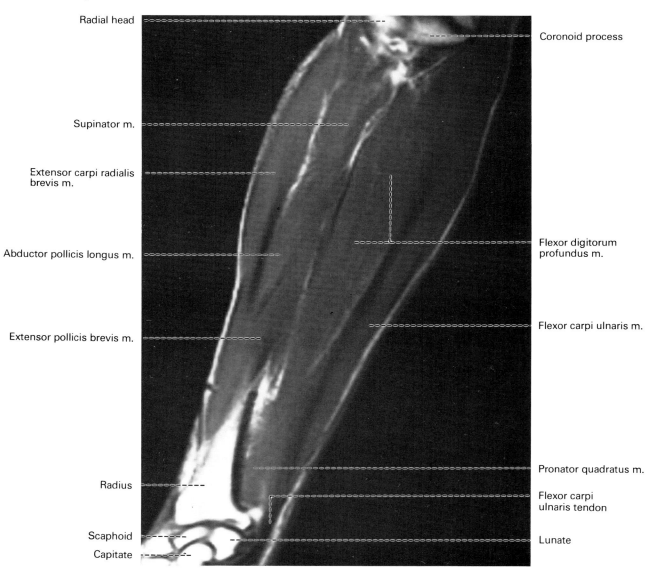

Radial head — Coronoid process

Supinator m.

Extensor carpi radialis brevis m.

Abductor pollicis longus m. — Flexor digitorum profundus m.

Extensor pollicis brevis m. — Flexor carpi ulnaris m.

Pronator quadratus m.

Radius — Flexor carpi ulnaris tendon

Scaphoid — Lunate

Capitate

Figure 4.2.6

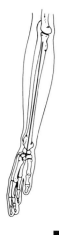

1. Abductor pollicis longus and extensor pollicis brevis tendons cross on the lateral aspect of the wrist toward their insertion on the thumb.

2. The supinator muscle covers the posterior, lateral, and part of the anterior portion of the proximal radius.

3. The distal end of brachialis is demonstrated as it approaches its insertion on the coronoid process.

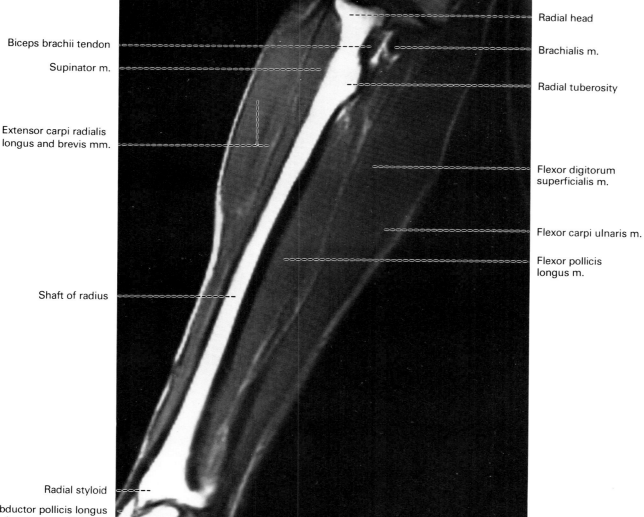

Figure 4.2.7

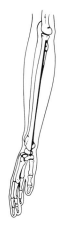

1. Note the insertion of the biceps tendon on the radial tuberosity.

2. The brachioradialis tendon is seen approaching its insertion on the lateral aspect of the distal radius.

3. Pronator teres inserts on the midpoint of the radius.

4. Flexor pollicis longus originates in part from the anterior surface of the radius.

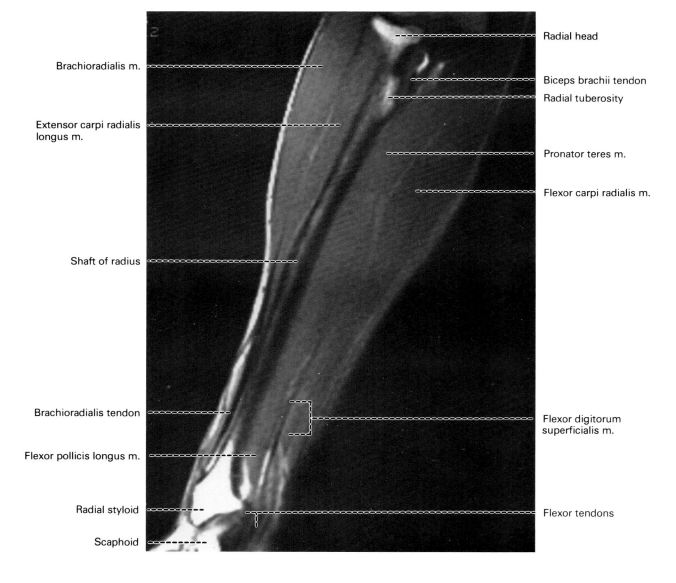

Figure 4.2.8

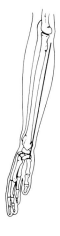

1. The three flexors seen in this section, pronator teres, flexor carpi radialis, and palmaris longus, all originate from the medial epicondyle.

2. Brachioradialis and extensor carpi radialis longus originate from the lateral supracondylar crest (ridge).

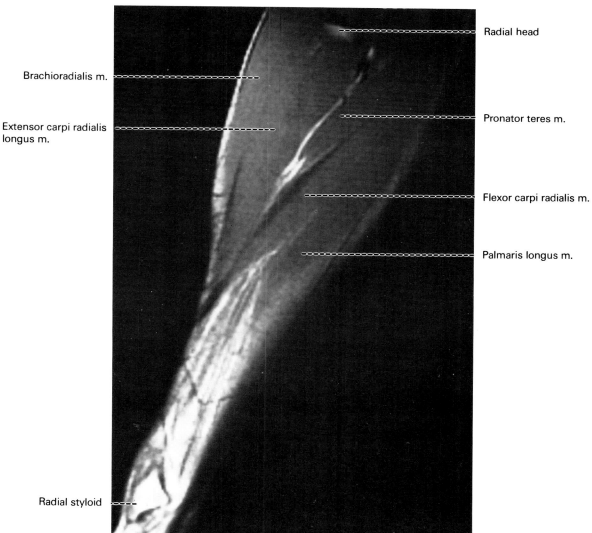

Brachioradialis m.

Extensor carpi radialis longus m.

Radial head

Pronator teres m.

Flexor carpi radialis m.

Palmaris longus m.

Radial styloid

Figure 4.2.9

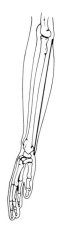

1. The cephalic vein is one of the larger superficial veins. It starts at the wrist and drains into the axillary vein at the deltopectoral groove.

2. Extensor carpi radialis longus is partially demonstrated adjacent to the brachioradialis muscle.

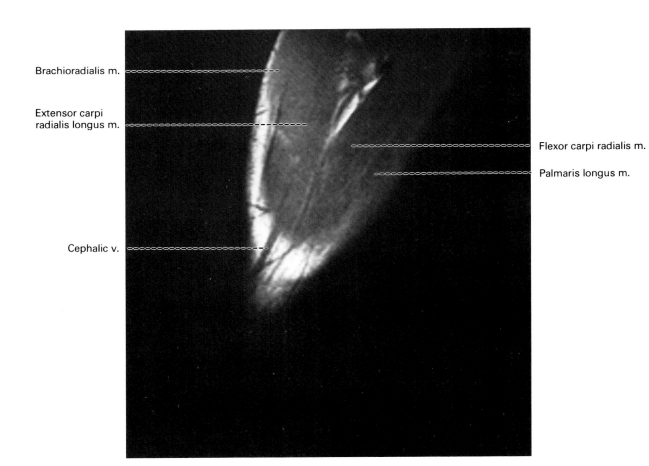

Brachioradialis m.

Extensor carpi radialis longus m.

Flexor carpi radialis m.

Palmaris longus m.

Cephalic v.

Figure 4.2.10

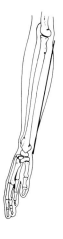

1. This is a superficial section through the anterior aspect of the forearm.

2. Brachioradialis on the extensor side of the forearm and flexor carpi radialis on the flexor side are only partially demonstrated.

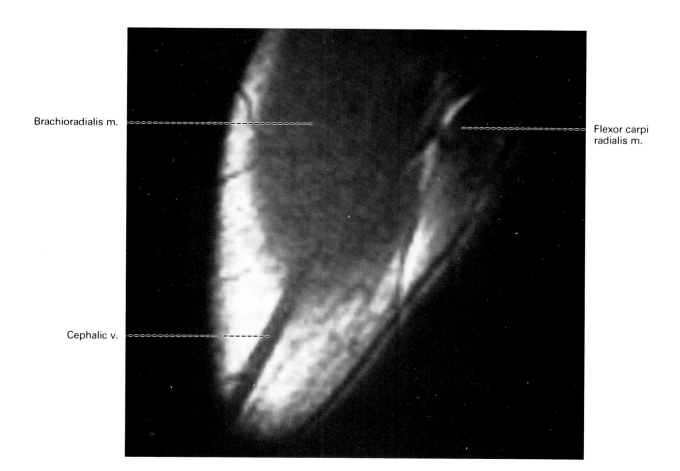

Brachioradialis m.

Flexor carpi radialis m.

Cephalic v.

Figure 4.3.1

1. This is the most medial sagittal section of the forearm. It passes through the medial epicondyle.

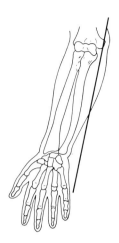

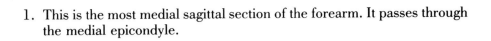

Medial epicondyle

Superficial flexors

Flexor carpi ulnaris and flexor digitorum profundus mm.

Figure 4.3.2

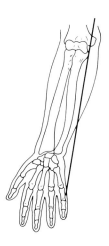

1. This section passes through the medial aspect of the trochlea and trochlear notch.

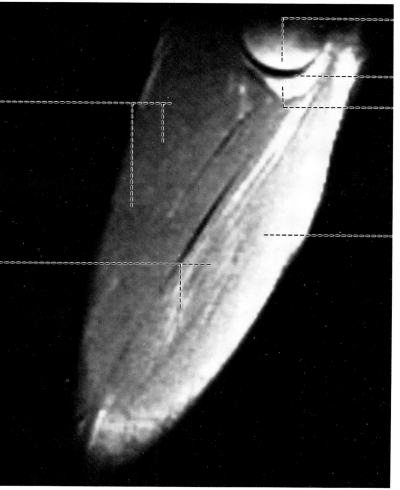

Trochlea

Trochlear notch

Coronoid process

Superficial flexor mm. (pronator teres, flexor carpi radialis, palmaris longus, flexor carpi ulnaris, and flexor digitorum superficialis)

Flexor carpi ulnaris m.

Flexor digitorum profundus m.

Figure 4.3.3

1. The superficial flexors originate from the medial epicondyle.

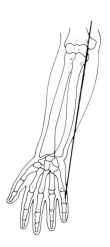

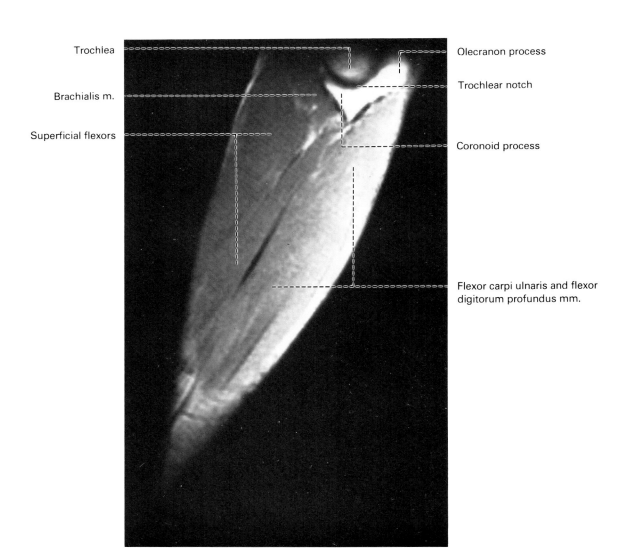

Trochlea

Brachialis m.

Superficial flexors

Olecranon process

Trochlear notch

Coronoid process

Flexor carpi ulnaris and flexor digitorum profundus mm.

Figure 4.3.4

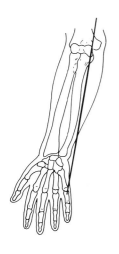

1. Brachialis inserts on the tuberosity of the ulna (part of the coronoid process).

2. The superficial flexors and flexor digitorum profundus constitute the muscular mass on the medial aspect of the forearm.

3. The coronoid and olecranon processes contribute to the depth of the trochlear notch.

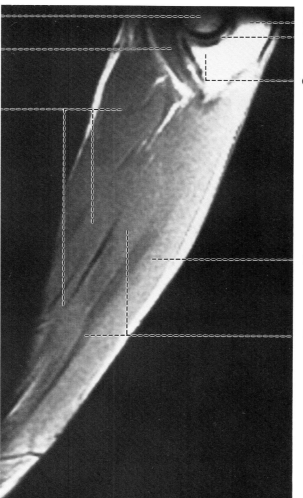

Trochlea

Brachialis m.

Superficial flexor mm. (pronator teres, flexor carpi radialis, palmaris longus, flexor carpi ulnaris, and flexor digitorum superficialis)

Olecranon process
Trochlear notch

Coronoid process

Flexor carpi ulnaris m.

Flexor digitorum profundus m.

Figure 4.3.5

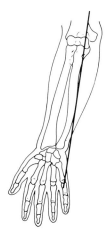

1. This section is just medial to the shaft of the ulna. Note the relationship of flexor carpi ulnaris and flexor digitorum profundus to the ulna.

2. The biceps tendon is clearly depicted in this section. It continues to insert on the radial tuberosity.

3. Note the trochlea within the trochlear notch.

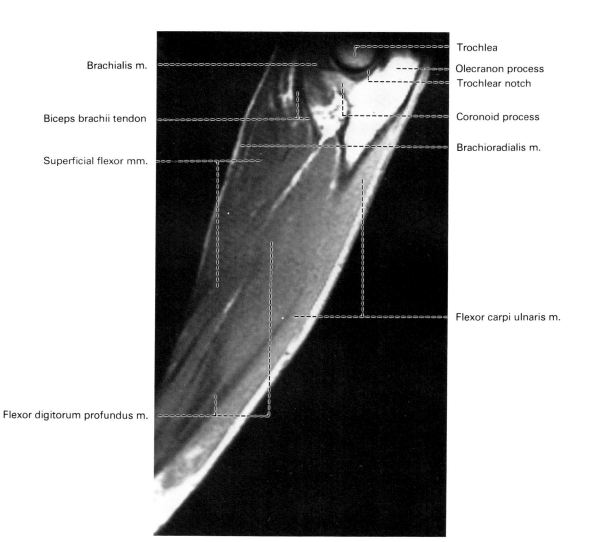

Brachialis m.

Biceps brachii tendon

Superficial flexor mm.

Flexor digitorum profundus m.

Trochlea

Olecranon process

Trochlear notch

Coronoid process

Brachioradialis m.

Flexor carpi ulnaris m.

Figure 4.3.6

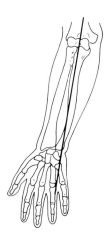

1. Flexor digitorum profundus surrounds the ulna on its posteromedial and anterior aspects.

2. Note that the radial tuberosity projects medially. It serves as the insertion site for the biceps tendon.

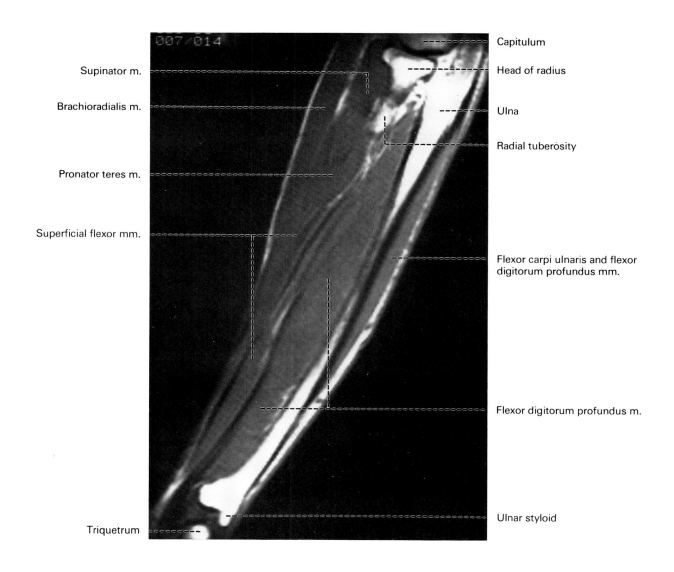

007/014

Supinator m.

Brachioradialis m.

Pronator teres m.

Superficial flexor mm.

Triquetrum

Capitulum

Head of radius

Ulna

Radial tuberosity

Flexor carpi ulnaris and flexor digitorum profundus mm.

Flexor digitorum profundus m.

Ulnar styloid

Figure 4.3.7

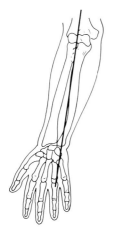

1. Anconeus is seen in this section. It originates from the lateral epicondyle and inserts on the lateral aspect of the olecranon.

2. The pronator teres is approaching its insertion on the lateral aspect of the radius at midshaft.

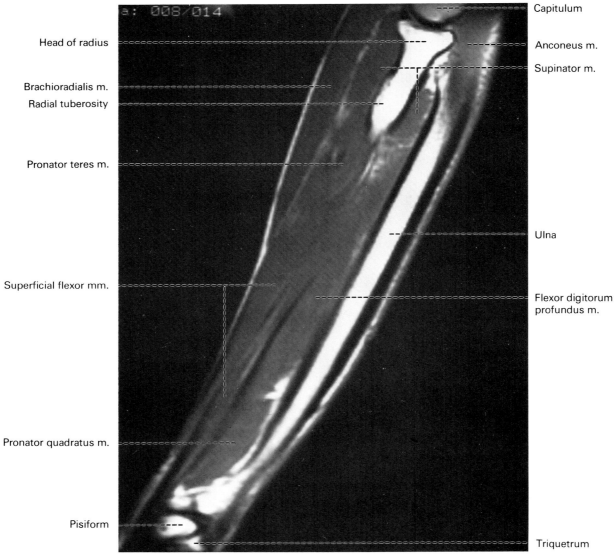

a: 008/014

Capitulum

Head of radius

Anconeus m.

Supinator m.

Brachioradialis m.

Radial tuberosity

Pronator teres m.

Ulna

Superficial flexor mm.

Flexor digitorum profundus m.

Pronator quadratus m.

Pisiform

Triquetrum

Figure 4.3.8

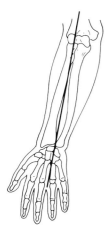

1. This section passes sagittally through the medial aspect of the radius and through the interosseous membrane.

2. The interosseous membrane serves as the origin for some deep flexor and extensor muscles.

3. The pronator quadratus lies deep to flexor pollicis longus and flexor digitorum profundus. It originates on the anterior surface of the distal ulna, runs transversely, and inserts on the anterior surface of the distal radius.

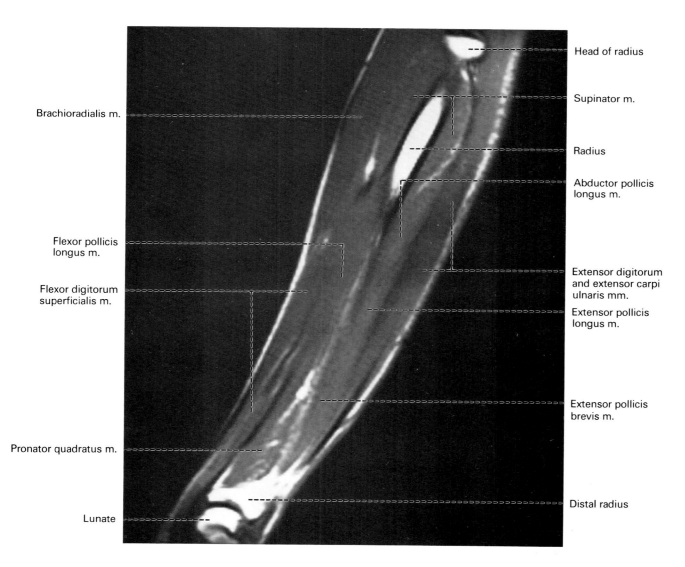

Figure 4.3.9

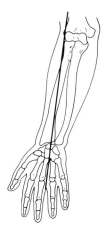

1. Pronator quadratus and supinator are demonstrated on either end of the radius.

2. Note the common extensor tendon, which originates from the lateral epicondyle.

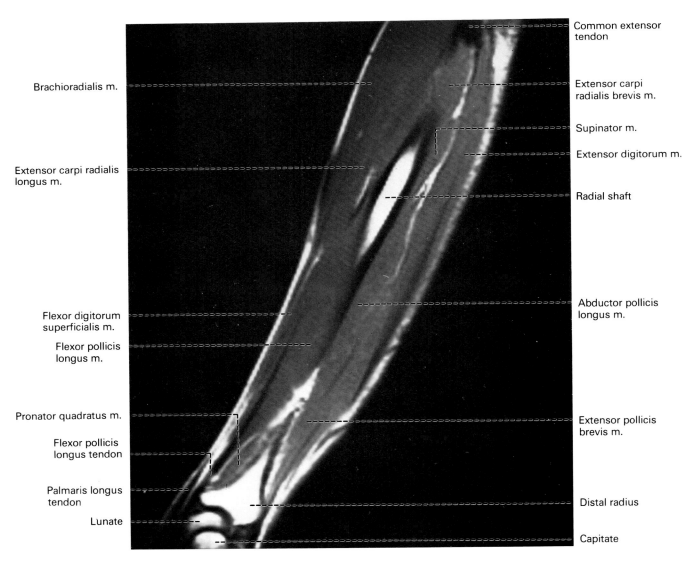

Figure 4.3.10

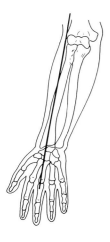

1. Brachioradialis and extensor carpi radialis longus originate from the lateral supracondylar crest (ridge).

2. Note the origin of flexor pollicis longus from the anterior surface of the radius.

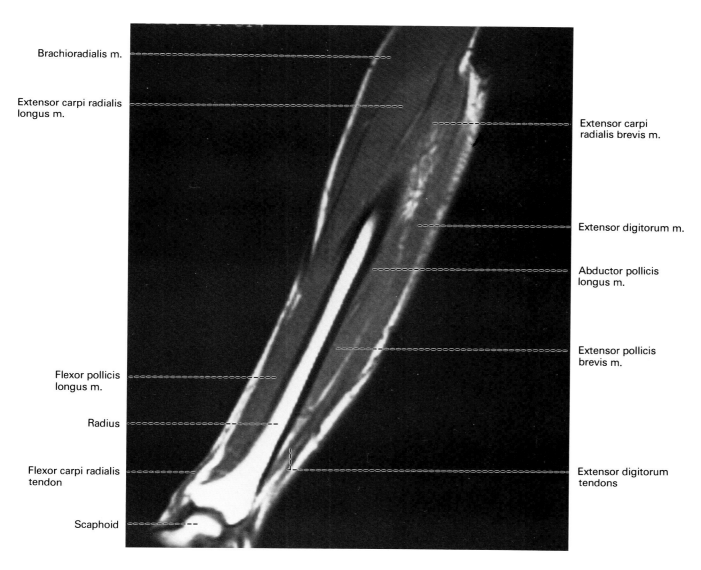

Brachioradialis m.

Extensor carpi radialis longus m.

Extensor carpi radialis brevis m.

Extensor digitorum m.

Abductor pollicis longus m.

Extensor pollicis brevis m.

Flexor pollicis longus m.

Radius

Flexor carpi radialis tendon

Extensor digitorum tendons

Scaphoid

Figure 4.3.11

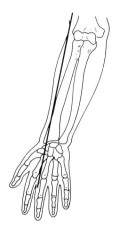

1. Note the origin of abductor pollicis longus and extensor pollicis brevis from the posterior surfaces of the radius. They also originate in part from the interosseous membrane.

2. Extensor carpi radialis brevis and extensor digitorum originate from the lateral epicondyle.

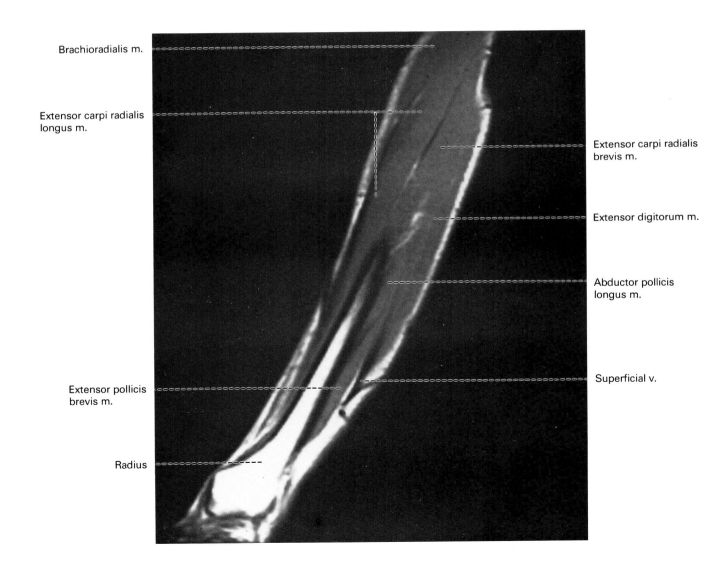

Brachioradialis m.

Extensor carpi radialis longus m.

Extensor carpi radialis brevis m.

Extensor digitorum m.

Abductor pollicis longus m.

Extensor pollicis brevis m.

Superficial v.

Radius

Figure 4.3.12

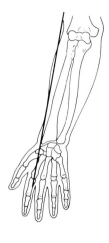

1. Abductor pollicis longus and extensor pollicis brevis cross the lateral aspect of the wrist to insert on the base of both the first metacarpal and proximal phalanx of the thumb, respectively.

2. This is the most lateral sagittal section of the forearm. It passes through some of the extensor muscles and tendons.

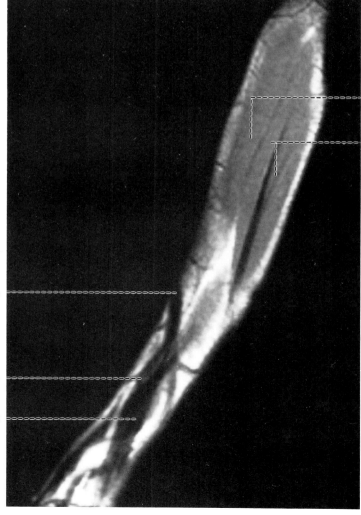

Extensor carpi radialis brevis m.

Extensor digitorum m.

Superficial v.

Abductor pollicis longus tendon

Extensor pollicis brevis tendon

Chapter 5

WRIST AND HAND

Figure 5.1.1

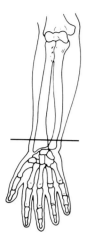

1. The tendon of palmaris longus flattens before it crosses the wrist superficial to the flexor retinaculum.

2. Palmaris longus terminates in the palmar aponeurosis (demonstrated in more distal sections).

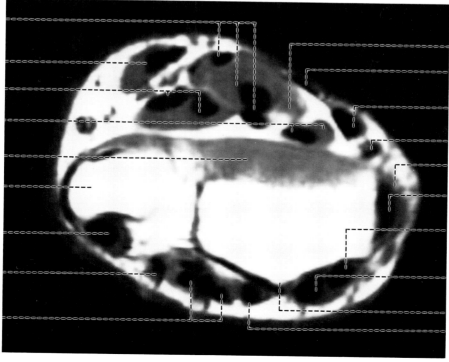

Flexor digitorum superficialis m. and tendon

Flexor carpi ulnaris tendon

Flexor digitorum profundus m.

Flexor pollicis longus m. and tendon

Pronator quadratus m.

Ulna

Extensor digiti minimi tendon

Extensor carpi ulnaris tendon

Extensor digitorum and extensor indicis tendons

Median nerve

Palmaris longus tendon

Flexor carpi radialis tendon

Radial a.

Abductor pollicis longus tendon

Extensor pollicis brevis tendon

Extensor carpi radialis longus tendon

Extensor carpi radialis brevis tendon

Tubercle of radius

Extensor pollicis longus tendon

Figure 5.1.2

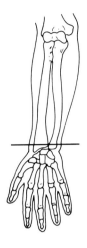

1. This section is through the distal radioulnar joint.

2. Note the groove on the dorsal surface of the distal ulna that houses the extensor carpi ulnaris tendon.

3. The extensor retinaculum is identified in this section; it is seen anchoring the tendons to the bone.

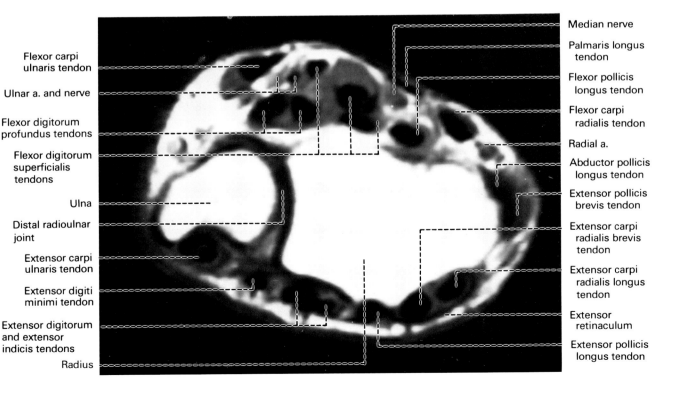

Labels (left):
- Flexor carpi ulnaris tendon
- Ulnar a. and nerve
- Flexor digitorum profundus tendons
- Flexor digitorum superficialis tendons
- Ulna
- Distal radioulnar joint
- Extensor carpi ulnaris tendon
- Extensor digiti minimi tendon
- Extensor digitorum and extensor indicis tendons
- Radius

Labels (right):
- Median nerve
- Palmaris longus tendon
- Flexor pollicis longus tendon
- Flexor carpi radialis tendon
- Radial a.
- Abductor pollicis longus tendon
- Extensor pollicis brevis tendon
- Extensor carpi radialis brevis tendon
- Extensor carpi radialis longus tendon
- Extensor retinaculum
- Extensor pollicis longus tendon

Figure 5.1.3

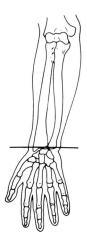

1. This section is through the radiocarpal joint.

2. Note the triangular fibrocartilage complex and its attachment to the distal radius.

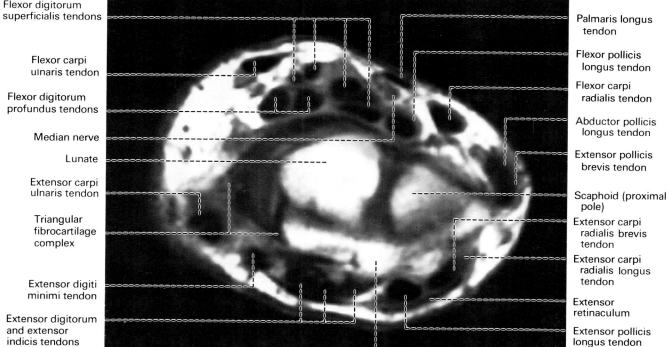

Flexor digitorum superficialis tendons

Flexor carpi ulnaris tendon

Flexor digitorum profundus tendons

Median nerve

Lunate

Extensor carpi ulnaris tendon

Triangular fibrocartilage complex

Extensor digiti minimi tendon

Extensor digitorum and extensor indicis tendons

Palmaris longus tendon

Flexor pollicis longus tendon

Flexor carpi radialis tendon

Abductor pollicis longus tendon

Extensor pollicis brevis tendon

Scaphoid (proximal pole)

Extensor carpi radialis brevis tendon

Extensor carpi radialis longus tendon

Extensor retinaculum

Extensor pollicis longus tendon

Radius

Figure 5.1.4

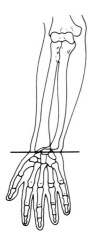

1. This section passes through the bones of the proximal carpal row.

2. Extensor pollicis longus tendon shifts its course laterally prior to crossing over the extensor carpi radialis longus and brevis tendons.

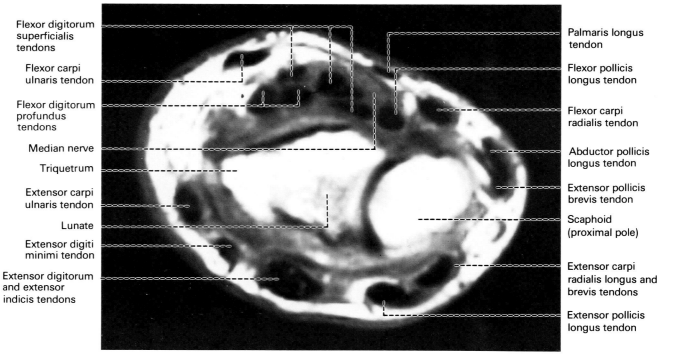

Flexor digitorum superficialis tendons

Flexor carpi ulnaris tendon

Flexor digitorum profundus tendons

Median nerve

Triquetrum

Extensor carpi ulnaris tendon

Lunate

Extensor digiti minimi tendon

Extensor digitorum and extensor indicis tendons

Palmaris longus tendon

Flexor pollicis longus tendon

Flexor carpi radialis tendon

Abductor pollicis longus tendon

Extensor pollicis brevis tendon

Scaphoid (proximal pole)

Extensor carpi radialis longus and brevis tendons

Extensor pollicis longus tendon

Figure 5.1.5

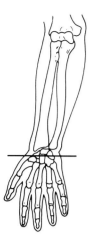

1. The flexor carpi ulnaris tendon inserts on the pisiform.

2. Note the flattened tendon of palmaris longus. It continues superficial to the flexor retinaculum and merges more distally with the palmar aponeurosis.

3. Note the position of the median nerve just beneath the flexor retinaculum.

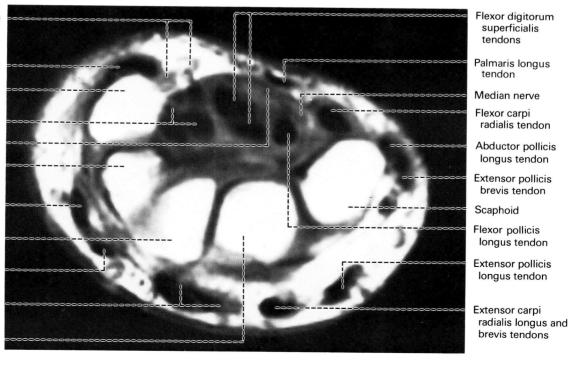

Ulnar a. and nerve

Flexor carpi ulnaris tendon

Pisiform

Flexor digitorum profundus tendons

Flexor retinaculum

Triquetrum

Extensor carpi ulnaris tendon

Hamate

Extensor digiti minimi tendon

Extensor digitorum and extensor indicis tendons

Capitate

Flexor digitorum superficialis tendons

Palmaris longus tendon

Median nerve

Flexor carpi radialis tendon

Abductor pollicis longus tendon

Extensor pollicis brevis tendon

Scaphoid

Flexor pollicis longus tendon

Extensor pollicis longus tendon

Extensor carpi radialis longus and brevis tendons

Figure 5.1.6

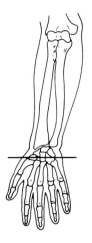

1. This section is through the proximal portion of the carpal tunnel.

2. Four bones form the boundaries on each side of the carpal tunnel. These are the pisiform and hamulus of the hamate on the medial side and scaphoid and trapezoid on the lateral side.

3. Extensor pollicis longus has completed its crossing of extensor carpi radialis longus and brevis tendons.

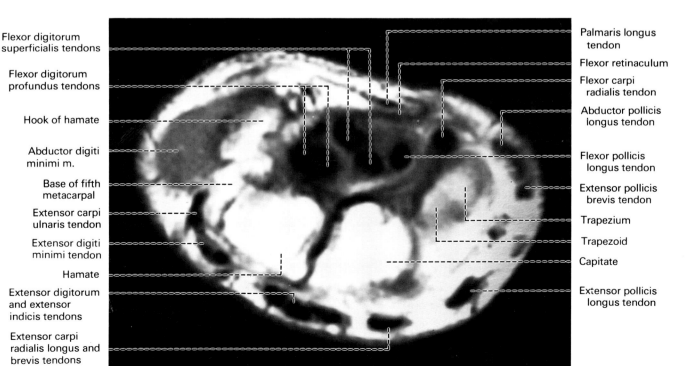

Flexor digitorum superficialis tendons

Flexor digitorum profundus tendons

Hook of hamate

Abductor digiti minimi m.

Base of fifth metacarpal

Extensor carpi ulnaris tendon

Extensor digiti minimi tendon

Hamate

Extensor digitorum and extensor indicis tendons

Extensor carpi radialis longus and brevis tendons

Palmaris longus tendon

Flexor retinaculum

Flexor carpi radialis tendon

Abductor pollicis longus tendon

Flexor pollicis longus tendon

Extensor pollicis brevis tendon

Trapezium

Trapezoid

Capitate

Extensor pollicis longus tendon

Figure 5.1.7

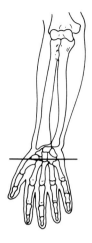

1. For the most part, this section is through the distal carpal row.

2. Extensor carpi radialis brevis inserts on the base of the third metacarpal.

3. Extensor carpi ulnaris inserts on the base of the fifth metacarpal.

4. Note the tubercle of the trapezium and hamulus of the hamate to which the flexor retinaculum attaches.

5. The proximal portions of the thenar and hypothenar muscles are seen at their origin from the flexor retinaculum and surrounding carpal bones.

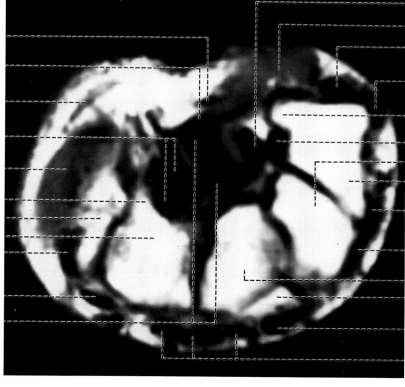

Palmaris longus tendon

Flexor retinaculum

Palmaris brevis m.

Flexor digitorum profundus tendons

Abductor digiti minimi m.

Hamulus of hamate

Base of fifth metacarpal

Hamate

Extensor carpi ulnaris tendon

Extensor digiti minimi tendon

Flexor digitorum superficialis tendons

Flexor pollicis longus tendon

Abductor pollicis brevis m.

Abductor pollicis longus tendon

Extensor pollicis brevis tendon

Tubercle of trapezium

Flexor carpi radialis tendon

Trapezoid

Trapezium

Extensor pollicis longus and brevis tendons

Extensor carpi radialis longus tendon

Capitate

Styloid process, third metacarpal

Extensor carpi radialis brevis tendon

Extensor digitorum and extensor indicis tendons

Figure 5.1.8

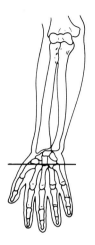

1. This section is through the bases of the metacarpals.

2. The abductor pollicis longus tendon inserts on the radial aspect of the base of the first metacarpal.

3. Note the thin fibers of palmaris brevis in subcutaneous fat overlying the hypothenar muscles.

4. The flexor carpi radialis tendon inserts at the base of the second metatarsal.

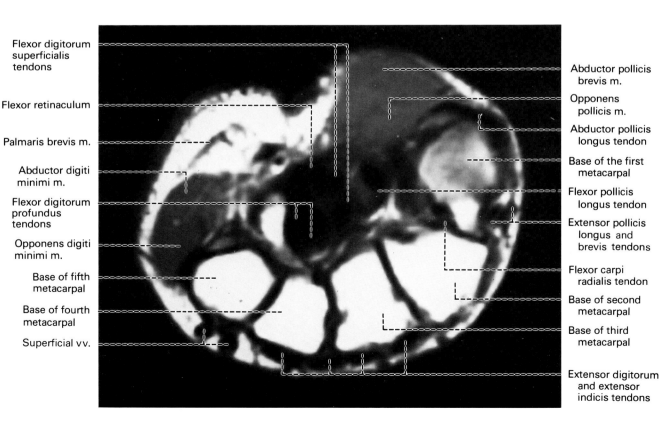

Flexor digitorum superficialis tendons

Flexor retinaculum

Palmaris brevis m.

Abductor digiti minimi m.

Flexor digitorum profundus tendons

Opponens digiti minimi m.

Base of fifth metacarpal

Base of fourth metacarpal

Superficial vv.

Abductor pollicis brevis m.

Opponens pollicis m.

Abductor pollicis longus tendon

Base of the first metacarpal

Flexor pollicis longus tendon

Extensor pollicis longus and brevis tendons

Flexor carpi radialis tendon

Base of second metacarpal

Base of third metacarpal

Extensor digitorum and extensor indicis tendons

Figure 5.1.9

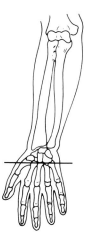

1. Note the origin of adductor pollicis from the shaft of the third metacarpal.

2. The extensor pollicis brevis and longus tendons proceed toward their insertion on the posterolateral aspect of the thumb.

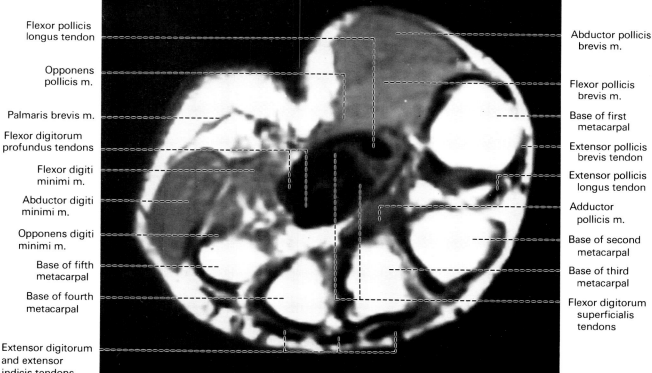

Flexor pollicis longus tendon

Opponens pollicis m.

Palmaris brevis m.

Flexor digitorum profundus tendons

Flexor digiti minimi m.

Abductor digiti minimi m.

Opponens digiti minimi m.

Base of fifth metacarpal

Base of fourth metacarpal

Extensor digitorum and extensor indicis tendons

Abductor pollicis brevis m.

Flexor pollicis brevis m.

Base of first metacarpal

Extensor pollicis brevis tendon

Extensor pollicis longus tendon

Adductor pollicis m.

Base of second metacarpal

Base of third metacarpal

Flexor digitorum superficialis tendons

Figure 5.1.10

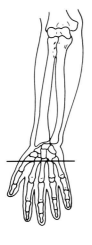

1. The flexor pollicis longus takes an independent course from the rest of the flexor tendons as it proceeds toward the thumb.

2. Some of the dorsal and palmar interosseous muscles are demonstrated on this section.

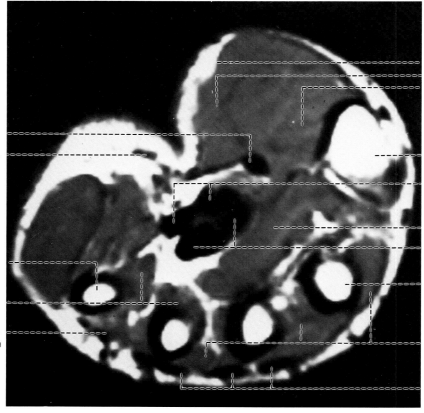

Flexor pollicis longus tendon

Palmaris brevis m.

Fifth metacarpal

Palmar interosseous mm.

Extensor digiti minimi tendon

Abductor pollicis brevis m.
Flexor pollicis brevis m.
Opponens pollicis m.
} Thenar mm.

First metacarpal

Flexor digitorum superficialis tendons

Adductor pollicis m.

Flexor digitorum profundus tendons

Second metacarpal

Dorsal interosseous mm.

Extensor digitorum and extensor indicis tendons

Figure 5.1.11

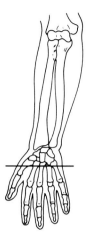

1. The intrinsic muscles of the hand are well demonstrated in this section.

2. The flexor pollicis longus tendon continues in its course toward the thumb. It lies between the thenar muscles and adductor pollicis.

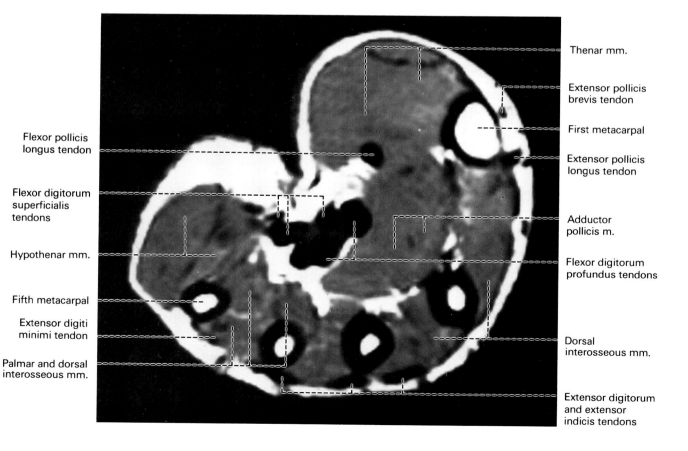

Flexor pollicis longus tendon

Flexor digitorum superficialis tendons

Hypothenar mm.

Fifth metacarpal

Extensor digiti minimi tendon

Palmar and dorsal interosseous mm.

Thenar mm.

Extensor pollicis brevis tendon

First metacarpal

Extensor pollicis longus tendon

Adductor pollicis m.

Flexor digitorum profundus tendons

Dorsal interosseous mm.

Extensor digitorum and extensor indicis tendons

Figure 5.1.12

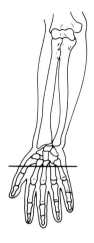

1. With the exception of the flexor pollicis longus tendon, all the flexor tendons travel in the center of the palm.

2. In this section as well as in several of the more proximal sections, the tendons of the flexor digitorum profundus appear as two structures rather than four. This is because the tendons to the little and ring fingers as well as the middle and index fingers are fused. These will split into four separate tendons in more distal sections.

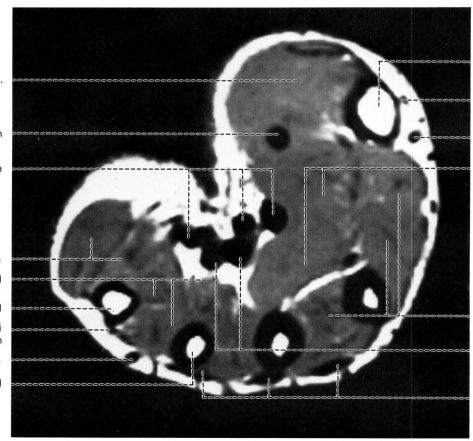

Thenar mm.

Flexor pollicis longus tendon

Flexor digitorum superficialis tendons

Hypothenar mm

Palmar and dorsal interosseous mm

Fifth metacarpal

Extensor digiti minimi tendon

Superficial v.

Fourth metacarpal

First metacarpal

Extensor pollicis brevis tendon

Extensor pollicis longus tendon

Adductor pollicis m.

Dorsal interosseous mm.

Flexor digitorum profundus tendons

Extensor digitorum and extensor indicis tendons

Figure 5.1.13

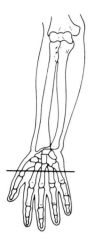

1. The thenar and hypothenar muscles diminish in size as they approach their insertion at the bases of the proximal phalanges of the thumb and little finger, respectively.

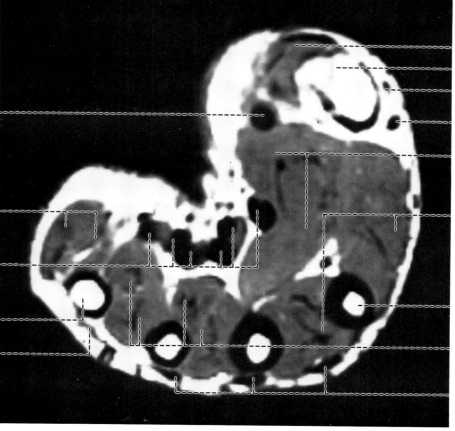

Flexor pollicis longus tendon

Hypothenar mm.

Flexor digitorum profundus and superficialis tendons

Fifth metacarpal

Extensor digiti minimi tendon

Thenar mm.

First metacarpal

Extensor pollicis brevis tendon

Extensor pollicis longus tendon

Adductor pollicis m.

Dorsal interosseous mm.

Second metacarpal

Palmar and dorsal interosseous mm.

Flexor digitorum and extensor indicis tendons

Figure 5.1.14

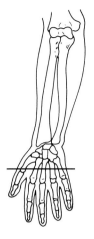

1. In this section the proximal portions of the lumbrical muscles can be identified. They originate on the surface of the flexor digitorum profundus tendons.

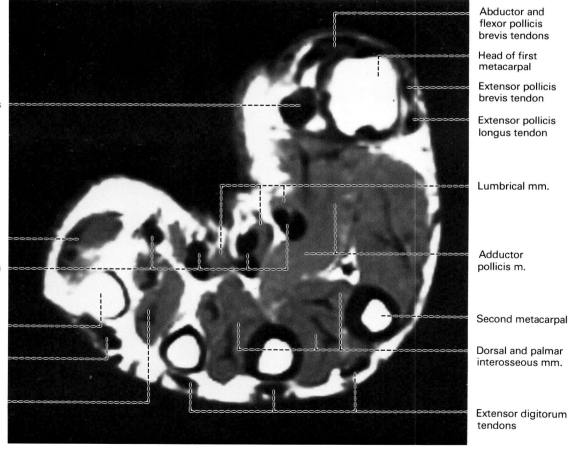

Flexor pollicis longus m.

Hypothenar mm.

Flexor digitorum profundus and superficialis tendons

Fifth metacarpal

Extensor digiti minimi tendon

Dorsal interosseous m.

Abductor and flexor pollicis brevis tendons

Head of first metacarpal

Extensor pollicis brevis tendon

Extensor pollicis longus tendon

Lumbrical mm.

Adductor pollicis m.

Second metacarpal

Dorsal and palmar interosseous mm.

Extensor digitorum tendons

Figure 5.1.15

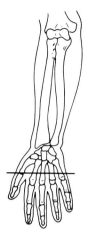

1. Extensor pollicis brevis inserts at the base of the proximal phalanx of the thumb.

2. The lumbricals continue distally in close relationship to the flexor tendons until their insertion on the dorsal expansions of the fingers.

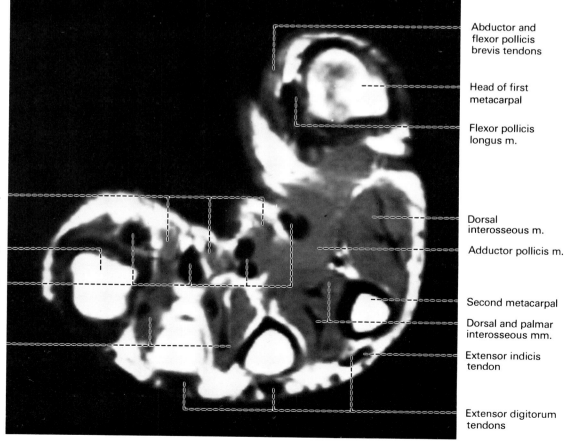

Figure 5.1.16

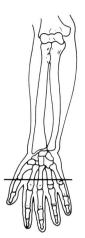

1. As the sections approach the fingers, the intrinsic muscles diminish in size and only tendons are prominently seen.

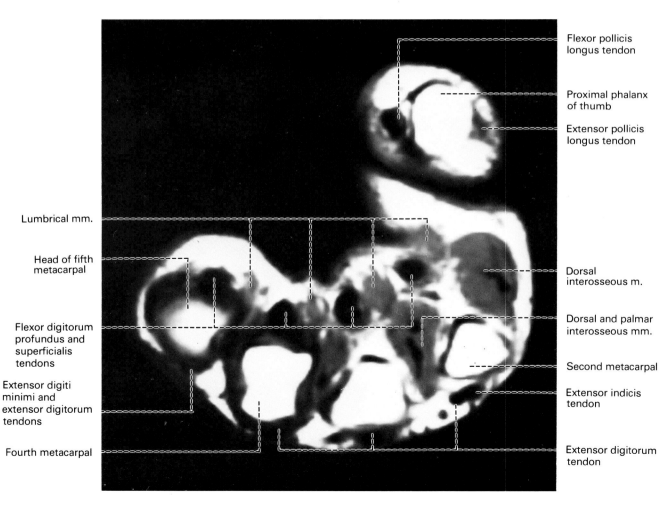

Figure 5.1.17

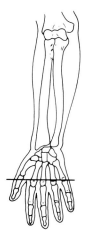

1. Note that the lumbrical muscles proceed distally on the radial side of the tendons.

2. The tendons of the flexor digitorum profundus and those of flexor digitorum superficialis are separable in the more distal sections.

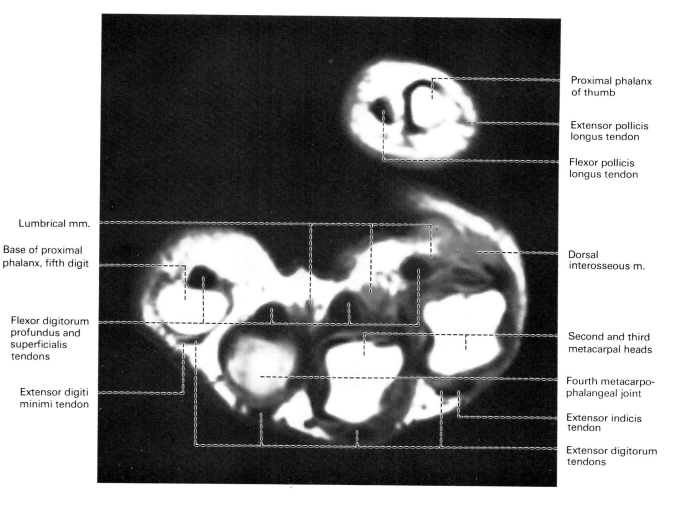

Proximal phalanx of thumb

Extensor pollicis longus tendon

Flexor pollicis longus tendon

Lumbrical mm.

Base of proximal phalanx, fifth digit

Flexor digitorum profundus and superficialis tendons

Extensor digiti minimi tendon

Dorsal interosseous m.

Second and third metacarpal heads

Fourth metacarpo-phalangeal joint

Extensor indicis tendon

Extensor digitorum tendons

Figure 5.1.18

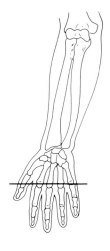

1. Note that beyond the metacarpophalangeal joints only tendons are present.

2. The extensor tendons are flat and small compared to the flexor tendons.

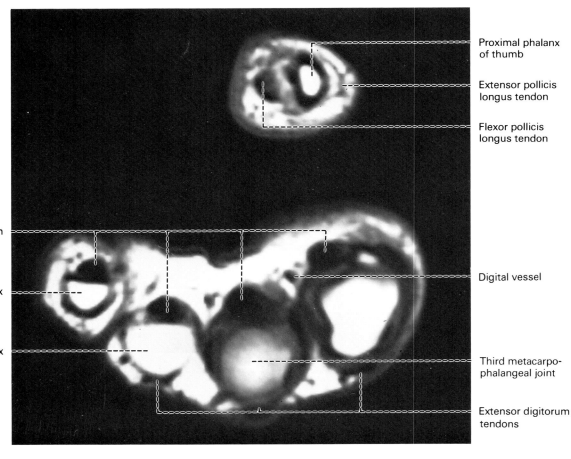

Proximal phalanx of thumb

Extensor pollicis longus tendon

Flexor pollicis longus tendon

Flexor digitorum profundus and superficialis tendons

Proximal phalanx of fifth digit

Proximal phalanx of fourth digit

Digital vessel

Third metacarpo-phalangeal joint

Extensor digitorum tendons

Figure 5.1.19

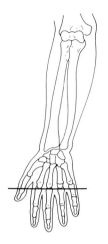

1. The dorsal expansions (hoods) on the dorsum of the proximal phalanges of the ring and little finger are seen as flattened fibrous structures adherent to the bone.

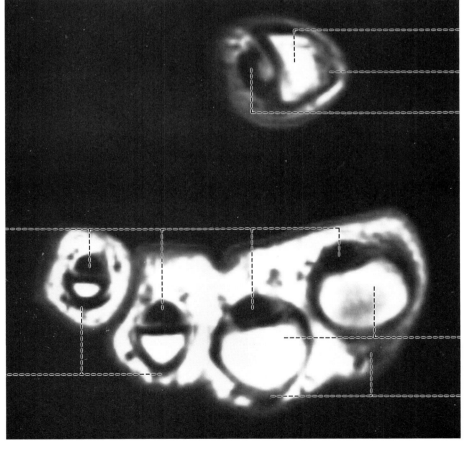

Proximal phalanx of thumb

Extensor pollicis longus tendon

Flexor pollicis longus tendon

Flexor digitorum profundus and superficialis tendons

Dorsal expansions (hoods)

Base of proximal phalanges, index and long (middle) fingers

Extensor digitorum tendons

Figure 5.1.20

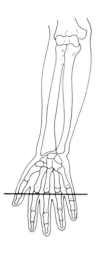

1. The flexor pollicis longus and extensor pollicis longus tendons insert on the base of the distal phalanx of the thumb.

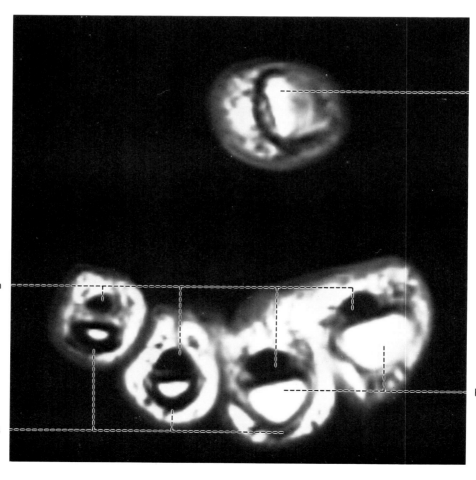

Figure 5.1.21

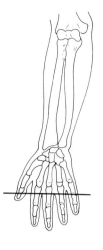

1. Part of the extensor tendon inserts on the base of the middle phalanx and the rest of the tendon inserts on the base of the distal phalanx.

2. The flexor digitorum superficialis tendons insert on the middle phalanges.

3. The flexor digitorum profundus tendons insert on the bases of the distal phalanges.

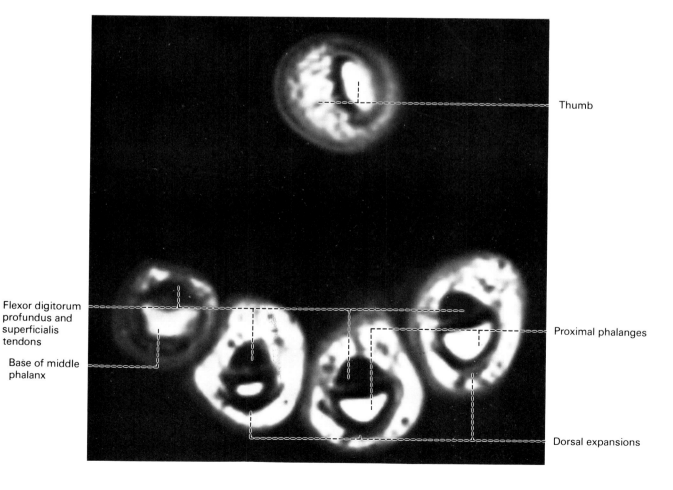

Thumb

Flexor digitorum profundus and superficialis tendons

Base of middle phalanx

Proximal phalanges

Dorsal expansions

Figure 5.2.1

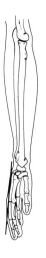

1. This coronal section is through the dorsum of the wrist and hand.

2. Some of the extensor tendons are clearly depicted.

3. Just distal to the radial tubercle the course of extensor pollicis longus angles radially toward the thumb and crosses over the tendons of extensor carpi radialis longus and brevis in the wrist.

4. Extensor digiti minimi tendon crosses the wrist on the radial aspect of the head of the ulna.

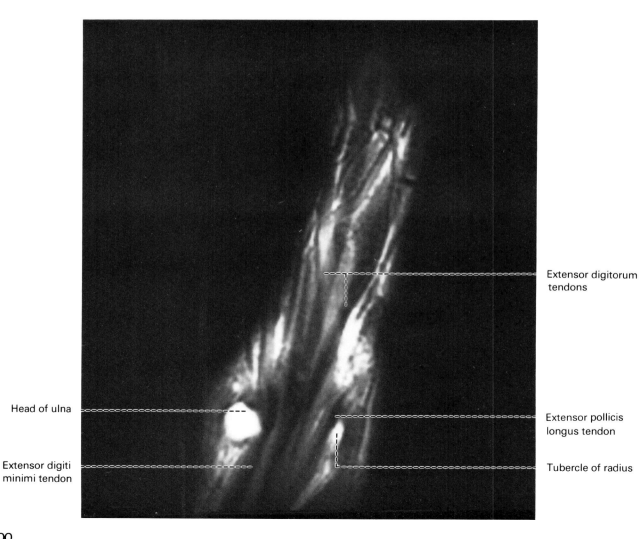

Extensor digitorum tendons

Head of ulna

Extensor pollicis longus tendon

Extensor digiti minimi tendon

Tubercle of radius

Figure 5.2.2

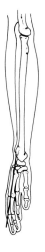

1. Extensor carpi radialis longus tendon inserts on the base of the second metacarpal.

2. The triangular fibrocartilage extends between the distal radius and ulnar styloid.

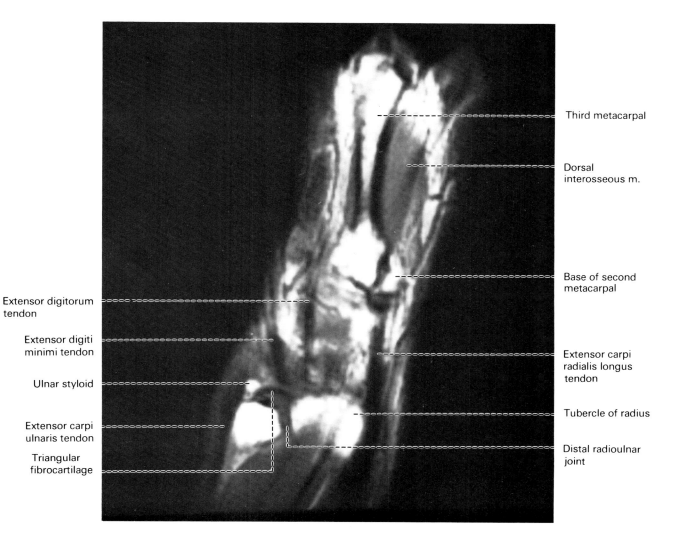

Third metacarpal

Dorsal interosseous m.

Base of second metacarpal

Extensor carpi radialis longus tendon

Tubercle of radius

Distal radioulnar joint

Extensor digitorum tendon

Extensor digiti minimi tendon

Ulnar styloid

Extensor carpi ulnaris tendon

Triangular fibrocartilage

Figure 5.2.3

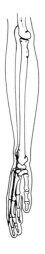

1. This section passes through the dorsal aspect of the carpal bones.

2. The distal radioulnar joint and part of the triangular fibrocartilage are demonstrated.

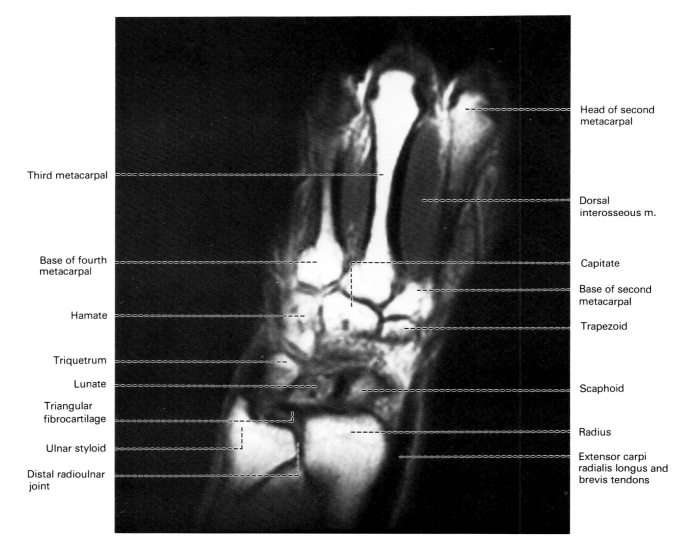

Third metacarpal

Base of fourth metacarpal

Hamate

Triquetrum

Lunate

Triangular fibrocartilage

Ulnar styloid

Distal radioulnar joint

Head of second metacarpal

Dorsal interosseous m.

Capitate

Base of second metacarpal

Trapezoid

Scaphoid

Radius

Extensor carpi radialis longus and brevis tendons

Figure 5.2.4

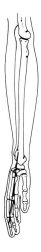

1. The interosseous muscles on either side of the third metacarpal are seen inserting on the proximal phalanx of the long (middle) finger. The interosseous muscles insert, in part, into the dorsal expansion.

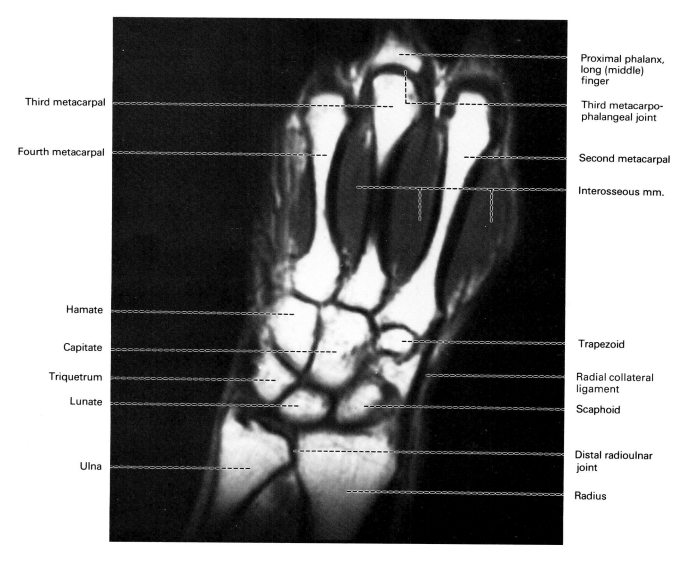

Third metacarpal

Fourth metacarpal

Hamate

Capitate

Triquetrum

Lunate

Ulna

Proximal phalanx, long (middle) finger

Third metacarpophalangeal joint

Second metacarpal

Interosseous mm.

Trapezoid

Radial collateral ligament

Scaphoid

Distal radioulnar joint

Radius

Figure 5.2.5

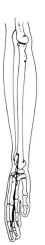

1. The radiocarpal, midcarpal, and carpometacarpal as well as some of the metacarpophalangeal joints are well seen in this section.

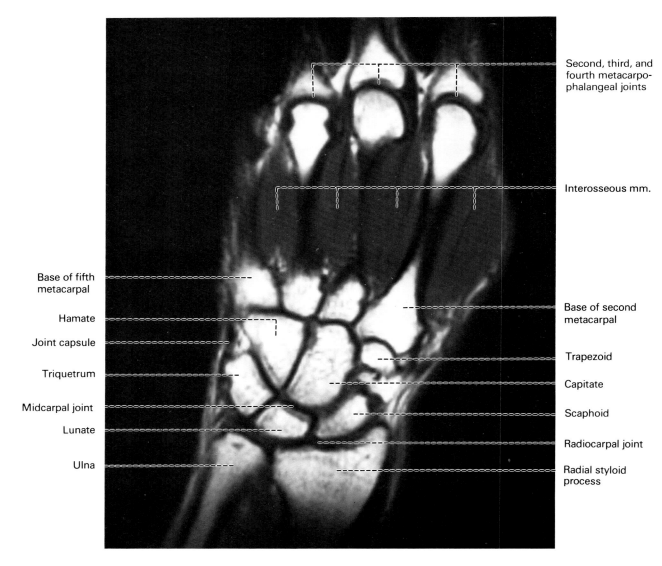

Second, third, and fourth metacarpo-phalangeal joints

Interosseous mm.

Base of fifth metacarpal

Hamate

Joint capsule

Triquetrum

Midcarpal joint

Lunate

Ulna

Base of second metacarpal

Trapezoid

Capitate

Scaphoid

Radiocarpal joint

Radial styloid process

Figure 5.2.6

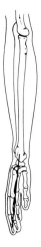

1. Abductor pollicis longus and extensor pollicis brevis tendons course in the direction of the thumb. They are demonstrated on the radial aspect of the wrist.

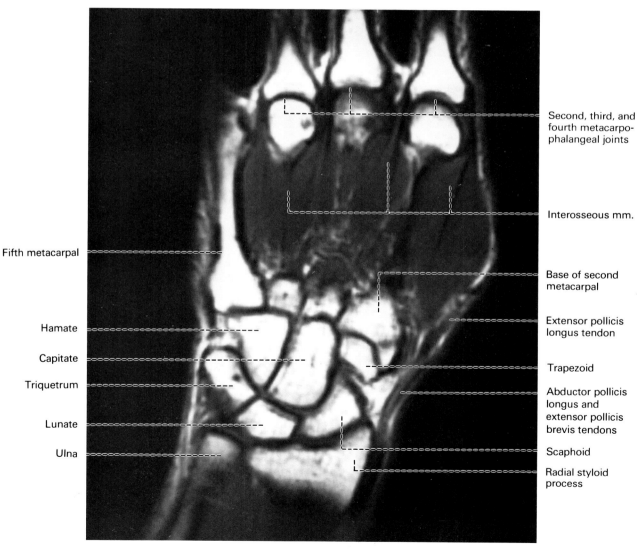

Second, third, and fourth metacarpo-phalangeal joints

Interosseous mm.

Fifth metacarpal

Base of second metacarpal

Hamate

Extensor pollicis longus tendon

Capitate

Trapezoid

Triquetrum

Abductor pollicis longus and extensor pollicis brevis tendons

Lunate

Ulna

Scaphoid

Radial styloid process

Figure 5.2.7

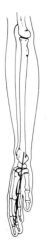

1. The adductor pollicis originates from the third metacarpal and capitate.

2. Note the insertion of the interosseous muscles at the base of the proximal phalanges of the second and third fingers.

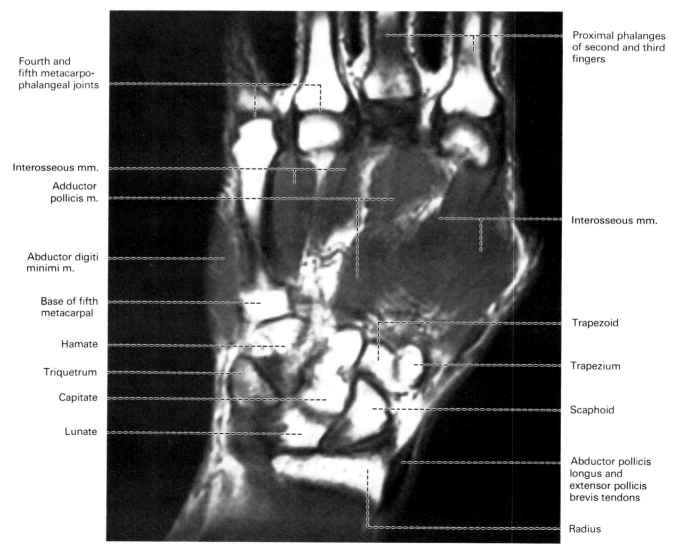

Fourth and fifth metacarpophalangeal joints

Interosseous mm.

Adductor pollicis m.

Abductor digiti minimi m.

Base of fifth metacarpal

Hamate

Triquetrum

Capitate

Lunate

Proximal phalanges of second and third fingers

Interosseous mm.

Trapezoid

Trapezium

Scaphoid

Abductor pollicis longus and extensor pollicis brevis tendons

Radius

Figure 5.2.8

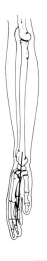

1. This section passes through the carpal tunnel and volar aspect of the palm.

2. Abductor digiti minimi originates from the pisiform.

3. Note the four bones forming the boundary of the carpal tunnel; they are the hamulus of the hamate, pisiform, trapezium, and scaphoid tubercle.

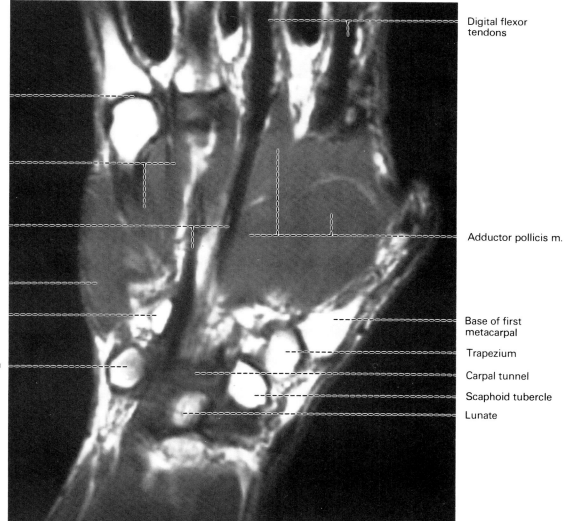

Figure 5.2.9

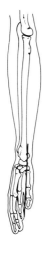

1. All the hypothenar muscles are depicted in this section. Flexor digiti minimi brevis and opponens digiti minimi originate from the flexor retinaculum.

2. Along with digital flexor tendons, the median nerve passes through the carpal tunnel into the palm.

3. The lumbrical muscles originate from the flexor digitorum profundus tendons.

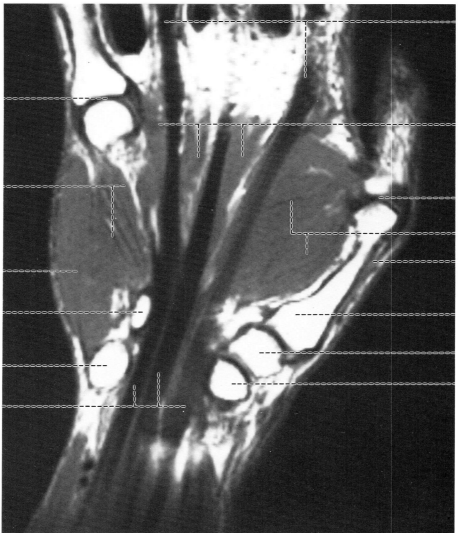

Figure 5.2.10

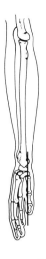

1. Flexor pollicis longus tendon courses between flexor pollicis brevis and adductor pollicis muscles.

2. Note the extensor pollicis longus tendon inserting at the base of the distal phalanx of the thumb.

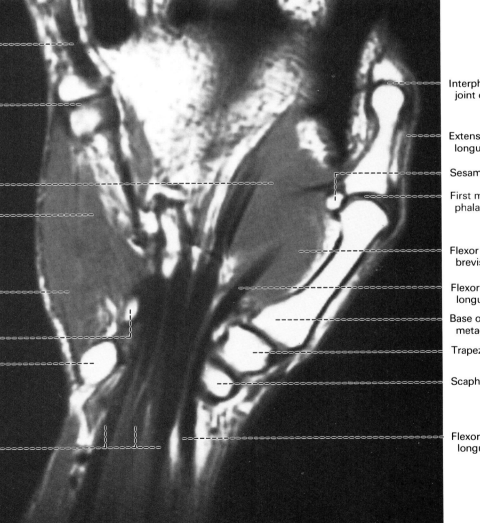

Flexor tendon, fifth digit

Fifth metacarpo- phalangeal joint

Adductor pollicis m.

Flexor digiti minimi brevis and opponens digiti minimi mm.

Abductor digiti minimi m.

Hamulus of hamate

Pisiform

Digital flexor tendons

Interphalangeal joint of thumb

Extensor pollicis longus tendon

Sesamoid bone

First metacarpo- phalangeal joint

Flexor pollicis brevis m.

Flexor pollicis longus tendon

Base of first metacarpal

Trapezium

Scaphoid tubercle

Flexor pollicis longus tendon

Figure 5.2.11

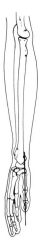

1. Some of the thenar and hypothenar muscles are clearly demonstrated in this section.

2. Flexor carpi radialis courses in the groove of the trapezium to reach its insertion at the base of the second metacarpal.

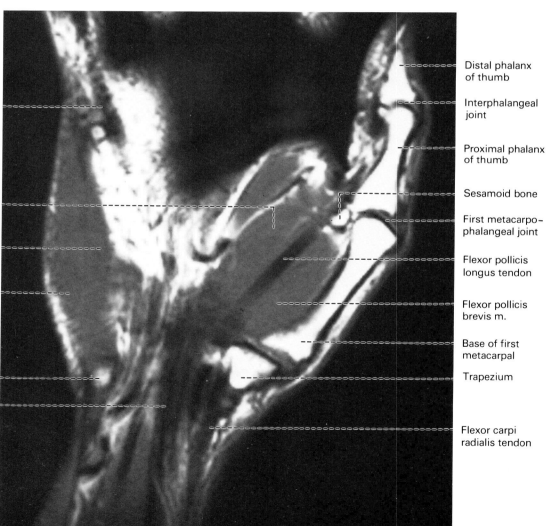

Flexor tendon, fifth finger

Adductor pollicis m.

Flexor digiti minimi brevis m.

Abductor digiti minimi m.

Pisiform

Palmaris longus tendon

Distal phalanx of thumb

Interphalangeal joint

Proximal phalanx of thumb

Sesamoid bone

First metacarpo-phalangeal joint

Flexor pollicis longus tendon

Flexor pollicis brevis m.

Base of first metacarpal

Trapezium

Flexor carpi radialis tendon

Figure 5.2.12

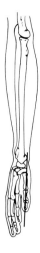

1. The fibers of palmaris brevis are quite superficial in the hypothenar aspect of the palm.

2. Note the insertion of the flexor pollicis longus tendon onto the base of the distal phalanx of the thumb.

3. Note the insertion of the flexor carpi ulnaris tendon onto the pisiform.

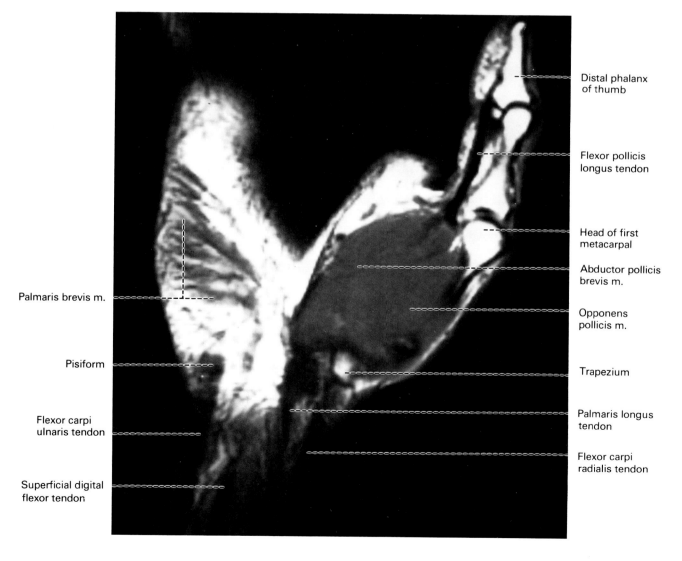

Palmaris brevis m.

Pisiform

Flexor carpi
ulnaris tendon

Superficial digital
flexor tendon

Distal phalanx
of thumb

Flexor pollicis
longus tendon

Head of first
metacarpal

Abductor pollicis
brevis m.

Opponens
pollicis m.

Trapezium

Palmaris longus
tendon

Flexor carpi
radialis tendon

Figure 5.2.13

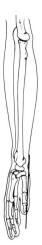

1. This parasagittal section is through the thenar muscles. They are not separable into individual components.

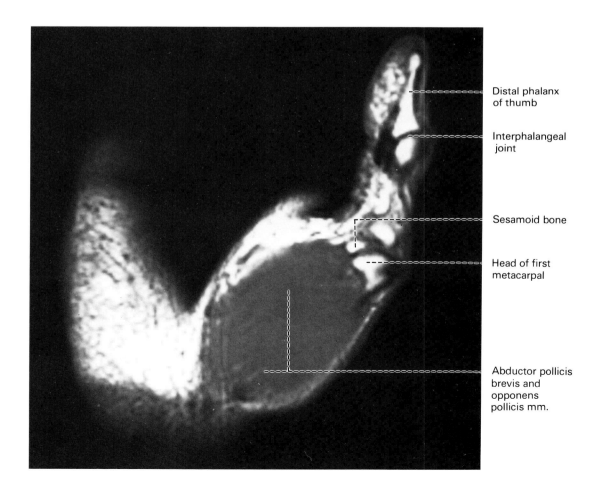

Distal phalanx of thumb

Interphalangeal joint

Sesamoid bone

Head of first metacarpal

Abductor pollicis brevis and opponens pollicis mm.

SAGITTAL

Figure 5.3.1

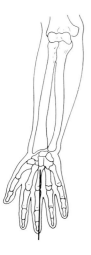

1. This parasagittal section is just off the midline.

2. The extensor mechanism is not demonstrated beyond the metacarpo-phalangeal joint because it is relatively much thinner than the flexor mechanism.

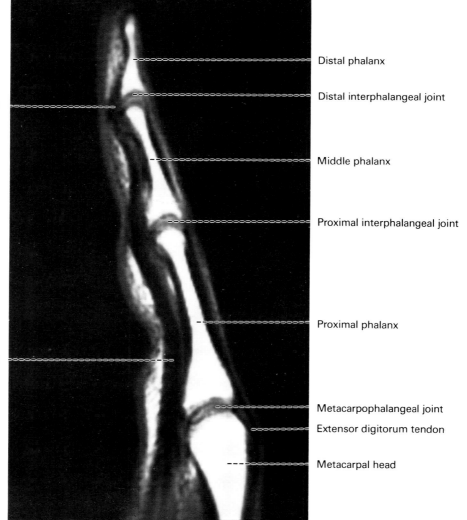

Flexor digitorum profundus tendon

Flexor digitorum profundus and superficialis tendons

Distal phalanx

Distal interphalangeal joint

Middle phalanx

Proximal interphalangeal joint

Proximal phalanx

Metacarpophalangeal joint

Extensor digitorum tendon

Metacarpal head

Figure 5.3.2

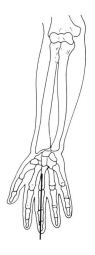

1. This is a midsagittal section through the long or middle finger.

2. On the palmar aspect of the finger, flexor digitorum profundus and flexor digitorum superficialis tendons course together to the middle phalanx.

3. Flexor digitorum superficialis inserts on the middle phalanx.

4. Flexor digitorum profundus continues distally to insert on the palmar aspect of the distal phalanx.

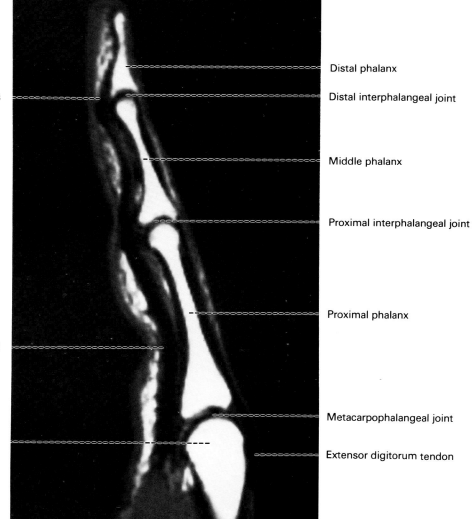

Flexor digitorum profundus tendon

Distal phalanx

Distal interphalangeal joint

Middle phalanx

Proximal interphalangeal joint

Proximal phalanx

Flexor digitorum profundus and superficialis tendons

Metacarpophalangeal joint

Metacarpal head

Extensor digitorum tendon

THORAX

Chapter 6

CARDIAC AND GREAT VESSEL ANATOMY

AXIAL

Figure 6.1.1

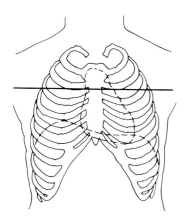

1. This section is through the aortic arch.

2. The azygos vein is arching anteriorly toward the superior vena cava.

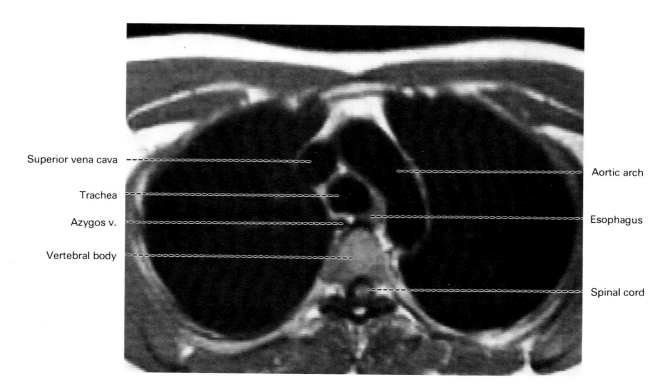

Superior vena cava

Trachea

Azygos v.

Vertebral body

Aortic arch

Esophagus

Spinal cord

Figure 6.1.2

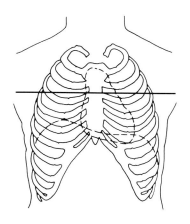

1. This section is through the left pulmonary artery.

2. The truncus anterior branch of the right pulmonary artery lies anterior to the right mainstem bronchus.

3. The azygos vein ascends adjacent to the esophagus.

4. Note the small pericardial recess posterior to the ascending aorta.

5. Because of the more cephalad location of the left pulmonary artery (when compared to the right), it appears falsely asymmetric in size.

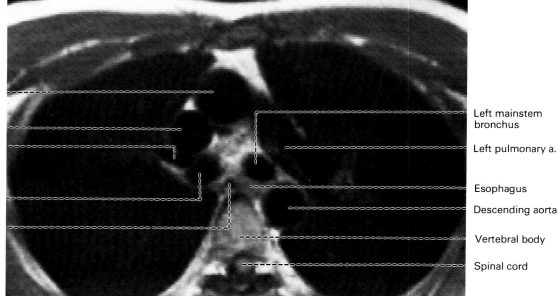

Figure 6.1.3

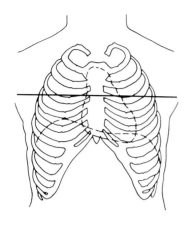

1. This section is through the main pulmonary artery.

2. A moderate-sized pericardial recess is noted, anterior to the aorta.

3. The azygos vein lies directly posterior to the right mainstem bronchus.

4. The left pulmonary artery arches over the left mainstem bronchus, while the right pulmonary artery passes anterior to the right mainstem bronchus.

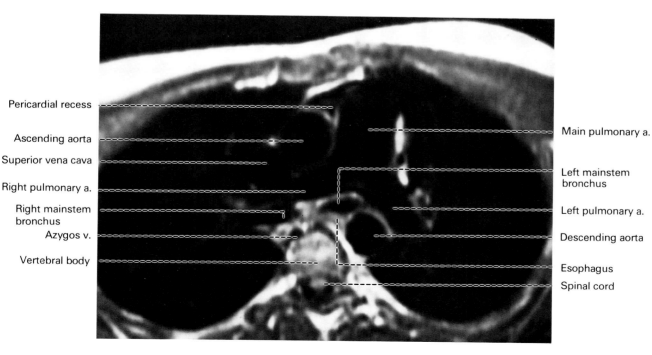

Pericardial recess

Ascending aorta

Superior vena cava

Right pulmonary a.

Right mainstem bronchus

Azygos v.

Vertebral body

Main pulmonary a.

Left mainstem bronchus

Left pulmonary a.

Descending aorta

Esophagus

Spinal cord

Figure 6.1.4

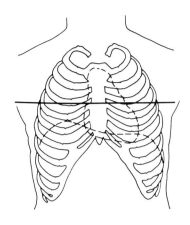

1. This section is through the right pulmonary artery.

2. A prominent pericardial recess is noted anterior to the aorta.

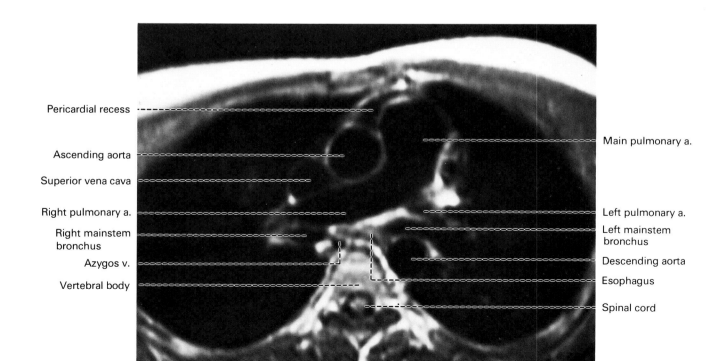

Pericardial recess

Ascending aorta

Superior vena cava

Right pulmonary a.

Right mainstem bronchus

Azygos v.

Vertebral body

Main pulmonary a.

Left pulmonary a.

Left mainstem bronchus

Descending aorta

Esophagus

Spinal cord

Figure 6.1.5

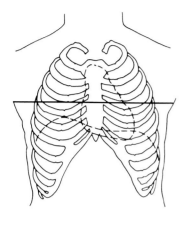

1. This section is through the proximal main pulmonary artery at the same level as the left atrial appendage.

2. The anterior pericardial recess may be mistaken for a right coronary artery.

3. The posterior right lung recess abuts the azygos vein.

4. Note the left pulmonary vein branch anterior to the left bronchus and the interlobar pulmonary artery posterior to the bronchus.

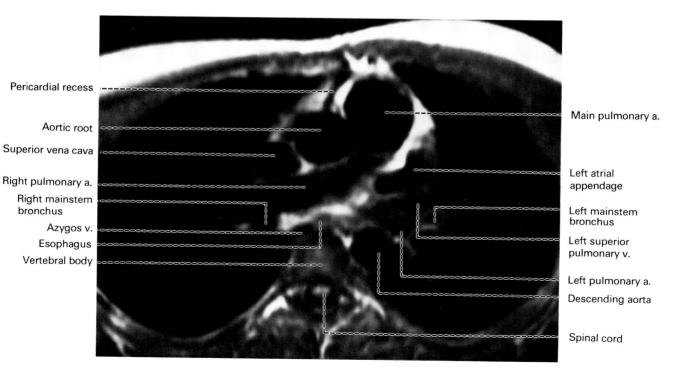

Pericardial recess

Aortic root

Superior vena cava

Right pulmonary a.

Right mainstem bronchus

Azygos v.

Esophagus

Vertebral body

Main pulmonary a.

Left atrial appendage

Left mainstem bronchus

Left superior pulmonary v.

Left pulmonary a.

Descending aorta

Spinal cord

Figure 6.1.6

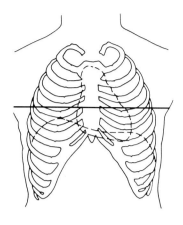

1. This section is through the aortic root at the origin of the left coronary artery.

2. A small portion of the left anterior descending branch of the left coronary artery is visualized as a low signal intensity structure surrounded by epicardial fat.

3. Note the orientation of the anterior pericardial recess; it is directed anteriorly from right to left. This can be distinguished from the right coronary artery, which is directed anteriorly from left to right.

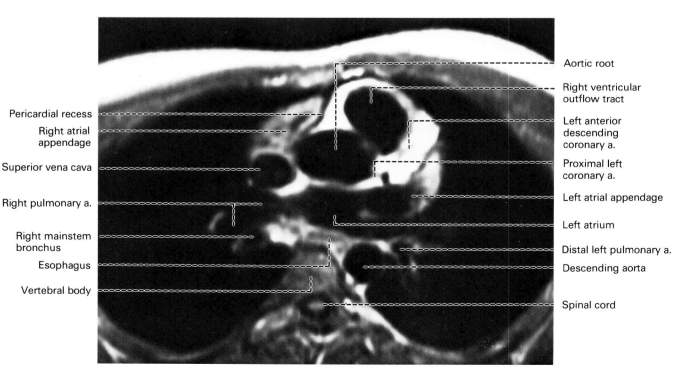

Figure 6.1.7

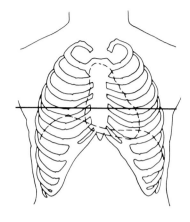

1. This section is through the aortic root at the origin of the right coronary artery.

2. The right atrial appendage demonstrates the internal architecture of the pectinate muscles.

3. Note the entrance of the superior vena cava into the right atrium at this level.

4. The roof of the left atrium is situated cephalad to the right atrium.

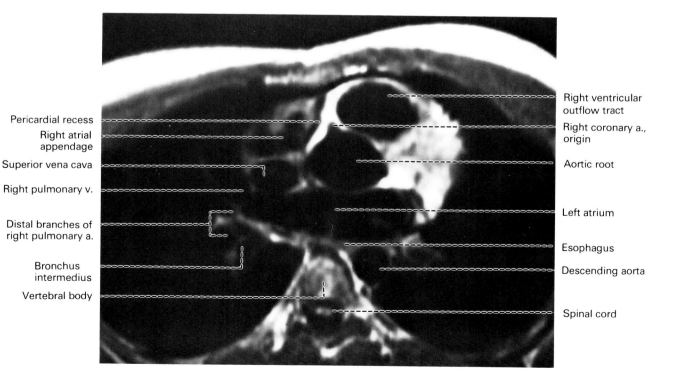

Figure 6.1.8

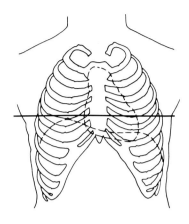

1. This section is through the left ventricular outflow tract.

2. Note the continuity of the anterior mitral valve leaflet with the posterior wall of the aorta — a normal relationship.

3. The ventricular septum is contiguous with the anterior wall of the aorta in a normal fashion.

4. Inferior pulmonary veins are seen entering the left atrium.

5. The proximal right coronary artery is surrounded by fat in the atrioventricular groove.

6. This section also shows the interatrial septum separating the right atrium from the left atrium.

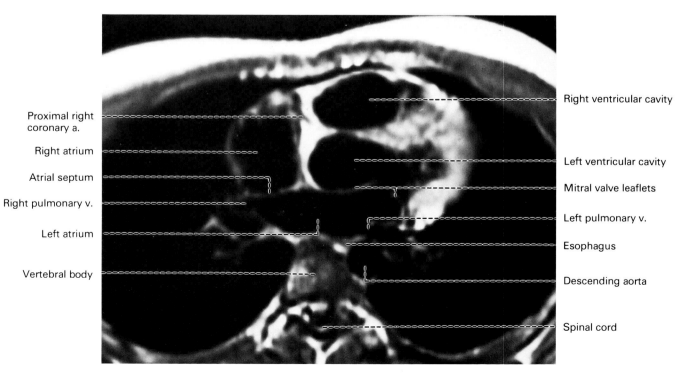

Figure 6.1.9

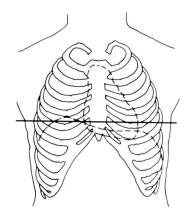

1. This section is through the plane of the atrioventricular valves.

2. Note the relationship of the posterior mitral valve leaflet with the posterior papillary muscle.

3. The atrial septum thins considerably at the level of the fossa ovalis and may become nearly indistinguishable.

4. The membranous ventricular septum is also thin at this level.

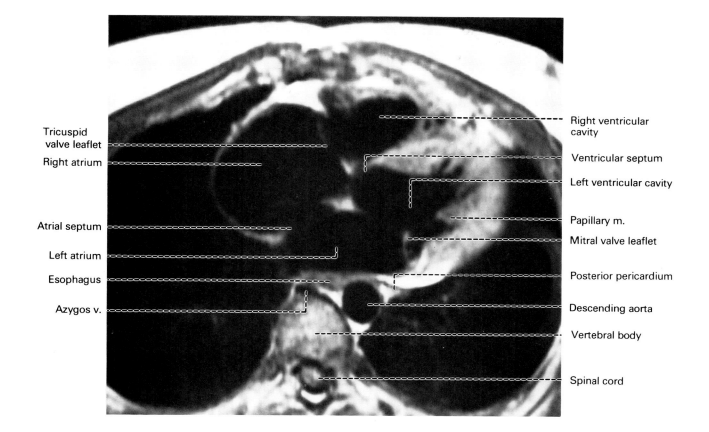

Tricuspid valve leaflet
Right atrium
Atrial septum
Left atrium
Esophagus
Azygos v.

Right ventricular cavity
Ventricular septum
Left ventricular cavity
Papillary m.
Mitral valve leaflet
Posterior pericardium
Descending aorta
Vertebral body
Spinal cord

Figure 6.1.10

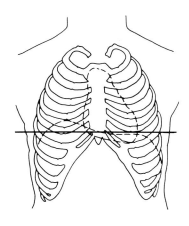

1. This section is through the inferior aspect of the atrioventricular valves.

2. The inferior vena cava is noted entering the right atrium. Blood flow is directed by the eustachian valve.

3. A short segment of pericardium is seen over the posterior left ventricle as a low signal intensity linear structure.

4. The left ventricular wall thickness is approximately three times the right ventricular wall thickness.

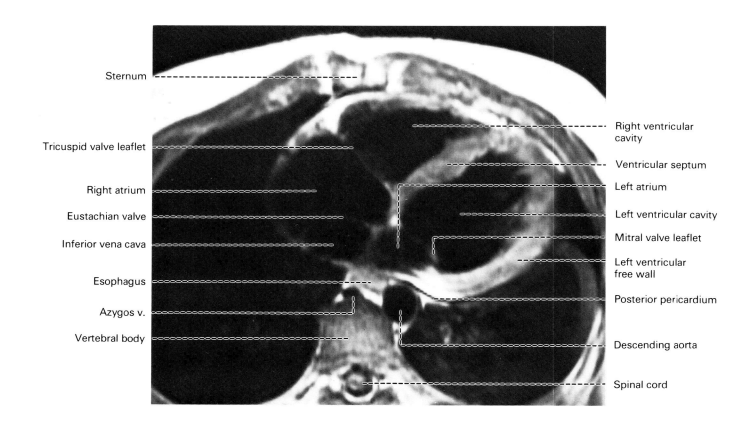

CORONAL

Figure 6.2.1

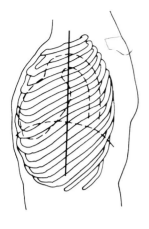

1. This section is through the posterior left atrium.

2. Note the right pulmonary artery lies immediately superior to the left atrium, in the same plane.

3. The coronary sinus is identified in the atrioventricular groove surrounded by high signal intensity fat.

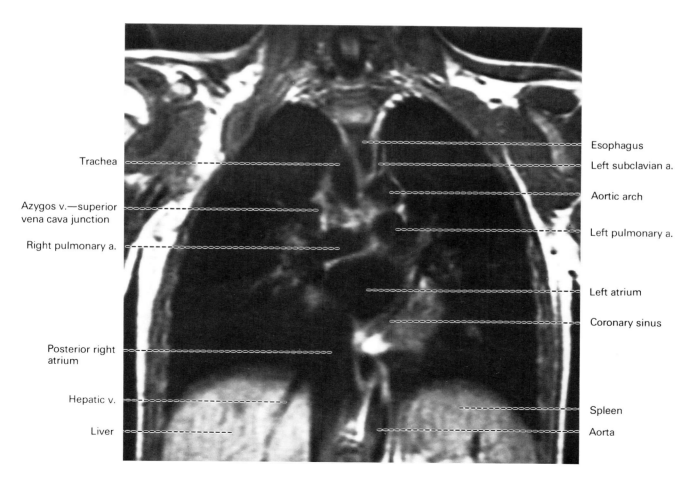

Figure 6.2.2

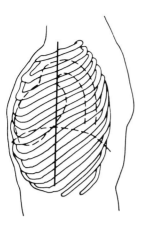

1. This section is through the atrial septum.

2. Note the middle hepatic vein joining the inferior vena cava **immediately** adjacent to its junction with the right atrium.

3. The right pulmonary artery passes under the aortic arch.

4. At this level the trachea and esophagus are in a side-by-side relationship.

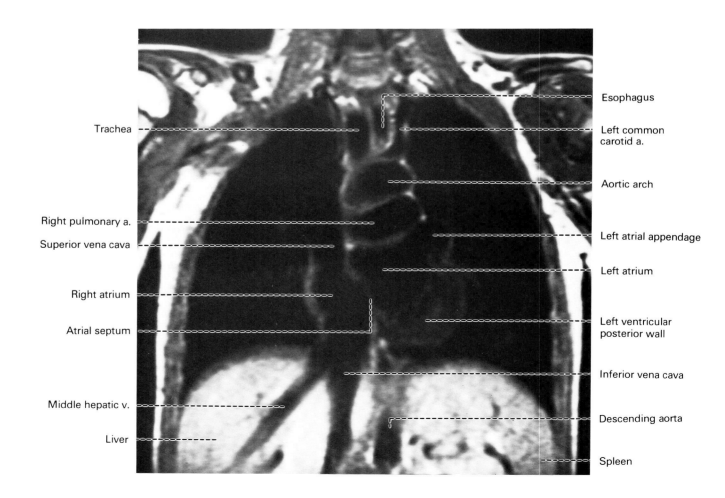

Figure 6.2.3

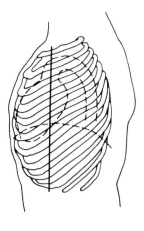

1. This section is through the ascending aorta.

2. The brachiocephalic trunk (innominate artery) ascends immediately posterior to the left brachiocephalic (innominate) vein (see subsequent sections). In younger patients this vessel crosses from left-to-right anterior to the trachea.

3. Note the slight outpouching at the level of the left sinus of Valsalva.

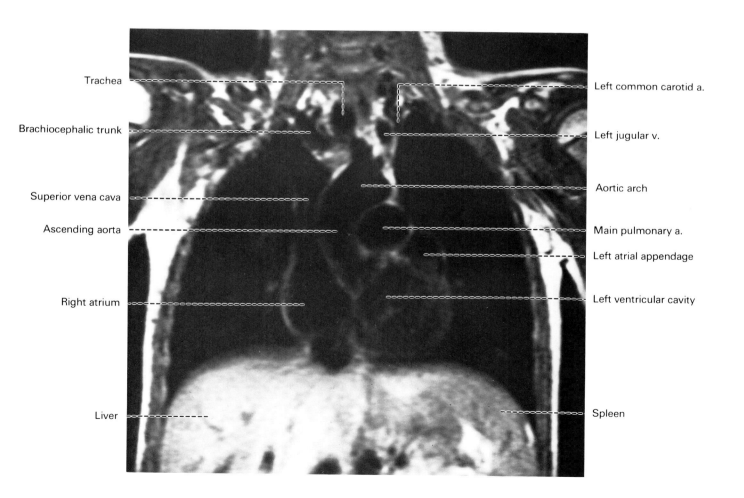

Figure 6.2.4

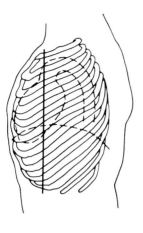

1. This section is through the left ventricular outflow tract (i.e., aortic valve).

2. Note how the brachiocephalic trunk (innominate artery) crosses left-to-right anterior to the trachea.

3. The right brachiocephalic vein joins the left brachiocephalic (innominate) vein to form the superior vena cava.

4. The aorticopulmonary window is positioned just above the main pulmonary artery, adjacent to the aortic arch.

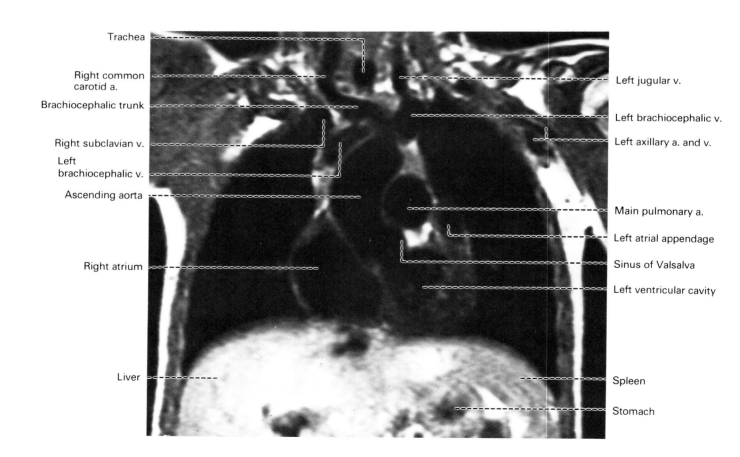

Trachea
Right common carotid a.
Brachiocephalic trunk
Right subclavian v.
Left brachiocephalic v.
Ascending aorta
Right atrium
Liver

Left jugular v.
Left brachiocephalic v.
Left axillary a. and v.
Main pulmonary a.
Left atrial appendage
Sinus of Valsalva
Left ventricular cavity
Spleen
Stomach

Figure 6.2.5

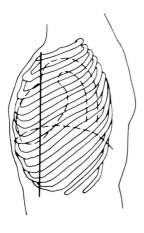

1. This section is through the left ventricular outflow tract.

2. Note the minimal separation between the right atrium and the right side of the ascending aorta.

3. The left atrial appendage projects anterior to the left atrial chamber.

4. Note the normal asymmetry between the right and left jugular veins.

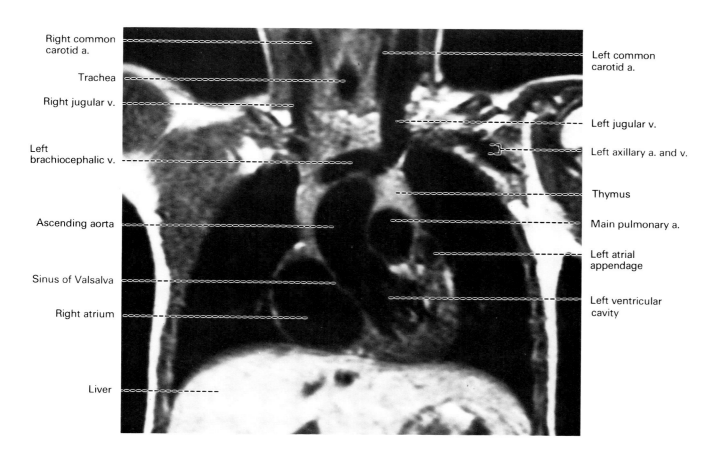

Right common carotid a.

Trachea

Right jugular v.

Left brachiocephalic v.

Ascending aorta

Sinus of Valsalva

Right atrium

Liver

Left common carotid a.

Left jugular v.

Left axillary a. and v.

Thymus

Main pulmonary a.

Left atrial appendage

Left ventricular cavity

Figure 6.2.6

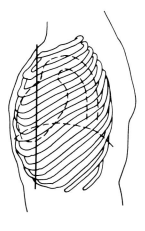

1. This section is through the midportion of the left ventricle at the level of the papillary muscles.

2. The left brachiocephalic (innominate) vein crosses from left-to-right in the superior mediastinum anterior to the aortic branch vessels to the head and neck.

3. Note that the main pulmonary artery is positioned to the left of the ascending aorta.

4. In this coronal section the right atrium and left ventricle are in the same plane.

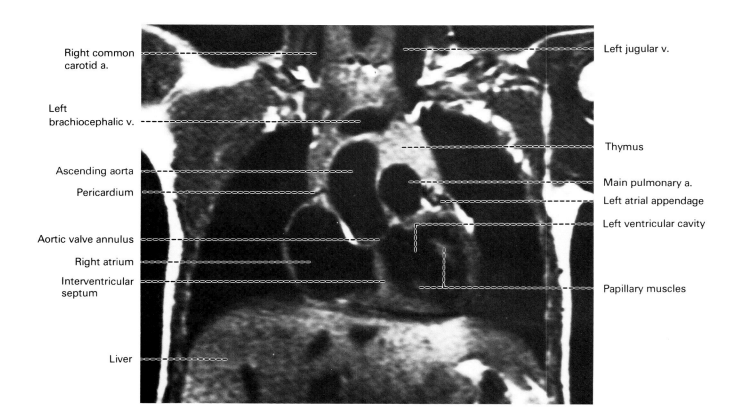

Right common carotid a.

Left brachiocephalic v.

Ascending aorta

Pericardium

Aortic valve annulus

Right atrium

Interventricular septum

Liver

Left jugular v.

Thymus

Main pulmonary a.

Left atrial appendage

Left ventricular cavity

Papillary muscles

Figure 6.2.7

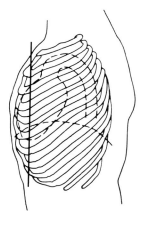

1. This section is through the pulmonic valve annulus.

2. The pericardium extends superiorly to attach on the main pulmonary artery.

3. On this coronal image note the left-of-midline position of the pulmonic valve.

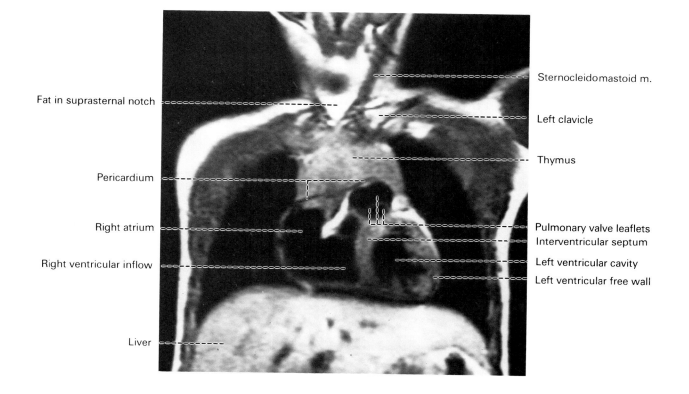

Figure 6.2.8

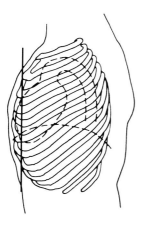

1. This section is through the right ventricular outflow tract.

2. Note the low signal intensity fibrous pericardium extending superiorly over the outflow tract.

3. The thymus is normal in size for a 10-year-old child.

4. The left ventricular wall thickness is approximately three times the right ventricular wall thickness.

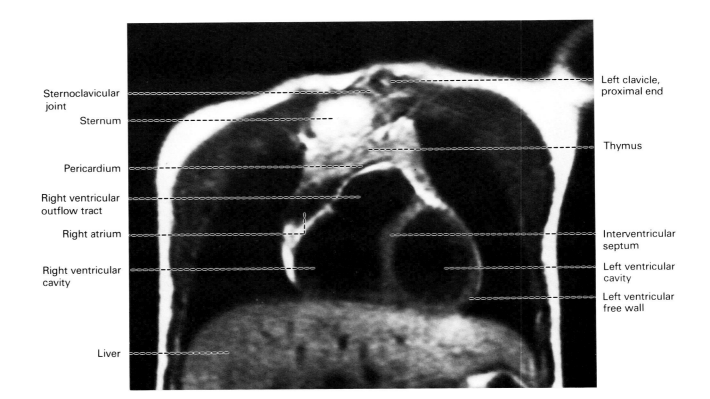

SAGITTAL

Figure 6.3.1

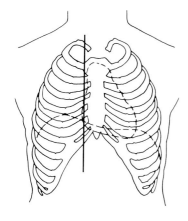

1. This section is through the body of the right atrium.

2. The azygos vein arches over the right mainstem bronchus to join the posterior aspect of the superior vena cava.

3. The right pulmonary artery is positioned anterior to the right mainstem bronchus.

4. Note how the inferior vena cava arches anteriorly to join the right atrium.

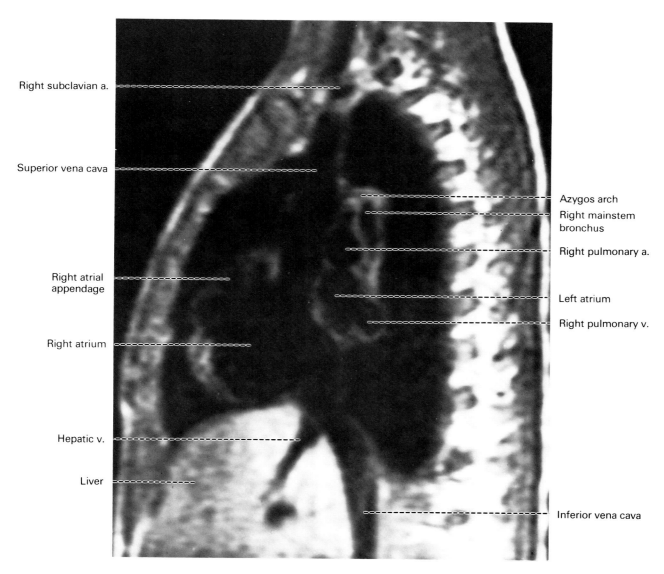

Right subclavian a.

Superior vena cava

Azygos arch

Right mainstem bronchus

Right pulmonary a.

Right atrial appendage

Left atrium

Right pulmonary v.

Right atrium

Hepatic v.

Liver

Inferior vena cava

Figure 6.3.2

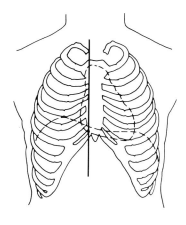

1. This section is through the bodies of the right and left atria.

2. Note the anteroposterior relationship of the two atria at this level.

3. The inferior vena cava enters the right atrium posteriorly.

4. At this level the left brachiocephalic (innominate) vein is seen joining the superior vena cava.

5. The right atrial appendage is an anterosuperior extension of the right atrium.

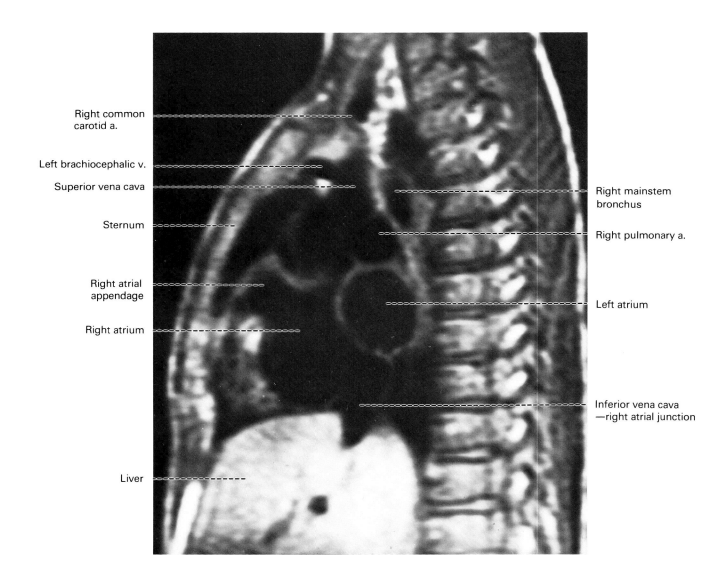

Figure 6.3.3

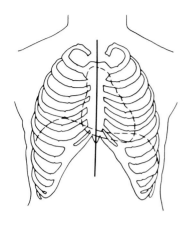

1. This section is through the aortic root.

2. Note that the brachiocephalic trunk (innominate artery) crosses anterior to the trachea causing a slight anterior indentation on the anterior wall of the trachea.

3. The right pulmonary artery crosses anterior to the carina.

4. The sinuses of Valsalva are demonstrated at the level of the aortic root.

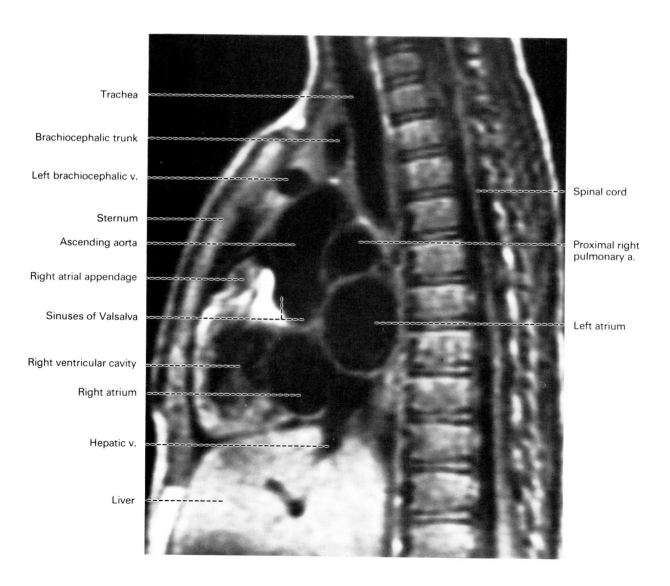

Figure 6.3.4

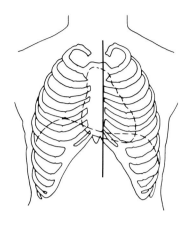

1. This section is through the aortic root.

2. The right pulmonary artery passes beneath the aortic arch superior to the left atrium.

3. The aorticopulmonary window is the small area of high signal intensity below the aortic arch and above the right pulmonary artery.

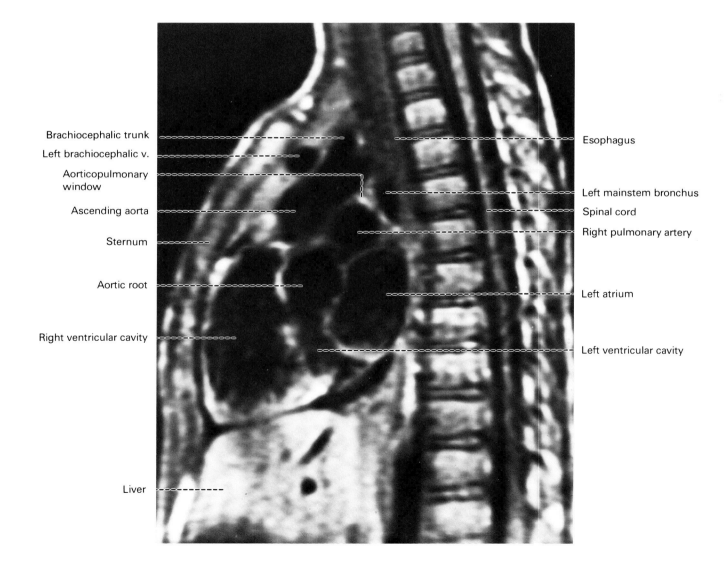

Brachiocephalic trunk
Left brachiocephalic v.
Aorticopulmonary window
Ascending aorta
Sternum
Aortic root
Right ventricular cavity
Liver

Esophagus
Left mainstem bronchus
Spinal cord
Right pulmonary artery
Left atrium
Left ventricular cavity

Figure 6.3.5

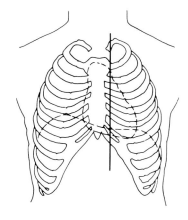

1. This section is through the right ventricular outflow tract and descending aorta.

2. Note that the main pulmonary artery is of larger caliber than the aorta.

3. The left mainstem bronchus is positioned between the descending aorta and the left atrium.

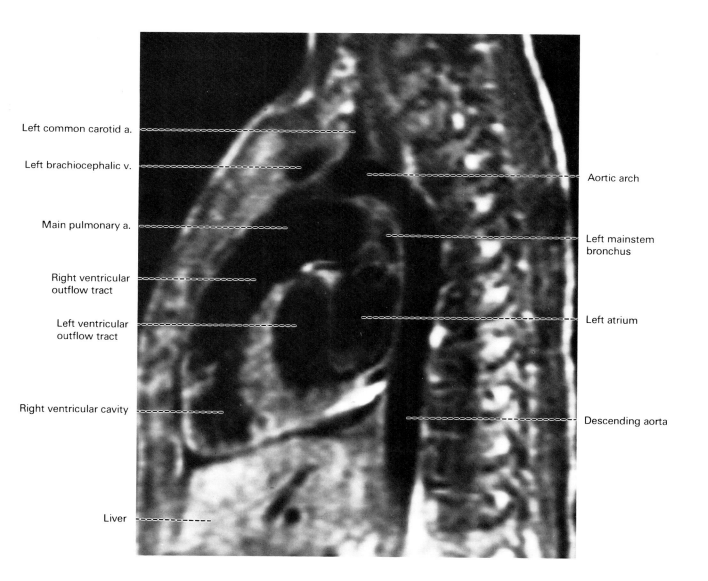

Left common carotid a.

Left brachiocephalic v.

Main pulmonary a.

Right ventricular outflow tract

Left ventricular outflow tract

Right ventricular cavity

Liver

Aortic arch

Left mainstem bronchus

Left atrium

Descending aorta

Figure 6.3.6

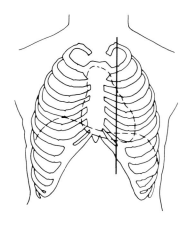

1. This section is through the axis of the main pulmonary artery.

2. The left brachiocephalic (innominate) vein is immediately deep to the distal clavicle.

3. The ventricular septum bulges anteriorly giving the left ventricle a spherical shape.

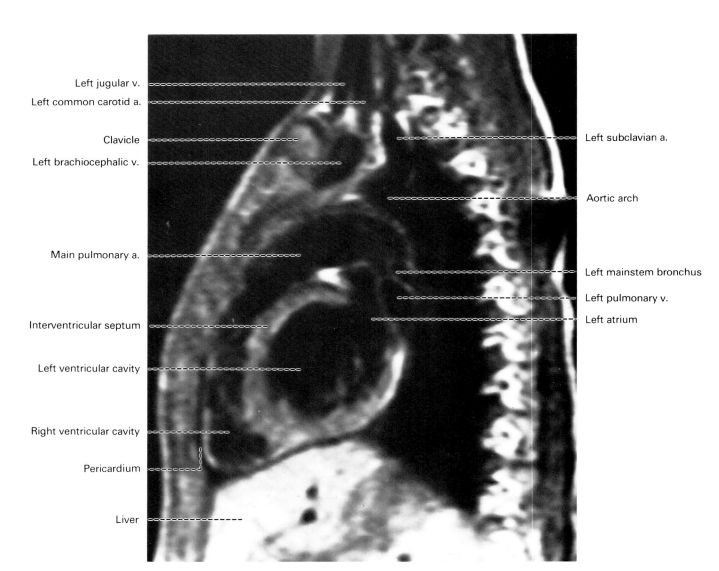

Left jugular v.
Left common carotid a.
Clavicle
Left brachiocephalic v.
Main pulmonary a.
Interventricular septum
Left ventricular cavity
Right ventricular cavity
Pericardium
Liver

Left subclavian a.
Aortic arch
Left mainstem bronchus
Left pulmonary v.
Left atrium

Figure 6.3.7

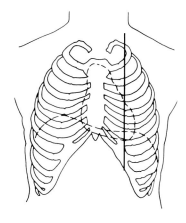

1. This section is through the left ventricular cavity.

2. The left ventricular apex is positioned anteroinferiorly.

3. Note that the liver lies anteriorly within the upper abdomen.

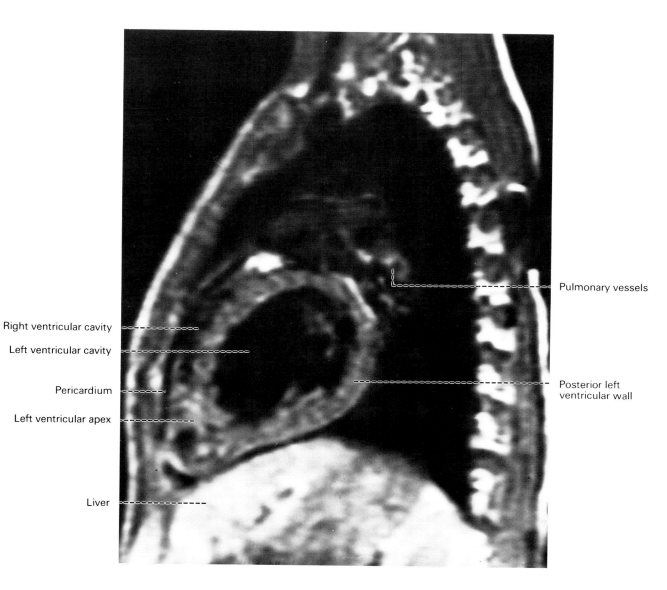

Chapter 7

CARDIAC AND GREAT VESSEL ANATOMY — ULTRAFAST CT (CINÉ)*

* All the CT images were taken supine with the patient's arms extended above the head.

AXIAL

Figure 7.1.1

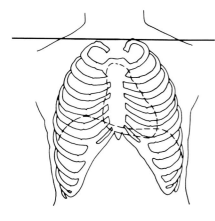

1. This section is at the level of the thoracic inlet.

2. At the thoracic inlet the trachea, thyroid gland, left common carotid artery, and left jugular veins are seen.

3. Contrast material is entering the chest through the left axillary and subclavian veins.

Right jugular v.
Pectoralis major m.
Pectoralis minor m.
Neurovascular bundle
Latissimus dorsi and teres major mm.
Humeral head
Glenoid
Deltoid m.
Scapular spine
Supraspinatus m.
Trapezius m.

Sternocleidomastoid m.
Trachea
Axillary v.
Left jugular v.
Left subclavian v.
Left lung, apex
Left common carotid a.
Thyroid gland

Figure 7.1.2

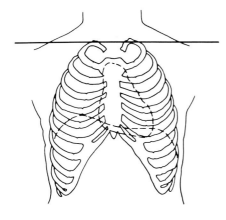

1. This section is through the lung apex. The section is somewhat oblique with the right side slightly higher than the left.

2. The left and right common carotid arteries are well opacified by contrast material.

3. At this level the innominate artery has divided into the right subclavian and right common carotid arteries.

4. The right jugular vein lies anterior to the right subclavian artery.

Right common carotid a.
Clavicle
Pectoralis major m.
Latissimus dorsi and teres major mm.
Neurovascular bundle
Pectoralis minor m.
Infraspinatus m.
Deltoid m.
Supraspinatus m.
Scapular spine
Trapezius m.

Sternocleidomastoid m.
Thyroid gland
Left common carotid a.
Axillary v.
Left jugular v.
Left lung, apex
Trachea
Erector spinae m.
Subclavian a.
Right jugular v.

Figure 7.1.3

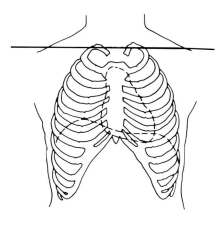

1. This section is through the lung apex.

2. Contrast material is entering the thorax through the left subclavian vein.

3. The left subclavian and jugular veins have joined to form the left brachiocephalic vein.

4. The left and right common carotid and left and right subclavian arteries are well opacified with contrast.

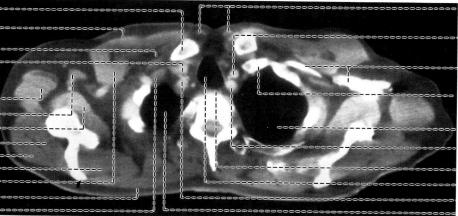

Clavicle
Pectoralis major m.
Right jugular v.
Right common carotid a.
Latissimus dorsi and teres major mm.
Neurovascular bundle
Subscapularis m.
Infraspinatus m.
Deltoid m.
Supraspinatus m.
Pectoralis minor m.
Trapezius m.
Right subclavian v.

Sternocleidomastoid mm.
Left common carotid a.
Left subclavian v.
Left brachiocephalic v.
Left lung
Left subclavian a.
Esophagus
Trachea
Right subclavian a.
Right lung, apex

Figure 7.1.4

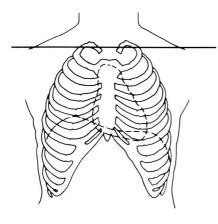

1. This section is through the lung apex at the level of the subclavian and common carotid arteries.

2. Contrast material is opacifying the left subclavian and left brachiocephalic veins.

3. The left and right subclavian and common carotid arteries are well opacified. They lie alongside the trachea.

4. The right subclavian vein is seen as it enters the thorax.

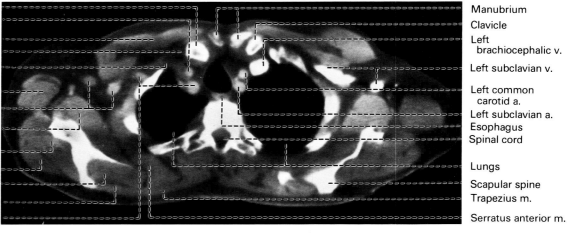

Clavicle (proximal end)
Right common carotid a.
Pectoralis major m.
Right jugular v.
Right subclavian v.
Latissimus dorsi and teres major mm.
Neurovascular bundle
Subscapularis m.
Infraspinatus m.
Deltoid m.
Supraspinatus m.
Pectoralis minor m.
Right subclavian a.

Manubrium
Clavicle
Left brachiocephalic v.
Left subclavian v.
Left common carotid a.
Left subclavian a.
Esophagus
Spinal cord
Lungs
Scapular spine
Trapezius m.
Serratus anterior m.

Figure 7.1.5

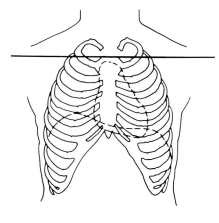

1. This section is through the lung apex above the bifurcation of the innominate artery into the right subclavian and right common carotid arteries.

2. The left and right subclavian and common carotid arteries are well opacified and lie alongside of the trachea.

3. The right subclavian and jugular veins have joined to form the right brachiocephalic vein.

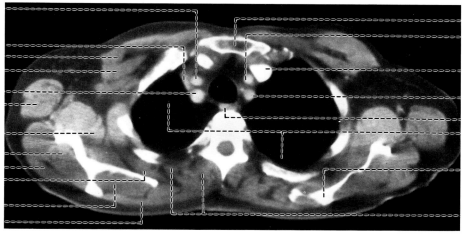

Right common carotid a.
Right brachiocephalic v.
Pectoralis major m.
Pectoralis minor m.

Right subclavian a.
Latissimus dorsi and teres major mm.

Subscapularis m.

Infraspinatus m.
Deltoid m.
Serratus anterior m.

Supraspinatus m.
Trapezius m.

Manubrium
Left common carotid a.

Left brachiocephalic v.
Left subclavian a.

Esophagus
Lungs

Scapular spine

Erector spinae m.

Figure 7.1.6

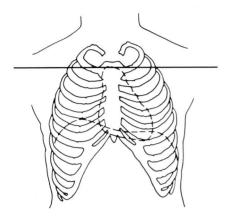

1. This section is at the level of the innominate artery.

2. In the anterior mediastinum, the left brachiocephalic vein courses from left to right prior to its merger with the right brachiocephalic vein to form the superior vena cava.

3. A tortuous innominate artery is superimposed on the right common carotid artery. The right subclavian artery is seen.

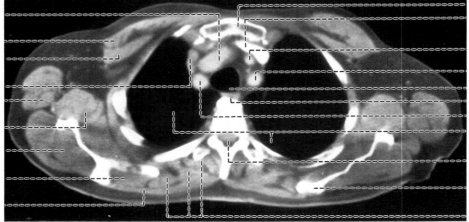

Right brachiocephalic trunk (innominate a.)

Pectoralis major m.

Pectoralis minor m.

Right brachiocephalic v.

Latissimus dorsi and teres major mm.

Subscapularis m.

Infraspinatus m.

Supraspinatus m.

Trapezius m.

Manubrium

Left brachiocephalic v.

Left common carotid a.

Left subclavian a.

Trachea

Esophagus

Right subclavian a.

Lungs

Spinal cord

Scapula

Erector spinae m.

Figure 7.1.7

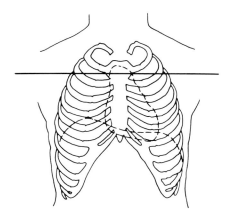

1. This section is at the top of the aortic arch.

2. The left brachiocephalic vein crosses the anterior mediastinum from left to right.

3. The innominate artery is dividing into the right common carotid and right subclavian arteries.

4. There is a small rim of calcification in the wall of the right common carotid artery.

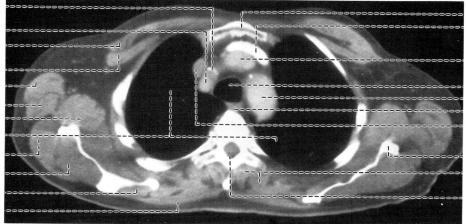

Right common carotid a.
Right subclavian a.
Pectoralis major m.

Pectoralis minor m.
Latissimus dorsi m.

Teres major m.
Subscapularis m.

Lungs

Teres minor m.

Infraspinatus m.

Supraspinatus m.

Trapezius m.

Manubrium
Left brachiocephalic v.

Brachiocephalic trunk (innominate a.)
Trachea
Aortic arch
Esophagus

Right brachiocephalic v.

Scapula
Erector spinae m.

Spinal cord

Figure 7.1.8

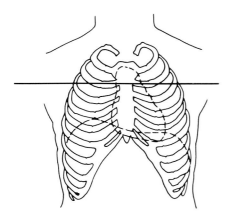

1. This section is through the aortic arch.

2. The left brachiocephalic (innominate) vein continues its crossing anterior to the aortic arch.

3. The right brachiocephalic (innominate) vein is identified just proximal to its merger with the left brachiocephalic (innominate) vein to form the superior vena cava.

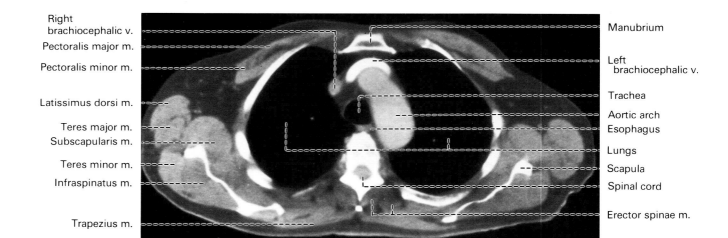

Right brachiocephalic v.
Pectoralis major m.
Pectoralis minor m.
Latissimus dorsi m.
Teres major m.
Subscapularis m.
Teres minor m.
Infraspinatus m.
Trapezius m.

Manubrium
Left brachiocephalic v.
Trachea
Aortic arch
Esophagus
Lungs
Scapula
Spinal cord
Erector spinae m.

Figure 7.1.9

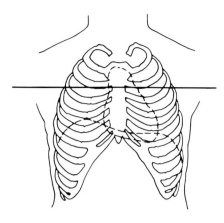

1. This section is at the undersurface of the aortic arch.

2. The trachea and esophagus lie to the right of the arch.

3. The right and left brachiocephalic (innominate) veins join at this level to form the superior vena cava.

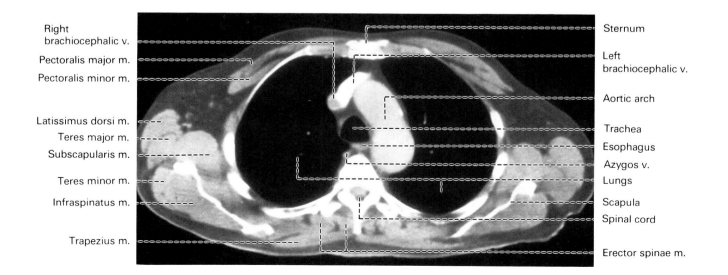

Right brachiocephalic v.

Pectoralis major m.

Pectoralis minor m.

Latissimus dorsi m.

Teres major m.

Subscapularis m.

Teres minor m.

Infraspinatus m.

Trapezius m.

Sternum

Left brachiocephalic v.

Aortic arch

Trachea

Esophagus

Azygos v.

Lungs

Scapula

Spinal cord

Erector spinae m.

Figure 7.1.10

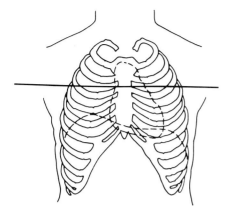

1. This section is at the level of the aorticopulmonary window.

2. There is intense opacification of the superior vena cava.

3. The azygos vein is coursing over the proximal right mainstem bronchus.

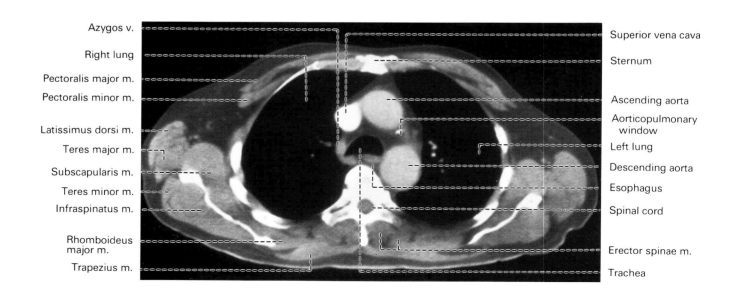

Azygos v.

Right lung

Pectoralis major m.

Pectoralis minor m.

Latissimus dorsi m.

Teres major m.

Subscapularis m.

Teres minor m.

Infraspinatus m.

Rhomboideus major m.

Trapezius m.

Superior vena cava

Sternum

Ascending aorta

Aorticopulmonary window

Left lung

Descending aorta

Esophagus

Spinal cord

Erector spinae m.

Trachea

Figure 7.1.11

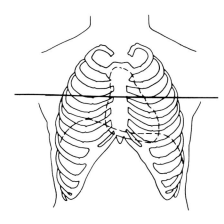

1. This section is just above the carina.

2. The azygos vein enters the dorsal aspect of the superior vena cava. The ascending portion of the azygos vein lies anterior to the vertebral body. The course of the azygos vein is from the posterior mediastinum over the right mainstem bronchus to enter the superior vena cava.

3. Superior aspect of the left pulmonary artery is visualized.

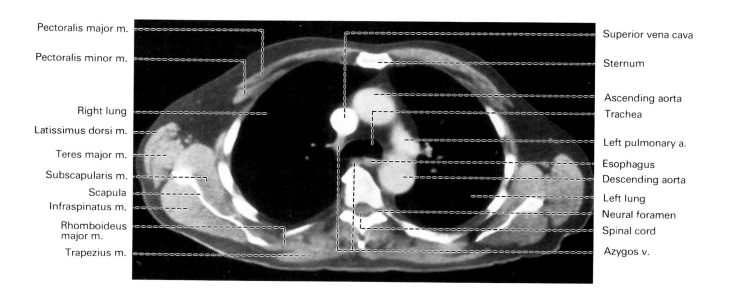

Pectoralis major m.
Pectoralis minor m.
Right lung
Latissimus dorsi m.
Teres major m.
Subscapularis m.
Scapula
Infraspinatus m.
Rhomboideus major m.
Trapezius m.

Superior vena cava
Sternum
Ascending aorta
Trachea
Left pulmonary a.
Esophagus
Descending aorta
Left lung
Neural foramen
Spinal cord
Azygos v.

Figure 7.1.12

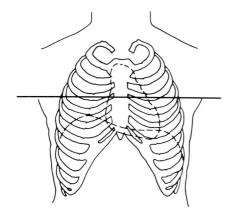

1. This level is at the carina showing the trachea bifurcating into the right and left mainstem bronchi.

2. The esophageal lumen is filled with air.

3. The azygos vein is ascending medial to the esophagus and anterior to the vertebral body.

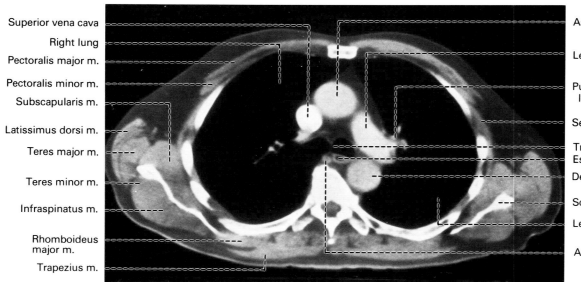

Superior vena cava — Right lung — Pectoralis major m. — Pectoralis minor m. — Subscapularis m. — Latissimus dorsi m. — Teres major m. — Teres minor m. — Infraspinatus m. — Rhomboideus major m. — Trapezius m. — Ascending aorta — Left pulmonary a. — Pulmonary v. of left upper lobe — Serratus anterior m. — Tracheal carina — Esophagus — Descending aorta — Scapula — Left lung — Azygos v.

Figure 7.1.13

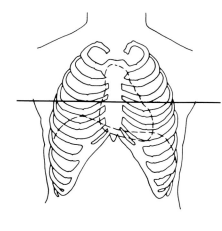

1. This section is at the level of the right pulmonary artery.

2. Note the location of the superior vena cava. It lies anterior to the right pulmonary artery.

3. The descending left pulmonary artery has crossed over the left mainstem bronchus and is lying dorsal to it.

4. Note the air-filled esophagus.

Right superior pulmonary v.

Pectoralis major m.

Pectoralis minor m.

Serratus anterior m.
Subscapularis m.
Latissimus dorsi m.

Teres major m.

Erector spinae m.

Infraspinatus m.

Rhomboideus major m.

Trapezius m.

Superior vena cava
Sternum

Ascending aorta

Main pulmonary a.

Right pulmonary a.

Left superior pulmonary v.

Left mainstem bronchus

Left descending pulmonary a.

Descending aorta

Esophagus

Azygos v.

Right mainstem bronchus

Figure 7.1.14

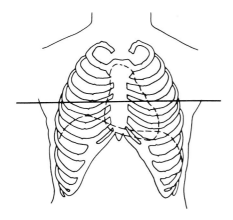

1. This section is through the undersurface of the right pulmonary artery.

2. The left mainstem bronchus has divided into branches to form the anterior and apical posterior segments of the upper lobe.

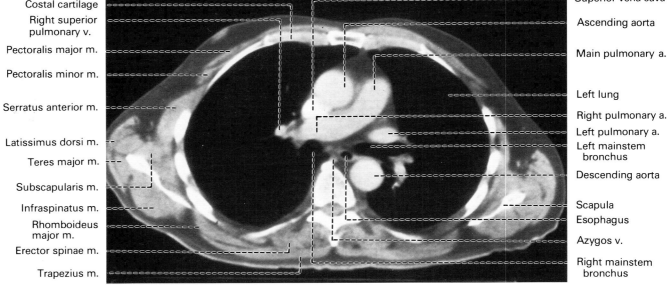

Costal cartilage
Right superior pulmonary v.
Pectoralis major m.
Pectoralis minor m.
Serratus anterior m.
Latissimus dorsi m.
Teres major m.
Subscapularis m.
Infraspinatus m.
Rhomboideus major m.
Erector spinae m.
Trapezius m.

Superior vena cava
Ascending aorta
Main pulmonary a.
Left lung
Right pulmonary a.
Left pulmonary a.
Left mainstem bronchus
Descending aorta
Scapula
Esophagus
Azygos v.
Right mainstem bronchus

Figure 7.1.15

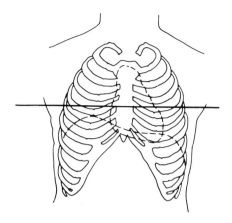

1. This section is at the level of the proximal main pulmonary artery.

2. The truncus anterior branch has arisen from the right pulmonary artery.

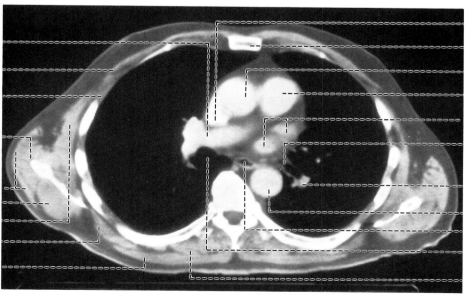

Truncus anterior branch, right pulmonary artery

Pectoralis major m.

Intercostal mm. (internal and external)

Teres major m.

Latissimus dorsi m.

Infraspinatus m.

Serratus anterior m.

Rhomboideus major m.

Trapezius m.

Superior vena cava

Sternum

Ascending aorta

Main pulmonary a.

Left atrium

Bronchus of left lower lobe

Left descending pulmonary a.

Descending aorta

Esophagus

Right mainstem bronchus

Erector spinae m.

Figure 7.1.16

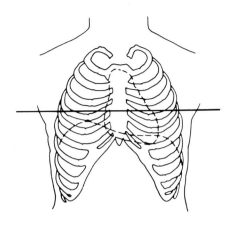

1. This section is through the superior aspect of the left atrium.

2. The descending right pulmonary artery is seen.

3. The right superior pulmonary vein is seen coursing laterally to the pulmonary artery.

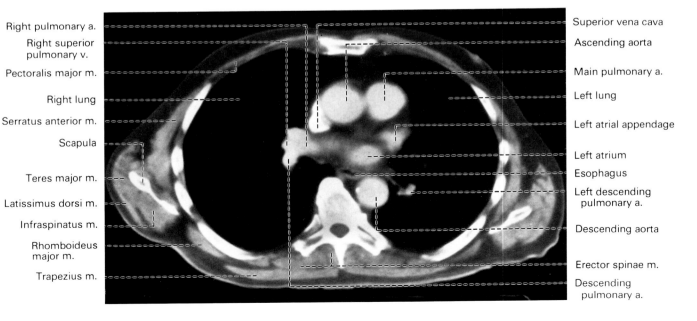

Right pulmonary a. — Superior vena cava

Right superior pulmonary v. — Ascending aorta

Pectoralis major m. — Main pulmonary a.

Right lung — Left lung

Serratus anterior m. — Left atrial appendage

Scapula — Left atrium

Teres major m. — Esophagus

Latissimus dorsi m. — Left descending pulmonary a.

Infraspinatus m. — Descending aorta

Rhomboideus major m. — Erector spinae m.

Trapezius m. — Descending pulmonary a.

Figure 7.1.17

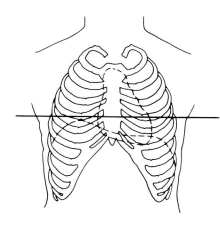

1. This section is at the level of the mid-left atrium.

2. The left superior pulmonary vein is seen entering the left atrium.

3. The circumflex coronary artery and a portion of the left anterior descending coronary artery are seen.

4. The right atrial appendage curves around the ascending aorta.

5. The superior vena cava is joining the right atrium.

Superior vena cava

Pectoralis major m.

Bronchus of right middle lobe

Right superior pulmonary v.

Serratus anterior m.

Right descending pulmonary a.

Teres major m.

Infraspinatus m.

Latissimus dorsi m.

Rhomboideus major m.

Right atrial appendage

Sternum

Right coronary a.

Right ventricular outflow tract

Ascending aorta

Left anterior descending coronary a.

Circumflex coronary a.

Left superior pulmonary v.

Descending aorta

Left atrium

Esophagus

Bronchus of right lower lobe

Trapezius m.

Figure 7.1.18

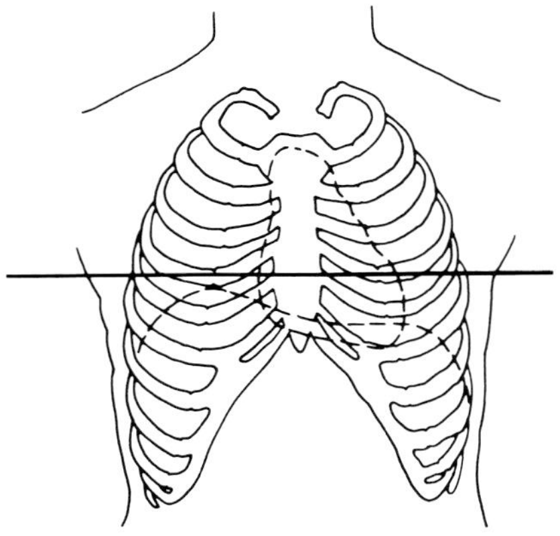

1. This section is through the outflow tract of the right ventricle.
2. Note the origin of the left coronary artery.
3. Note the relationship of the esophagus to the left atrium. The esophagus lies immediately posterior to the left atrium.
4. The circumflex coronary artery is seen coursing in the atrioventricular groove.

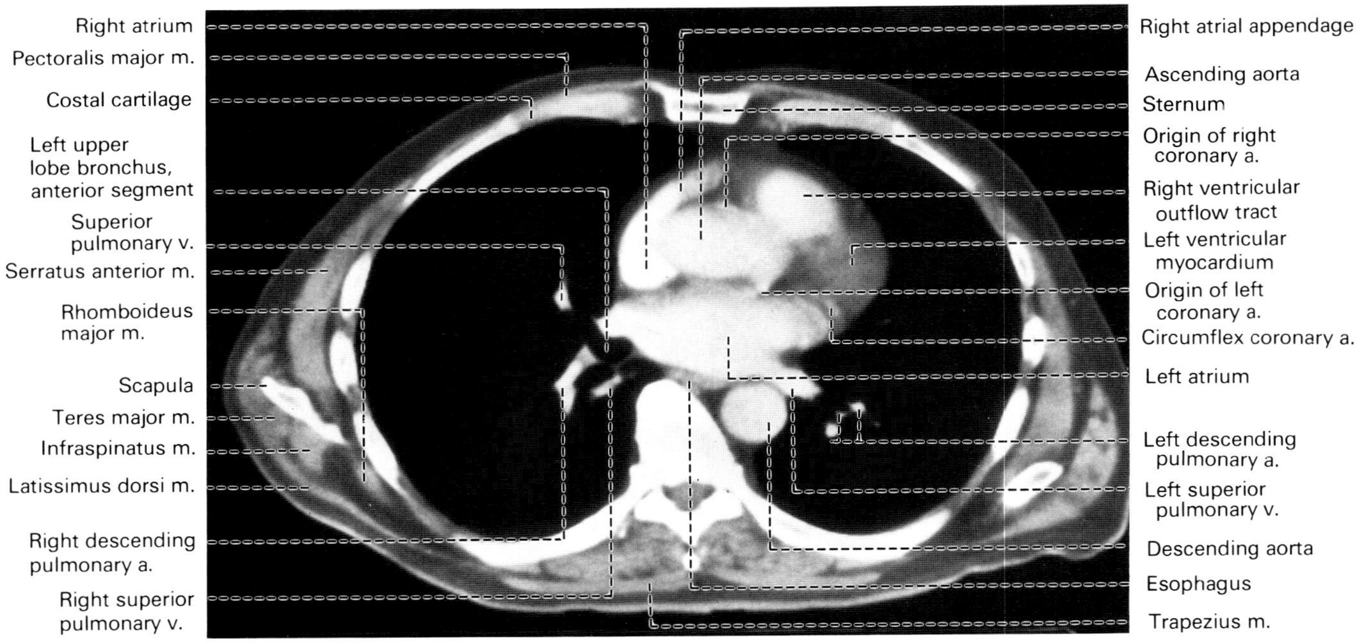
Right atrium
Pectoralis major m.
Costal cartilage
Left upper lobe bronchus, anterior segment
Superior pulmonary v.
Serratus anterior m.
Rhomboideus major m.
Scapula
Teres major m.
Infraspinatus m.
Latissimus dorsi m.
Right descending pulmonary a.
Right superior pulmonary v.
Right atrial appendage
Ascending aorta
Sternum
Origin of right coronary a.
Right ventricular outflow tract
Left ventricular myocardium
Origin of left coronary a.
Circumflex coronary a.
Left atrium
Left descending pulmonary a.
Left superior pulmonary v.
Descending aorta
Esophagus
Trapezius m.

Figure 7.1.19

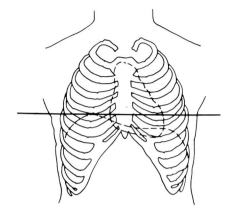

1. This section is at the level of the left ventricular outflow tract and root of the aorta.

2. The right ventricle forms the anterior border of the heart.

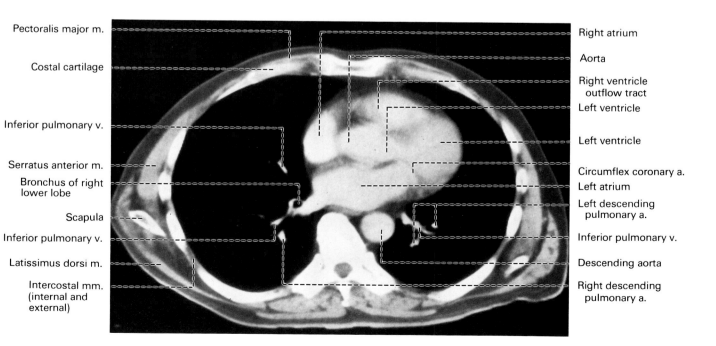

Pectoralis major m.

Costal cartilage

Inferior pulmonary v.

Serratus anterior m.

Bronchus of right lower lobe

Scapula

Inferior pulmonary v.

Latissimus dorsi m.

Intercostal mm. (internal and external)

Right atrium

Aorta

Right ventricle outflow tract

Left ventricle

Left ventricle

Circumflex coronary a.

Left atrium

Left descending pulmonary a.

Inferior pulmonary v.

Descending aorta

Right descending pulmonary a.

Figure 7.1.20

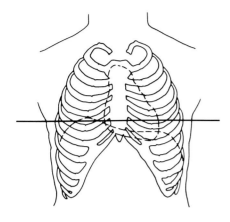

1. This section is at the level of the aortic valve.

2. The linear lucency between the right and left atrium is the interatrial septum.

3. Trabeculations in the wall of the right atrium are evident.

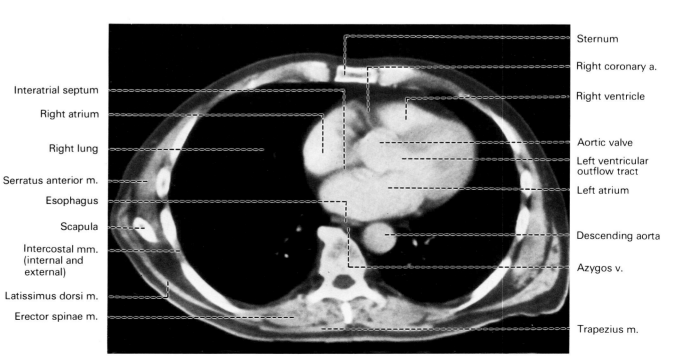

Figure 7.1.21

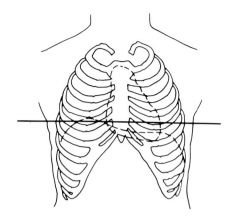

1. This section is through the upper part of the ventricles.

2. The right atrium, right ventricle, interventricular septum, and left ventricle are seen.

3. The mitral valve and left atrium can also be identified.

4. The pericardium can be seen anterior to the right ventricle and over the cardiac apex.

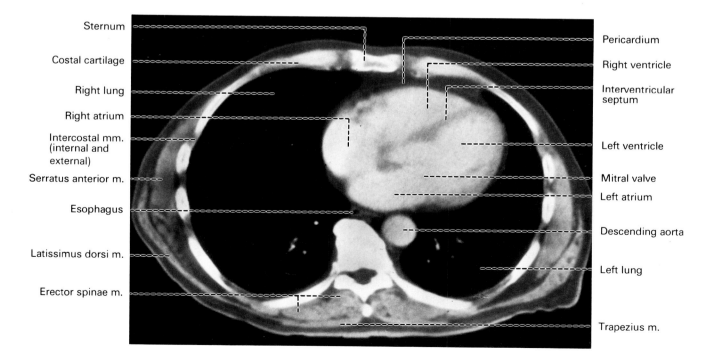

Figure 7.1.22

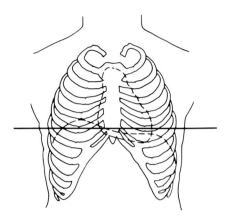

1. This section is through the mid-portion of the ventricles.

2. In this section the tricuspid valve can be faintly seen lying between the right atrium and the right ventricle.

3. The interventricular septum, left ventricle, mitral valve, and left atrium can be identified.

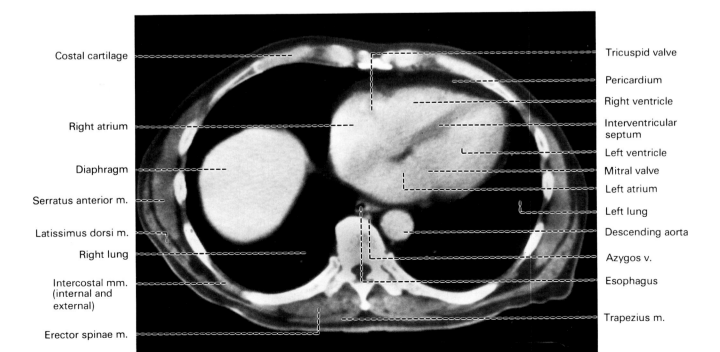

Figure 7.1.23

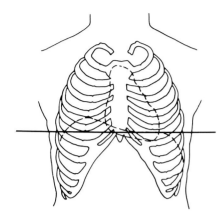

1. This section is at the inferior aspect of the left ventricular cavity.

2. The inferior vena cava can be seen at its junction with the right atrium.

3. The interventricular septum is identified.

4. The lucency overlying part of the left ventricle is myocardial muscle.

5. The coronary sinus drains into the right atrium.

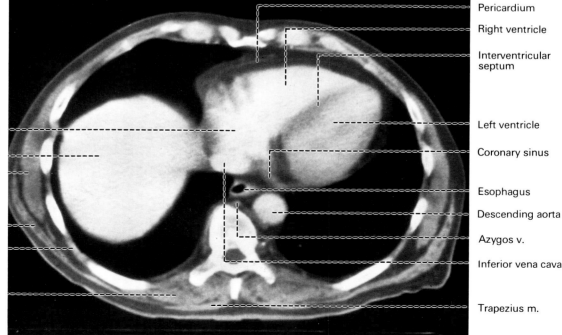

Figure 7.1.24

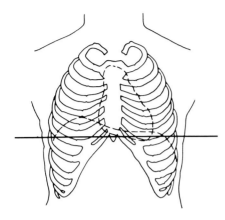

1. This section is through the inferior aspect of the right ventricular cavity.

2. The liver and inferior vena cava lie anterior and to the right of the esophagus.

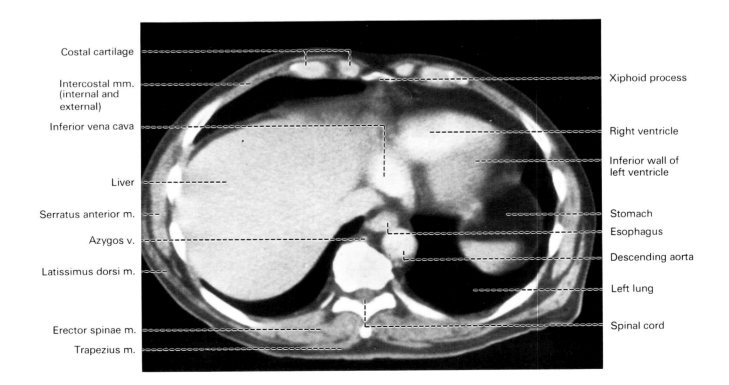

III
Abdomen

Chapter 8

MRI OF THE ABDOMEN

AXIAL

Figure 8.1.1

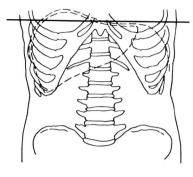

1. Note the three major hepatic veins (right, middle, and left) as they drain into the inferior vena cava at this level.

2. The distal esophagus is imaged just proximal to its junction with the stomach.

3. The base of each lung is concave and rests upon the diaphragm, which separates the right lung from the liver and the left lung from the liver, stomach, and spleen.

4. There are three large openings in the diaphragm: the aortic, esophageal, and vena caval.

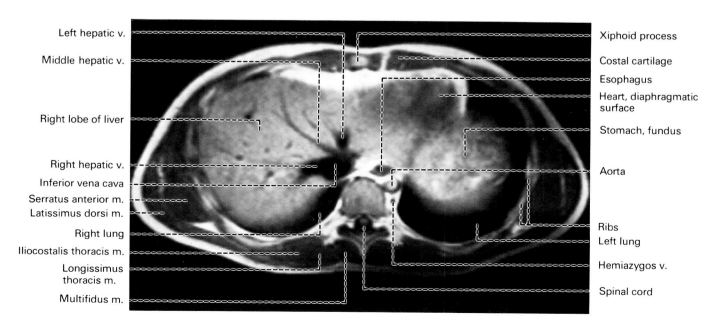

Left hepatic v.
Middle hepatic v.
Right lobe of liver
Right hepatic v.
Inferior vena cava
Serratus anterior m.
Latissimus dorsi m.
Right lung
Iliocostalis thoracis m.
Longissimus thoracis m.
Multifidus m.

Xiphoid process
Costal cartilage
Esophagus
Heart, diaphragmatic surface
Stomach, fundus
Aorta
Ribs
Left lung
Hemiazygos v.
Spinal cord

Figure 8.1.2

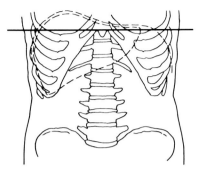

1. The hepatic veins are all intersegmental or interlobar.

2. Note the convergence of the hepatic veins into the intrahepatic portion of the inferior vena cava.

3. The esophagus can be seen as a low signal intensity structure anterior to the aorta between the left lobe of the liver and the vertebral body.

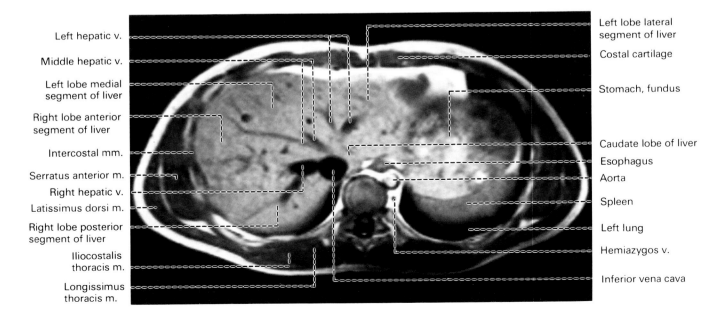

Left hepatic v.

Middle hepatic v.

Left lobe medial segment of liver

Right lobe anterior segment of liver

Intercostal mm.

Serratus anterior m.

Right hepatic v.

Latissimus dorsi m.

Right lobe posterior segment of liver

Iliocostalis thoracis m.

Longissimus thoracis m.

Left lobe lateral segment of liver

Costal cartilage

Stomach, fundus

Caudate lobe of liver

Esophagus

Aorta

Spleen

Left lung

Hemiazygos v.

Inferior vena cava

Figure 8.1.3

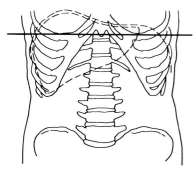

1. A portion of the caudate lobe can be appreciated as a triangular structure between the inferior vena cava, left lobe of the liver, and the vertebral body.

2. The spleen has a homogeneous and slightly lower signal intensity than the liver.

3. At this level the esophagus traverses the diaphragm through its hiatus and joins the cardia of the stomach.

4. The erector spinae complex of muscles is composed of three columns: the iliocostalis, longissimus, and spinalis.

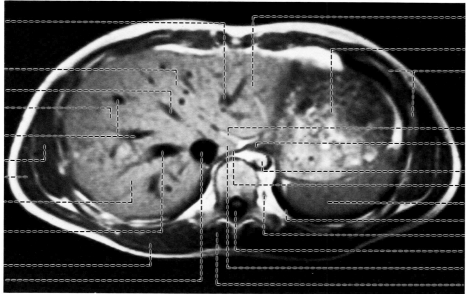

Left hepatic v.

Left lobe medial segment of liver

Middle hepatic v.

Right lobe anterior segment of liver

Branches of right portal vein

Serratus anterior m.

Latissimus dorsi m.

Right lobe posterior segment of liver

Right hepatic v.

Iliocostalis thoracis m.

Inferior vena cava

Left lobe lateral segment of liver

Stomach, fundus

Ribs

Fissure of ligamentum venosum

Gastroesophageal junction

Aorta

Crus of diaphragm

Spleen

Left lung

Hemiazygos v.

Spinal cord

Caudate lobe of liver

Multifidus m.

Figure 8.1.4

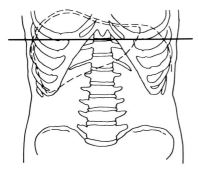

1. The visceral surface of the liver is related to the stomach, duodenum, hepatic flexure of the colon, right kidney, right adrenal gland, and gallbladder.

2. The spleen has a diaphragmatic and visceral surface. The visceral surface is related to the stomach, colon, tail of the pancreas, left adrenal gland, and kidney.

3. The right diaphragmatic crus lies posterior to the caudate lobe of the liver in this section.

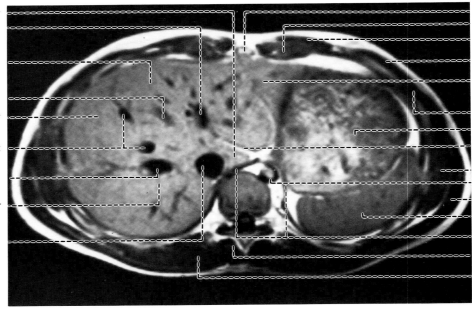

Caudate lobe of liver
Left branch of portal vein
Right lobe medial segment of liver
Middle hepatic v.
Right lobe anterior segment of liver
Branches of right portal vein
Right hepatic v.
Right lobe posterior segment of liver
Inferior vena cava

Xiphoid process
Costal cartilage
Rectus abdominis m.
External oblique m.
Left lobe lateral segment of liver
Intercostal mm.
Stomach, fundus
Fissure of ligamentum venosum
Serratus anterior m.
Aorta
Latissimus dorsi m.
Spleen
Crura of diaphragm
Multifidus m.
Longissimus thoracis m.

Figure 8.1.5

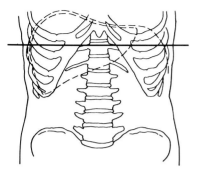

1. Splenic vessels are demonstrated within the spleen.

2. Note the position of the inferior vena cava in relationship to the caudate lobe of the liver and aorta.

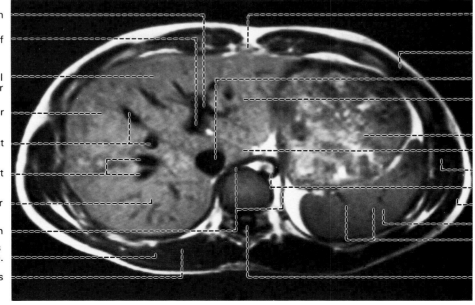

Left portal vein

Main trunk of portal vein

Left lobe medial segment of liver

Right lobe anterior segment of liver

Branches of right portal vein

Branches of right hepatic vein

Right lobe posterior segment of liver

Crura of diaphragm

Iliocostalis thoracis m.

Longissimus thoracis m.

Xiphoid process

External oblique m.

Inferior vena cava

Left lobe medial segment of liver

Stomach, fundus

Caudate lobe of liver

Serratus anterior m.

Aorta

Latissimus dorsi m.

Spleen

Branches of splenic vessels

Spinal cord

Figure 8.1.6

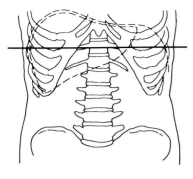

1. The lobes and segments of the liver are clearly depicted in this section.

2. The left lobe lateral segment of the liver is midsagittal or slightly to the right of midline in this section. It is separated from the left lobe medial segment by the left portal vein, which is located in the fissure of ligamentum teres.

3. The portal vein divides into right and left portal veins and caudate vein.

4. Each portal vein runs in the center of each segment along with branches of the hepatic artery and biliary duct.

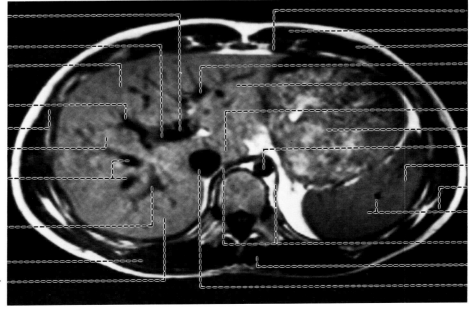

Main trunk of portal vein

Right portal vein

Left lobe medial segment of liver

Right anterior branch of portal vein

Intercostal mm.

Right lobe anterior segment of liver

Branches of right hepatic vein

Right posterior branch of portal vein

Iliocostalis thoracis m.

Right lobe posterior segment of liver

Costal cartilage

Rectus abdominis m.

External oblique m.

Left portal vein

Left lobe lateral segment of liver

Caudate lobe of liver

Stomach, fundus

Aorta

Spleen

Latissimus dorsi m.

Branches of splenic vessels

Crura of diaphragm

Multifidus m.

Inferior vena cava

Figure 8.1.7

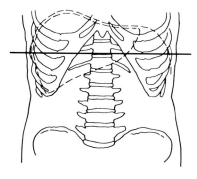

1. The left adrenal gland has an inverted Y-shaped configuration.

2. Note the fat in the fissure of ligamentum teres that is associated with a remnant of the umbilical vein, coursing between medial and lateral segments of the left lobe.

3. The main portal vein, posterior branches of the right portal vein, and distal branches of the left portal vein are all depicted in this section.

4. The high signal intensity fat surrounding the main portal vein represents the fatty materials within the fissure of the ligamentum venosum.

5. The tail of the caudate lobe forms the roof of the epiploic foramen (foramen of Winslow) that is the mouth of the lesser sac and lies between the upper part of the portal vein and inferior vena cava.

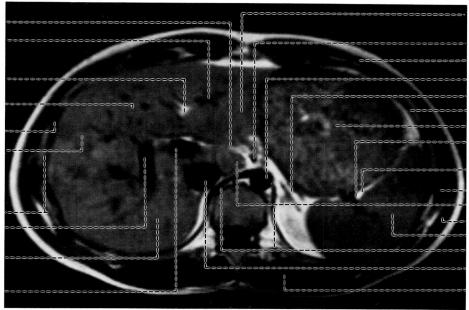

Left side labels:
- Fissure of ligamentum venosum
- Branch of left portal v.
- Fissure of ligamentum teres
- Left lobe medial segment of liver
- Intercostal mm.
- Right lobe anterior segment of liver
- Ribs
- Posterior branch of right portal v.
- Right lobe posterior segment of liver
- Main trunk of portal v.

Right side labels:
- Left lobe medial segment of liver
- Left gastric a.
- External oblique m.
- Aorta
- Left adrenal gland
- Diaphragm
- Stomach, fundus
- Branch of splenic vessel
- Splenic hilum
- Serratus anterior m.
- Caudate lobe of liver
- Latissimus dorsi m.
- Spleen
- Crura of diaphragm
- Inferior vena cava
- Longissimus thoracis m.

Figure 8.1.8

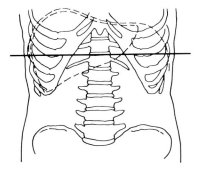

1. The main portal vein is located within the fissure of the ligamentum venosum. The hepatic triad consists of the bile duct (not demonstrated), portal vein, and hepatic artery.

2. Both left and right adrenal glands are situated within the fat-filled perirenal space.

3. Note that the right adrenal gland is posterior to the inferior vena cava and is seen as a linear structure.

4. The splenic vessels can be identified as curvilinear structures between the stomach and the spleen.

5. The curvilinear structure parallel to the main portal vein within the fissure of the ligamentum venosum represents the hepatic artery.

6. Diaphragmatic crura can be readily demonstrated as linear structures that surround the aorta and the vertebral body.

Fissure of ligamentum venosum

Costal cartilage

Left lobe medial segment of liver

Fissure of ligamentum teres

Hepatic a.

Right lobe of liver

Posterior branch of right portal v.

Main trunk of portal v.

Right adrenal gland

Inferior vena cava

Left lobe lateral segment of liver

Rectus abdominis m.
External oblique m.

Left gastric a.

Aorta

Stomach, body

Left adrenal gland

Splenic a.

Diaphragm

Crura of diaphragm

Spleen

Latissimus dorsi m.

Left upper pole of kidney

Spinal cord

Multifidus m.

Figure 8.1.9

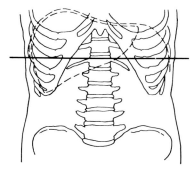

1. The corticomedullary junction in both kidneys is distinctly seen.

2. The spleen has a relatively lower signal intensity than the liver probably due to higher iron and/or water content.

3. The right adrenal gland is located cephalad to the upper pole of the right kidney and just dorsal to the inferior vena cava.

4. The left adrenal gland is located lateral to the crus of the left diaphragm.

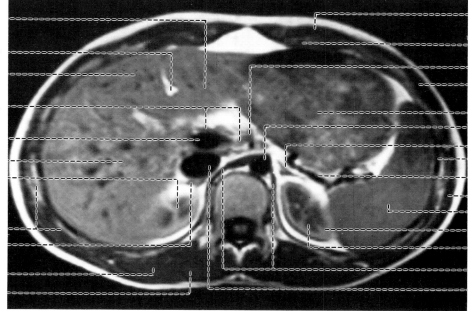

Left lobe lateral segment of liver

Fissure of ligamentum teres

Left lobe medial segment of liver

Hepatic a.

Portal v.

Right lobe of liver

Upper pole of kidney

Ribs

Right adrenal gland

Iliocostalis thoracis m.

Longissimus thoracis m.

External oblique m.

Costal cartilage

Left gastric a.

Serratus anterior m.

Stomach, body
Aorta

Left adrenal gland
Diaphragm

Splenic a.

Latissimus dorsi m.
Spleen

Cortex of left kidney

Medulla of left kidney

Crura of diaphragm

Inferior vena cava

Figure 8.1.10

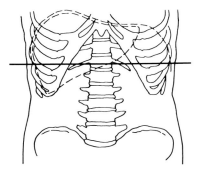

1. The splenic vein drains into the portal vein.

2. The following structures are related to the posterior wall of the stomach: spleen, splenic artery and vein, pancreas, left adrenal gland, and left kidney.

3. The celiac axis, which is the first unpaired branch of the abdominal aorta, divides to form the left gastric, common hepatic, and splenic arteries.

4. The splenic artery is more tortuous than the splenic vein and is located cephalad to the splenic vein.

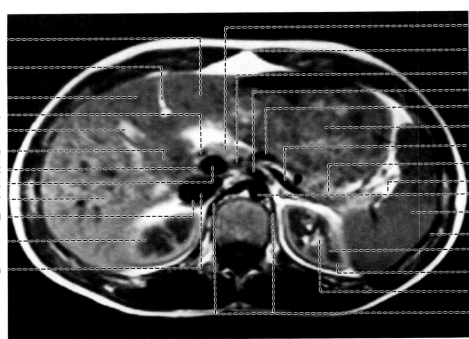

Left lobe lateral segment of liver
Fissure of ligamentum teres
Left lobe medial segment of liver
Gastroduodenal a.
Gallbladder
Stomach, antrum
Common bile duct
Portal v.
Right lobe of liver
Right adrenal gland
Right kidney
Inferior vena cava

Pancreas, head
Linea alba
Hepatic a.
Celiac a.
Splenic a.
Stomach, body
Splenic v.
Pancreas, tail
Splenic hilum
Aorta
Spleen
Diaphragm
Medulla of left kidney
Cortex of left kidney
Left renal sinus
Crura of diaphragm

Figure 8.1.11

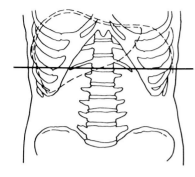

1. The splenic vein is demonstrated as it drains into the portal vein.

2. Anterior to the splenic vein, the tortuous splenic artery is partially depicted.

3. There is an accessory spleen near the hilum of the spleen proper.

4. The second portion of the duodenum is located lateral to the inferior vena cava.

5. The potential space between the pancreas and the stomach represents the lesser sac. The mouth of the lesser sac is called the epiploic foramen (foramen of Winslow) and is bounded dorsally by the inferior vena cava, superiorly by the caudate lobe of the liver, and inferiorly by the duodenum.

6. The pancreas lies just anterior to the portal and splenic veins. The tail of the pancreas extends to the hilum of the spleen and is situated within the splenorenal ligament.

7. The head of the pancreas surrounds the portal vein and is located within the concavity formed by the stomach and duodenum (the C-loop).

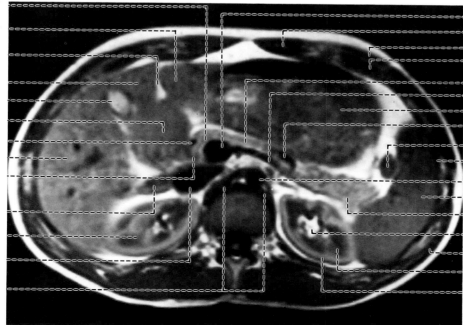

Pancreas, head
Left lobe lateral segment of liver
Fissure of ligamentum teres
Left lobe medial segment of liver
Gallbladder
Stomach, antrum
Gastroduodenal a.
Right lobe of liver
Common bile duct
Duodenum, second portion
Right kidney
Inferior vena cava
Crura of diaphragm

Portal v.
Rectus abdominis m.
External oblique m.
Transversus abdominis m.
Pancreas, body
Splenic v.
Stomach, body
Splenic a.
Accessory spleen
Diaphragm
Aorta
Spleen
Pancreas, tail
Left renal sinus
Latissimus dorsi m.
Medulla of left kidney
Cortex of left kidney

Figure 8.1.12

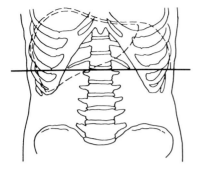

1. The tail, body, and a part of the head of the pancreas are well demonstrated.

2. Note the left renal vein draining into the inferior vena cava.

3. The superior mesenteric artery is the second unpaired branch of the abdominal aorta, and it branches off from the aorta 0.5 to 2 cm caudal to the celiac artery.

4. The splenic and superior mesenteric veins merge to become the portal vein.

5. The retroperitoneum is divided into three spaces: the anterior pararenal, the perirenal, and the posterior pararenal space. These three spaces are separated by renal fascia (Gerota's capsule).

6. The gallbladder is closely related to the anterior abdominal wall. It lies in a fossa on the visceral surface of the liver.

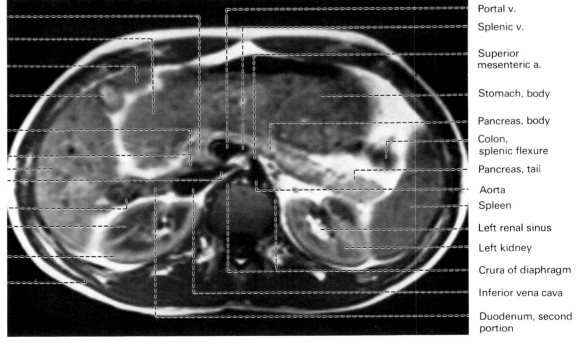

Figure 8.1.13

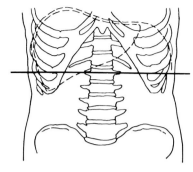

1. Both the hepatic and splenic flexures of the colon are depicted in this section.

2. The relationships of the superior mesenteric artery to the aorta and to the pancreas are anatomically important. The superior mesenteric artery arises dorsal to the body of the pancreas and splenic vein and runs down in front of the left renal vein and third portion of the duodenum.

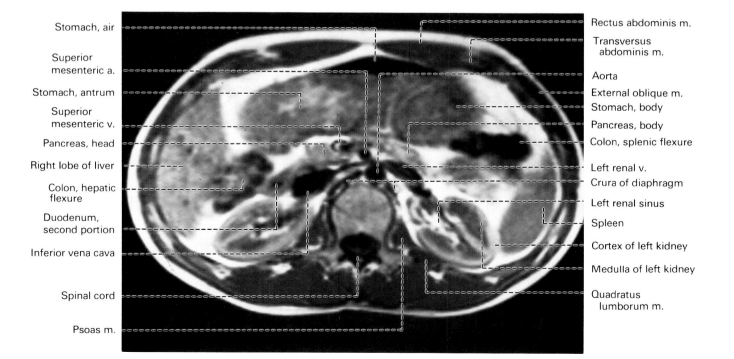

Stomach, air

Superior mesenteric a.

Stomach, antrum

Superior mesenteric v.

Pancreas, head

Right lobe of liver

Colon, hepatic flexure

Duodenum, second portion

Inferior vena cava

Spinal cord

Psoas m.

Rectus abdominis m.

Transversus abdominis m.

Aorta

External oblique m.

Stomach, body

Pancreas, body

Colon, splenic flexure

Left renal v.

Crura of diaphragm

Left renal sinus

Spleen

Cortex of left kidney

Medulla of left kidney

Quadratus lumborum m.

Figure 8.1.14

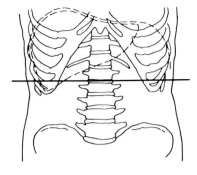

1. Note the right and left renal arteries as they originate from the abdominal aorta.

2. The right renal vein is demonstrated as it drains into the inferior vena cava.

3. The left renal vein courses cephalad to the third portion of the duodenum.

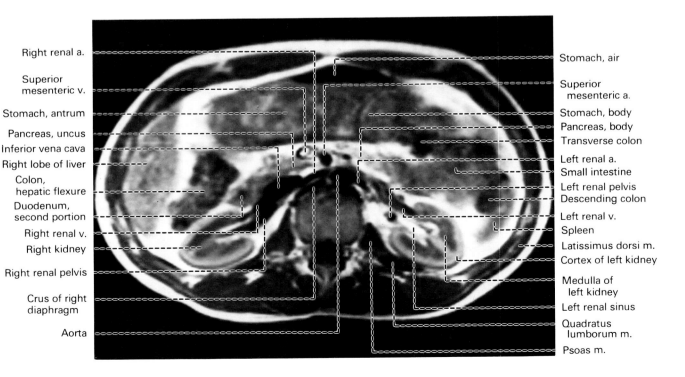

Right renal a.

Superior mesenteric v.

Stomach, antrum

Pancreas, uncus

Inferior vena cava

Right lobe of liver

Colon, hepatic flexure

Duodenum, second portion

Right renal v.

Right kidney

Right renal pelvis

Crus of right diaphragm

Aorta

Stomach, air

Superior mesenteric a.

Stomach, body

Pancreas, body

Transverse colon

Left renal a.

Small intestine

Left renal pelvis

Descending colon

Left renal v.

Spleen

Latissimus dorsi m.

Cortex of left kidney

Medulla of left kidney

Left renal sinus

Quadratus lumborum m.

Psoas m.

Figure 8.1.15

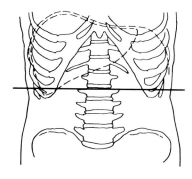

1. Note the ascending and descending colon on either side of the abdomen.

2. A portion of the jejunum can be identified in the left side of the abdomen.

3. The uncus is an extension of the head of the pancreas that hooks around the superior mesenteric vessels.

4. The renal pelvis is partly inside and partly outside of the kidney. The extrarenal portion tapers and becomes the ureter.

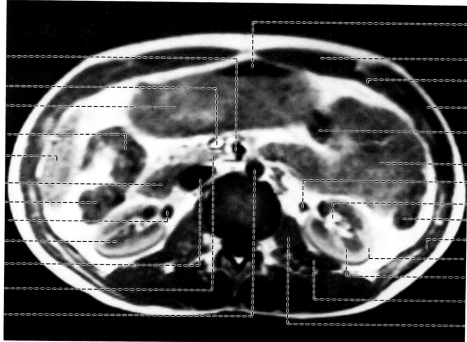

Left labels:
Superior mesenteric a.
Superior mesenteric v.
Stomach, antrum
Colon, hepatic flexure
Right lobe of liver
Duodenum, second portion
Ascending colon
Right renal pelvis
Right kidney
Inferior vena cava
Pancreas, uncus
Aorta

Right labels:
Stomach, air
Rectus abdominis m.
Transversus abdominis m.
External oblique m.
Transverse colon
Jejunum
Left renal pelvis
Left renal sinus
Descending colon
Latissimus dorsi m.
Cortex of left kidney
Medulla of left kidney
Quadratus lumborum m.
Psoas m.

Figure 8.1.16

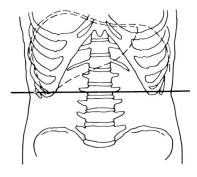

1. This section is at the level of the inferior edge of the liver.

2. The proximal ureters are clearly depicted in this section.

3. The third part of the duodenum courses to the left between the aorta and the superior mesenteric artery.

4. All four abdominal muscles are distinctly seen — rectus abdominis, external oblique, internal oblique, and transversus abdominis muscles.

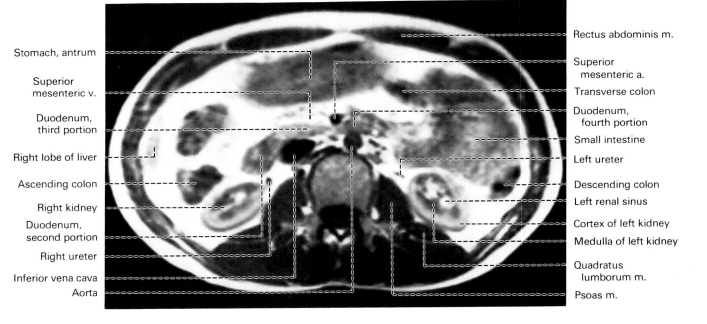

Stomach, antrum

Superior mesenteric v.

Duodenum, third portion

Right lobe of liver

Ascending colon

Right kidney

Duodenum, second portion

Right ureter

Inferior vena cava

Aorta

Rectus abdominis m.

Superior mesenteric a.

Transverse colon

Duodenum, fourth portion

Small intestine

Left ureter

Descending colon

Left renal sinus

Cortex of left kidney

Medulla of left kidney

Quadratus lumborum m.

Psoas m.

CORONAL

Figure 8.2.1

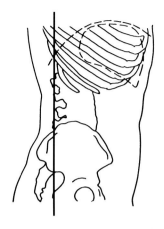

1. This section passes through the back muscles.

2. Note the quadratus lumborum muscle inserting on the twelfth rib.

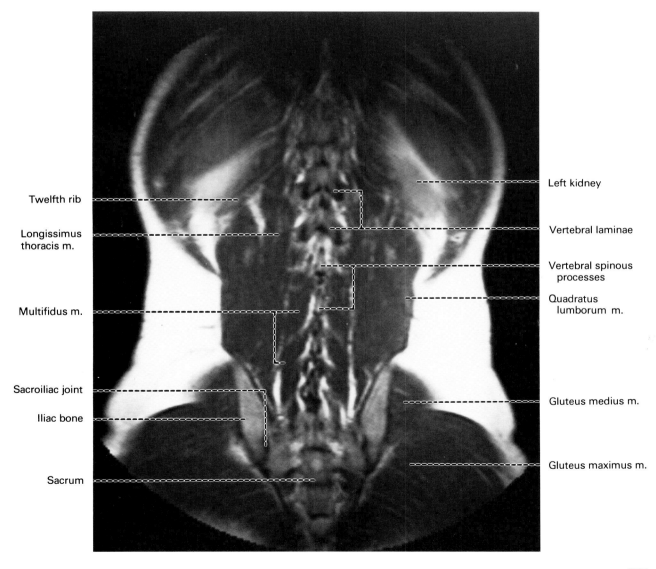

Twelfth rib

Longissimus thoracis m.

Multifidus m.

Sacroiliac joint

Iliac bone

Sacrum

Left kidney

Vertebral laminae

Vertebral spinous processes

Quadratus lumborum m.

Gluteus medius m.

Gluteus maximus m.

Figure 8.2.2

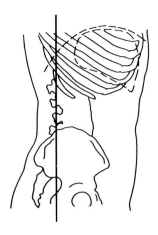

1. This section is through the thoracic portion of the spinal canal.

2. This aspect of the liver is not covered with peritoneum and therefore is called the "bare area" of the liver.

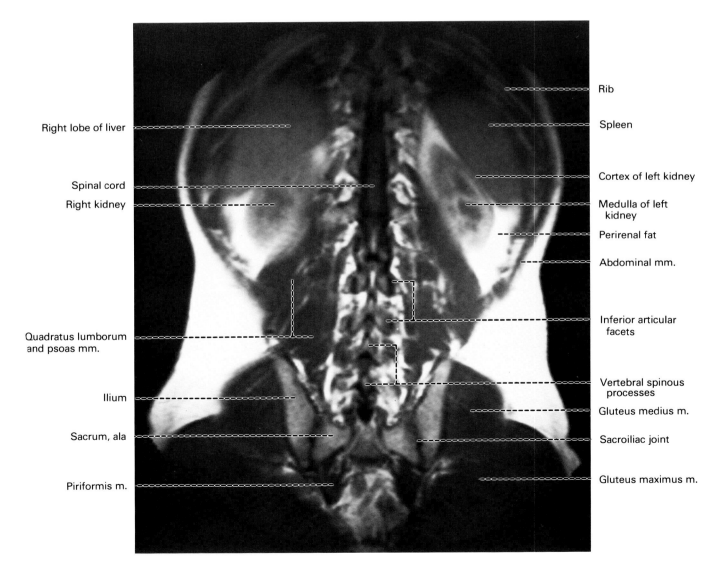

Right lobe of liver

Spinal cord

Right kidney

Quadratus lumborum and psoas mm.

Ilium

Sacrum, ala

Piriformis m.

Rib

Spleen

Cortex of left kidney

Medulla of left kidney

Perirenal fat

Abdominal mm.

Inferior articular facets

Vertebral spinous processes

Gluteus medius m.

Sacroiliac joint

Gluteus maximus m.

Figure 8.2.3

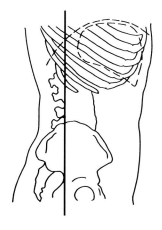

1. Note that the retroperitoneal organs extend posteriorly behind the vertebral bodies.

2. The potential space between the inferior surface of the liver and right kidney is called the hepatorenal recess (Morison's pouch).

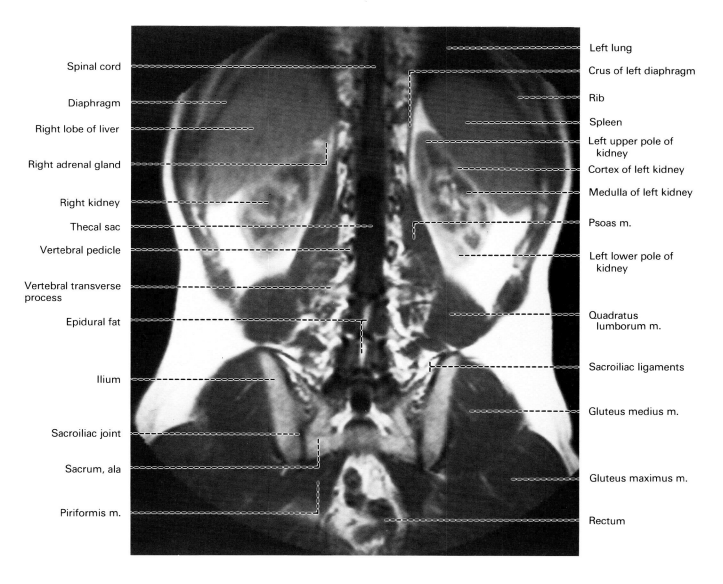

Spinal cord

Diaphragm

Right lobe of liver

Right adrenal gland

Right kidney

Thecal sac

Vertebral pedicle

Vertebral transverse process

Epidural fat

Ilium

Sacroiliac joint

Sacrum, ala

Piriformis m.

Left lung

Crus of left diaphragm

Rib

Spleen

Left upper pole of kidney

Cortex of left kidney

Medulla of left kidney

Psoas m.

Left lower pole of kidney

Quadratus lumborum m.

Sacroiliac ligaments

Gluteus medius m.

Gluteus maximus m.

Rectum

Figure 8.2.4

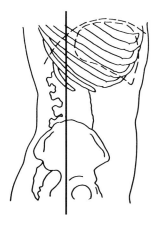

1. This section passes through the spinal canal in the lumbar region.

2. Note the thecal sac and nerve sleeves exiting under the pedicles.

3. The kidneys are embedded in the perirenal fat.

4. The retroperitoneal space is divided into three parts by the anterior and posterior pararenal fascia.

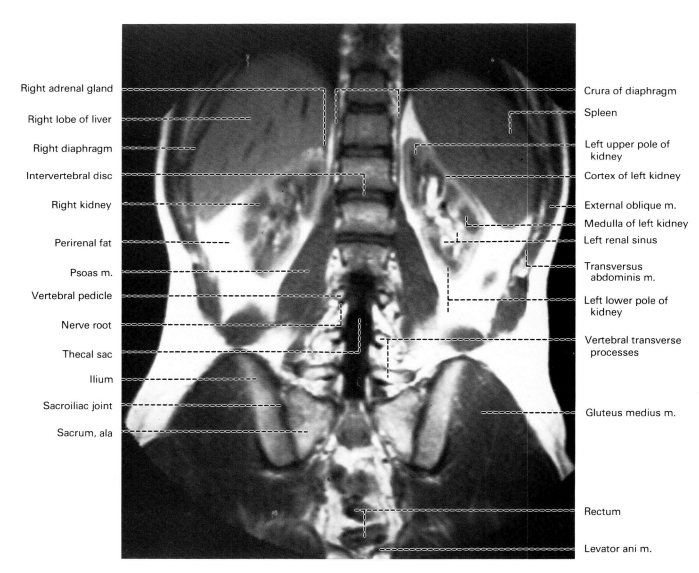

Right adrenal gland

Right lobe of liver

Right diaphragm

Intervertebral disc

Right kidney

Perirenal fat

Psoas m.

Vertebral pedicle

Nerve root

Thecal sac

Ilium

Sacroiliac joint

Sacrum, ala

Crura of diaphragm

Spleen

Left upper pole of kidney

Cortex of left kidney

External oblique m.

Medulla of left kidney

Left renal sinus

Transversus abdominis m.

Left lower pole of kidney

Vertebral transverse processes

Gluteus medius m.

Rectum

Levator ani m.

Figure 8.2.5

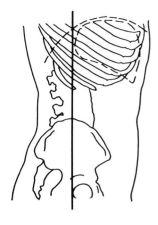

1. Both adrenal glands can be noted as inverted Y-shaped structures above the kidneys.

2. The kidneys show distinct corticomedullary differentiation.

3. The anterior portion of the sacroiliac articulation is a synovial (diarthrodial) joint.

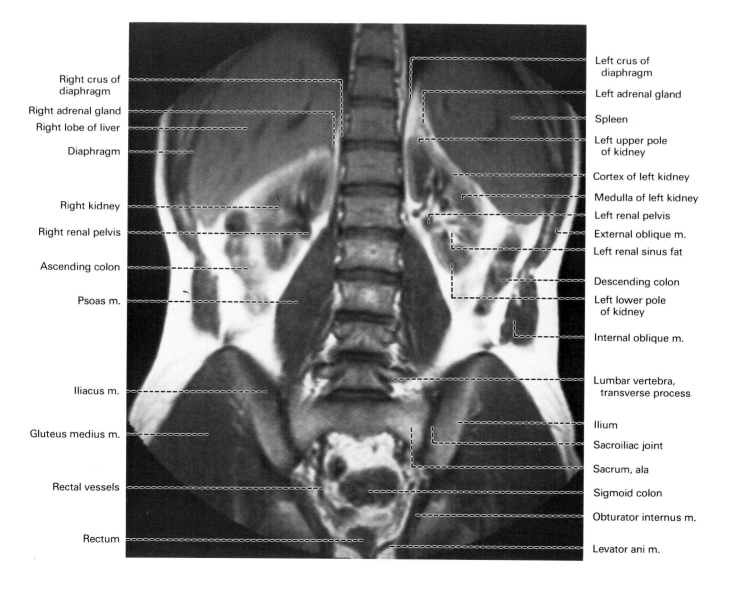

Right crus of diaphragm
Right adrenal gland
Right lobe of liver
Diaphragm
Right kidney
Right renal pelvis
Ascending colon
Psoas m.
Iliacus m.
Gluteus medius m.
Rectal vessels
Rectum

Left crus of diaphragm
Left adrenal gland
Spleen
Left upper pole of kidney
Cortex of left kidney
Medulla of left kidney
Left renal pelvis
External oblique m.
Left renal sinus fat
Descending colon
Left lower pole of kidney
Internal oblique m.
Lumbar vertebra, transverse process
Ilium
Sacroiliac joint
Sacrum, ala
Sigmoid colon
Obturator internus m.
Levator ani m.

Figure 8.2.6

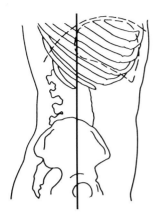

1. The left crus of the diaphragm is depicted in this section.

2. The right and left crura lie on either side of the aortic hiatus and they are joined anterior to the hiatus by the median arcuate ligament.

3. Note the haustral pattern that characterizes the colon.

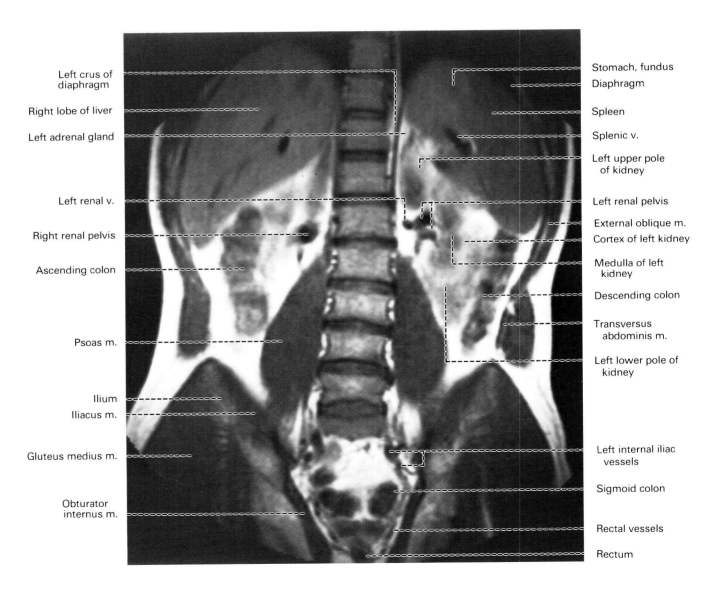

Left crus of diaphragm

Right lobe of liver

Left adrenal gland

Left renal v.

Right renal pelvis

Ascending colon

Psoas m.

Ilium

Iliacus m.

Gluteus medius m.

Obturator internus m.

Stomach, fundus

Diaphragm

Spleen

Splenic v.

Left upper pole of kidney

Left renal pelvis

External oblique m.

Cortex of left kidney

Medulla of left kidney

Descending colon

Transversus abdominis m.

Left lower pole of kidney

Left internal iliac vessels

Sigmoid colon

Rectal vessels

Rectum

Figure 8.2.7

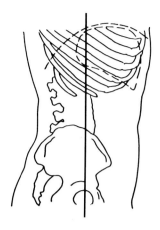

1. The splenic artery and vein course on the posterosuperior aspect of the pancreas. The splenic artery is more tortuous than the vein.

2. The right hepatic vein divides the right lobe of the liver into anterior and posterior segments.

3. The psoas and iliacus muscles are clearly depicted in this section. They merge in the pelvis to form the iliopsoas muscle.

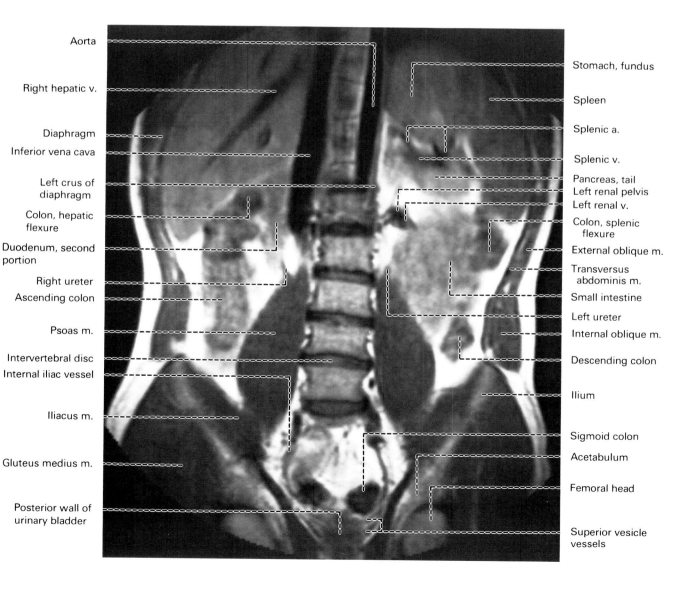

Aorta

Right hepatic v.

Diaphragm
Inferior vena cava

Left crus of diaphragm

Colon, hepatic flexure

Duodenum, second portion

Right ureter
Ascending colon

Psoas m.

Intervertebral disc
Internal iliac vessel

Iliacus m.

Gluteus medius m.

Posterior wall of urinary bladder

Stomach, fundus

Spleen

Splenic a.

Splenic v.

Pancreas, tail
Left renal pelvis
Left renal v.

Colon, splenic flexure

External oblique m.

Transversus abdominis m.

Small intestine

Left ureter

Internal oblique m.

Descending colon

Ilium

Sigmoid colon

Acetabulum

Femoral head

Superior vesicle vessels

Figure 8.2.8

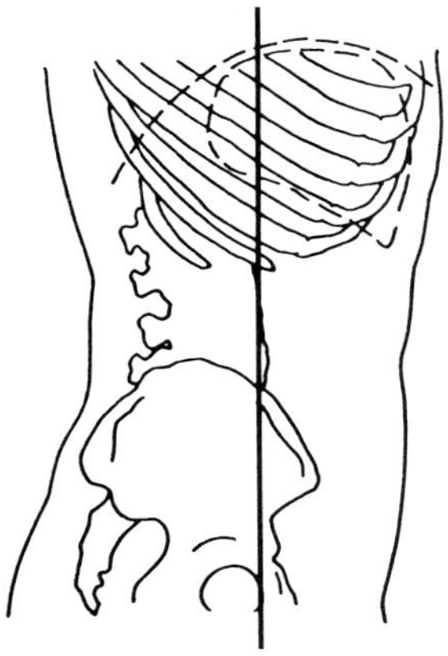

1. Note the relationship of the tail of the pancreas to the splenic hilum. The tail of the pancreas is located in the splenorenal ligament.

2. The right hepatic vein is demonstrated draining into the inferior vena cava.

3. After leaving the aorta, the right renal artery crosses the midline between the inferior vena cava and vertebral body.

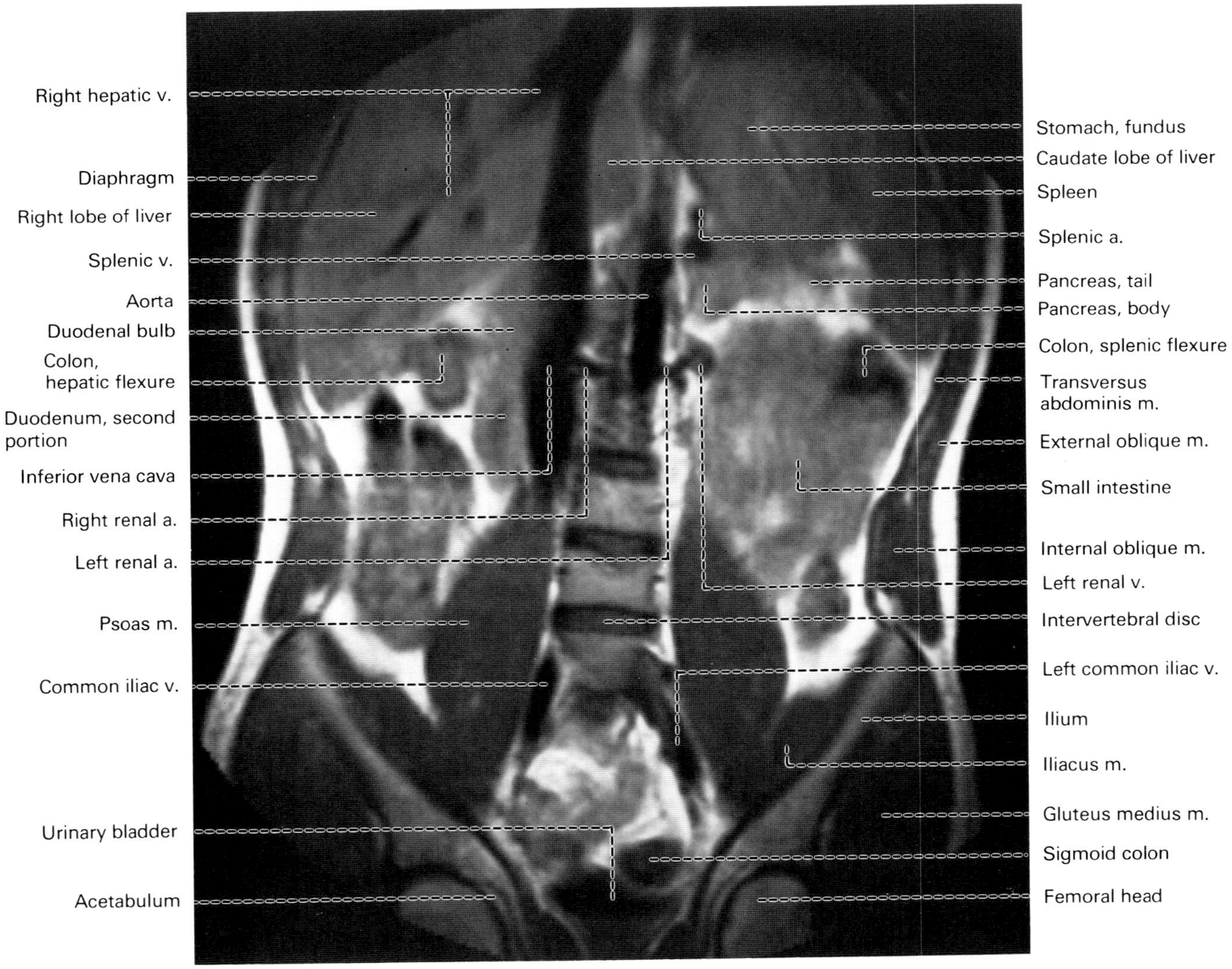
Right hepatic v.
Diaphragm
Right lobe of liver
Splenic v.
Aorta
Duodenal bulb
Colon, hepatic flexure
Duodenum, second portion
Inferior vena cava
Right renal a.
Left renal a.
Psoas m.
Common iliac v.
Urinary bladder
Acetabulum
Stomach, fundus
Caudate lobe of liver
Spleen
Splenic a.
Pancreas, tail
Pancreas, body
Colon, splenic flexure
Transversus abdominis m.
External oblique m.
Small intestine
Internal oblique m.
Left renal v.
Intervertebral disc
Left common iliac v.
Ilium
Iliacus m.
Gluteus medius m.
Sigmoid colon
Femoral head

Figure 8.2.9

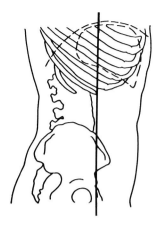

1. The portal vein courses obliquely toward the liver in the gastrohepatic ligament.

2. Note the celiac artery as it divides into the hepatic, splenic, and left gastric arteries. The celiac artery originates from the anterior aspect of the aorta at the level of T12-L1.

3. Distal to the celiac artery, the superior mesenteric artery is seen originating from the aorta.

4. Just caudal to the superior mesenteric artery, the origin of the renal arteries from the aorta can be seen at the level of L1-L2.

5. The inferior vena cava is of larger caliber than the aorta.

6. The pancreas is divided into a head with the uncinate process, body, and tail. The head is located within the loop of duodenum. The caudal and left portion of the head hooks around the superior mesenteric vessels forming the uncinate process.

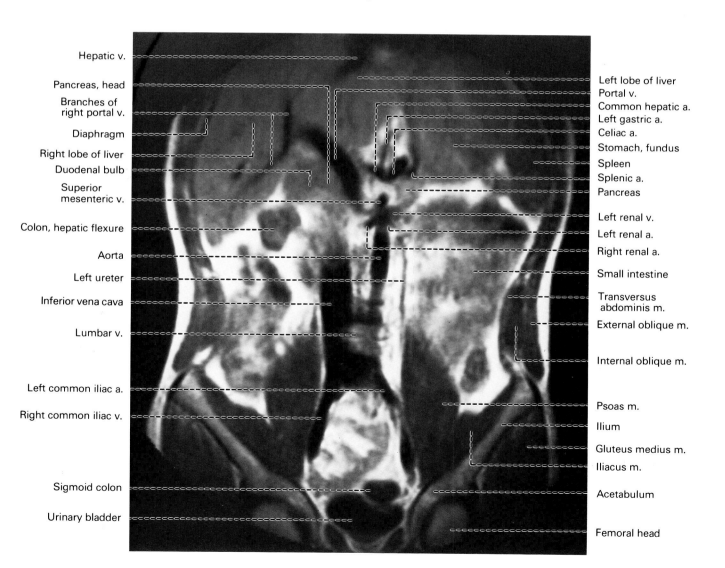

Hepatic v.
Pancreas, head
Branches of right portal v.
Diaphragm
Right lobe of liver
Duodenal bulb
Superior mesenteric v.
Colon, hepatic flexure
Aorta
Left ureter
Inferior vena cava
Lumbar v.
Left common iliac a.
Right common iliac v.
Sigmoid colon
Urinary bladder

Left lobe of liver
Portal v.
Common hepatic a.
Left gastric a.
Celiac a.
Stomach, fundus
Spleen
Splenic a.
Pancreas
Left renal v.
Left renal a.
Right renal a.
Small intestine
Transversus abdominis m.
External oblique m.
Internal oblique m.
Psoas m.
Ilium
Gluteus medius m.
Iliacus m.
Acetabulum
Femoral head

Figure 8.2.10

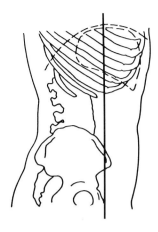

1. This section passes through portions of the aorta and portal vein.

2. Note the merger of the splenic and superior mesenteric veins contributing to the formation of the portal vein.

3. Note the relation between the superior mesenteric artery and vein. The superior mesenteric vein is located to the right of the superior mesenteric artery.

4. The left hepatic vein is demonstrated between the lateral and medial segments of the left lobe.

5. The middle hepatic vein is seen between the medial segment of the left lobe and right lobe of the liver.

6. The gastroduodenal artery is demonstrated originating from the common hepatic artery.

7. The ureters can be seen crossing the iliac vessels.

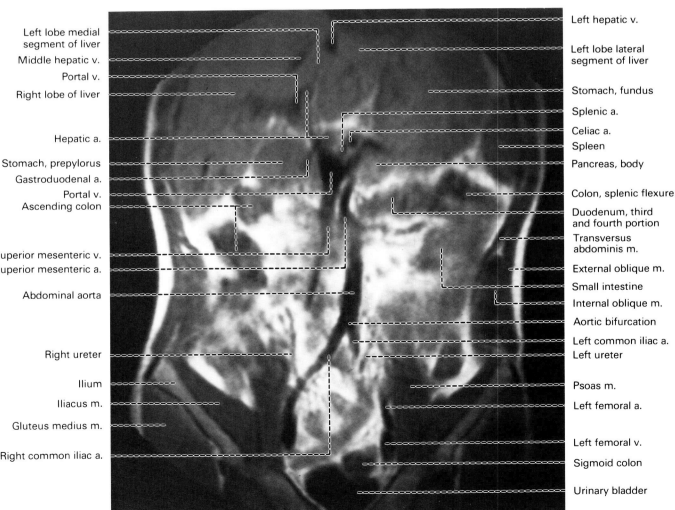

Left lobe medial segment of liver
Middle hepatic v.
Portal v.
Right lobe of liver
Hepatic a.
Stomach, prepylorus
Gastroduodenal a.
Portal v.
Ascending colon
Superior mesenteric v.
Superior mesenteric a.
Abdominal aorta
Right ureter
Ilium
Iliacus m.
Gluteus medius m.
Right common iliac a.

Left hepatic v.
Left lobe lateral segment of liver
Stomach, fundus
Splenic a.
Celiac a.
Spleen
Pancreas, body
Colon, splenic flexure
Duodenum, third and fourth portion
Transversus abdominis m.
External oblique m.
Small intestine
Internal oblique m.
Aortic bifurcation
Left common iliac a.
Left ureter
Psoas m.
Left femoral a.
Left femoral v.
Sigmoid colon
Urinary bladder

Figure 8.2.11

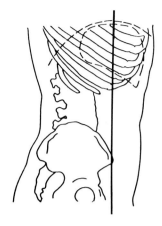

1. The branches of the superior and inferior mesenteric veins are seen in the midabdomen.

2. The inferior mesenteric vein drains blood from the left hemicolon.

3. The urinary bladder is located in the true pelvis, and its superior surface is covered by peritoneum.

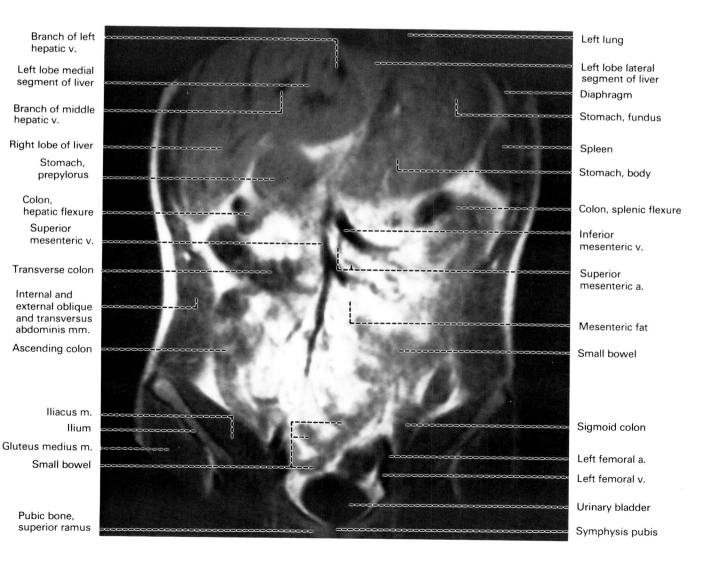

Branch of left hepatic v.
Left lobe medial segment of liver
Branch of middle hepatic v.
Right lobe of liver
Stomach, prepylorus
Colon, hepatic flexure
Superior mesenteric v.
Transverse colon
Internal and external oblique and transversus abdominis mm.
Ascending colon
Iliacus m.
Ilium
Gluteus medius m.
Small bowel
Pubic bone, superior ramus

Left lung
Left lobe lateral segment of liver
Diaphragm
Stomach, fundus
Spleen
Stomach, body
Colon, splenic flexure
Inferior mesenteric v.
Superior mesenteric a.
Mesenteric fat
Small bowel
Sigmoid colon
Left femoral a.
Left femoral v.
Urinary bladder
Symphysis pubis

Figure 8.2.12

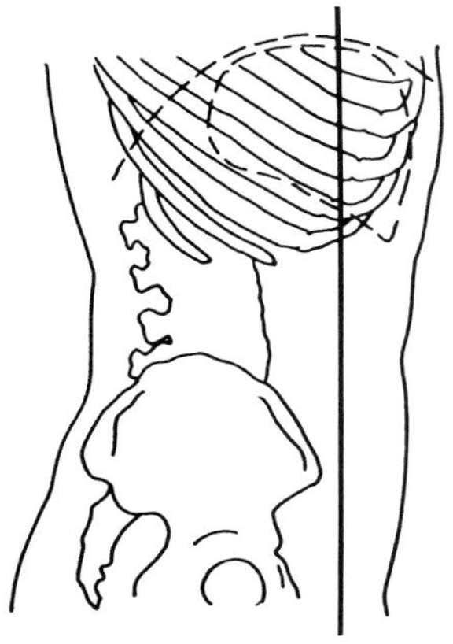

1. This section passes through the anterior portion of the urinary bladder.
2. The hepatic and splenic flexures of the colon are demonstrated caudal to the inferior surface of the liver and spleen.
3. Both femoral artery and vein are demonstrated as tubular structures. Note that the vein is medial to the artery.
4. The iliopsoas muscle leaves the pelvis to insert on the lesser trochanter.

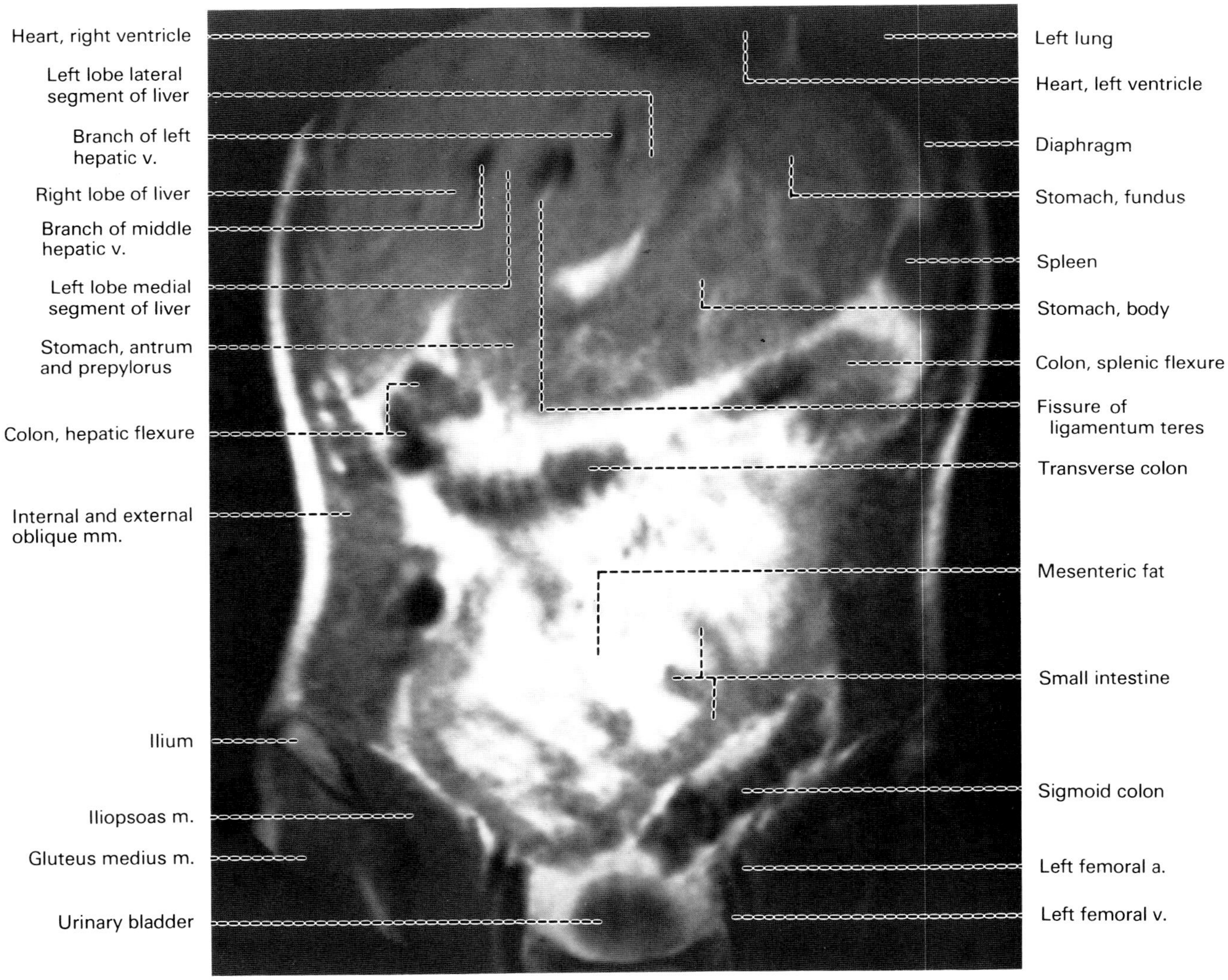
Heart, right ventricle
Left lobe lateral segment of liver
Branch of left hepatic v.
Right lobe of liver
Branch of middle hepatic v.
Left lobe medial segment of liver
Stomach, antrum and prepylorus
Colon, hepatic flexure
Internal and external oblique mm.
Ilium
Iliopsoas m.
Gluteus medius m.
Urinary bladder
Left lung
Heart, left ventricle
Diaphragm
Stomach, fundus
Spleen
Stomach, body
Colon, splenic flexure
Fissure of ligamentum teres
Transverse colon
Mesenteric fat
Small intestine
Sigmoid colon
Left femoral a.
Left femoral v.

Figure 8.2.13

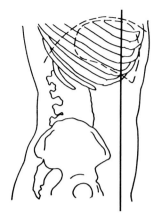

1. Between the diaphragm and liver surface there is a potential space called the subphrenic space. It is divided into right and left subphrenic spaces by the falciform ligament.

2. The transverse colon is demonstrated as a tubular structure inferior to the greater curvature of the stomach.

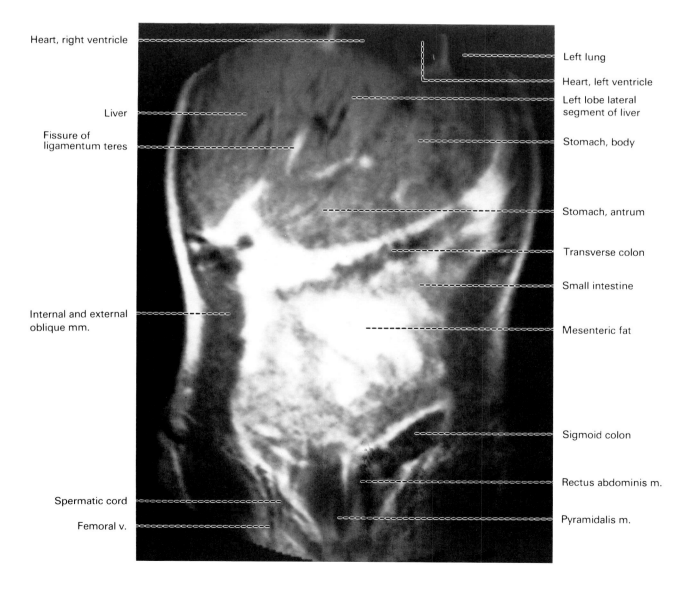

Heart, right ventricle

Liver

Fissure of ligamentum teres

Internal and external oblique mm.

Spermatic cord

Femoral v.

Left lung

Heart, left ventricle

Left lobe lateral segment of liver

Stomach, body

Stomach, antrum

Transverse colon

Small intestine

Mesenteric fat

Sigmoid colon

Rectus abdominis m.

Pyramidalis m.

Figure 8.2.14

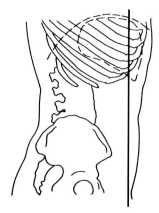

1. The fibers of the external oblique muscle course inferomedially, whereas the fibers of the internal oblique course in the opposite direction.

2. The external oblique, internal oblique, and transversus abdominis muscles all insert into the linea alba.

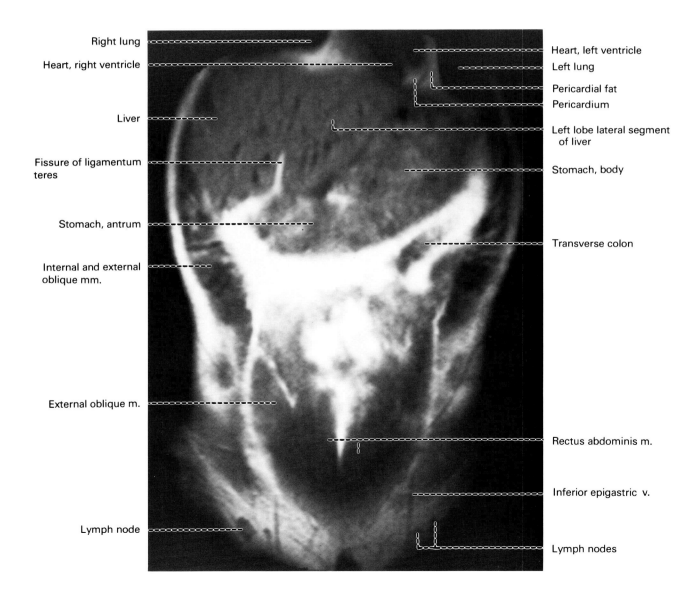

Right lung

Heart, right ventricle

Liver

Fissure of ligamentum teres

Stomach, antrum

Internal and external oblique mm.

External oblique m.

Lymph node

Heart, left ventricle

Left lung

Pericardial fat

Pericardium

Left lobe lateral segment of liver

Stomach, body

Transverse colon

Rectus abdominis m.

Inferior epigastric v.

Lymph nodes

Figure 8.2.15

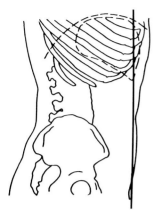

1. The most anterior portions of the liver and stomach are partially demonstrated.

2. The xiphoid and part of the inferior sternum can be seen as high signal intensity structures due to the fat-containing bone marrow.

3. Note the fissure of ligamentum teres. This fissure contains the falciform ligament, ligamentum teres, sagittal portion of the left branch of the portal vein, and corresponding branches of the hepatic artery.

4. The fissure of ligamentum teres lies between the medial and lateral segments of the left lobe of the liver.

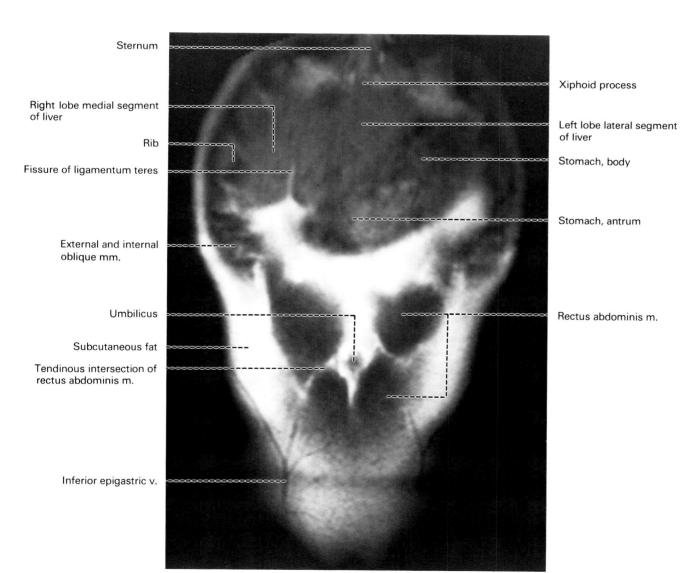

Sternum

Right lobe medial segment of liver

Rib

Fissure of ligamentum teres

External and internal oblique mm.

Umbilicus

Subcutaneous fat

Tendinous intersection of rectus abdominis m.

Inferior epigastric v.

Xiphoid process

Left lobe lateral segment of liver

Stomach, body

Stomach, antrum

Rectus abdominis m.

Figure 8.2.16

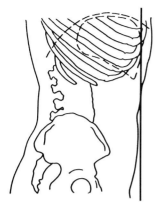

1. Ribs with cartilage and intercostal muscles can be seen as low signal intensity structures.

2. Note that the ribs do not articulate directly with the sternum but rather with costal cartilage.

3. The rectus abdominis muscle is distinguished by its transversely oriented tendinous intersections.

4. The umbilicus typically lies at the level of the aortic bifurcation and lumbar vertebrae L3-L4.

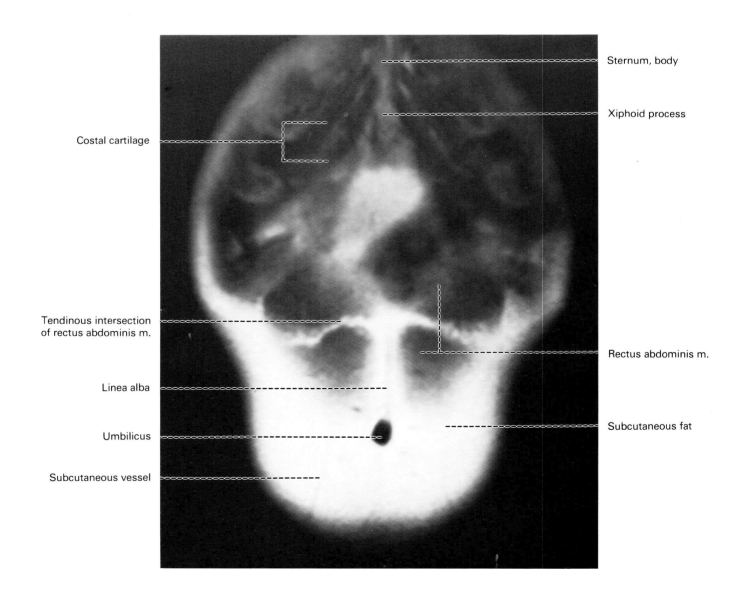

SAGITTAL

Figure 8.3.1

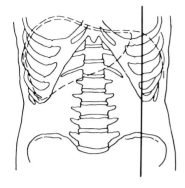

1. This section is through the left abdomen and it passes through the left kidney and spleen.

2. The splenic artery and vein course on the posterior superior surface of the pancreas.

3. Note the psoas and iliacus muscles as they merge in the pelvis to form the iliopsoas muscle.

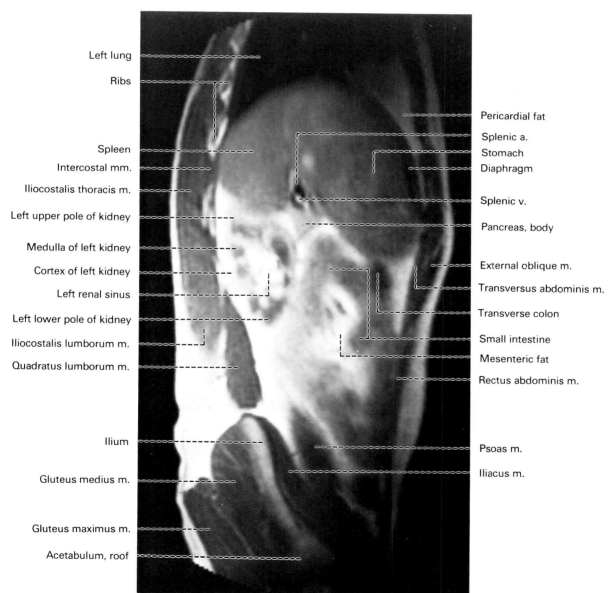

Left lung
Ribs
Spleen
Intercostal mm.
Iliocostalis thoracis m.
Left upper pole of kidney
Medulla of left kidney
Cortex of left kidney
Left renal sinus
Left lower pole of kidney
Iliocostalis lumborum m.
Quadratus lumborum m.
Ilium
Gluteus medius m.
Gluteus maximus m.
Acetabulum, roof

Pericardial fat
Splenic a.
Stomach
Diaphragm
Splenic v.
Pancreas, body
External oblique m.
Transversus abdominis m.
Transverse colon
Small intestine
Mesenteric fat
Rectus abdominis m.
Psoas m.
Iliacus m.

Figure 8.3.2

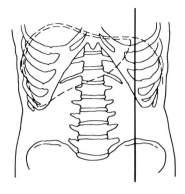

1. Note the posterior position of the spleen.

2. The anterior surface of the kidney is related to the spleen, stomach, jejunum, pancreas, and descending colon. The upper pole of the kidney is usually wider than the lower pole.

3. The quadratus lumborum lines the posterior abdominal wall. It arises from the iliac crest and transverse processes of the lower three lumbar vertebrae. It inserts on the transverse process of the upper three lumbar vertebrae and proximal part of the twelfth rib.

4. Iliocostalis lumborum is part of the erector spinae group. It originates from the posterior surface of the sacrum and inserts on the lower six ribs.

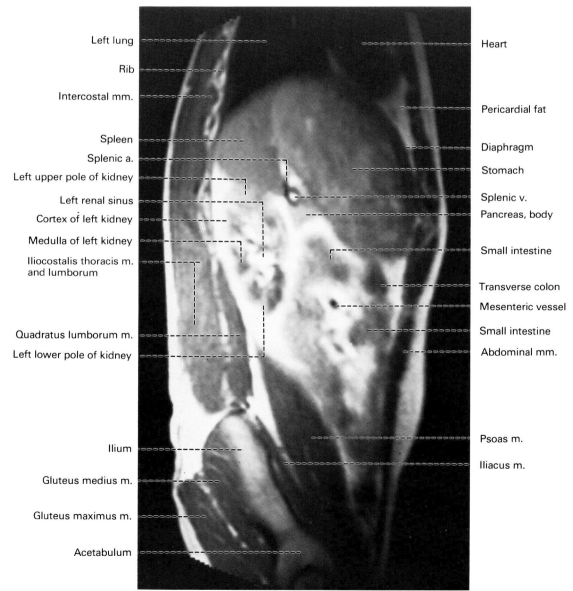

Left lung — Rib — Intercostal mm. — Spleen — Splenic a. — Left upper pole of kidney — Left renal sinus — Cortex of left kidney — Medulla of left kidney — Iliocostalis thoracis m. and lumborum — Quadratus lumborum m. — Left lower pole of kidney — Ilium — Gluteus medius m. — Gluteus maximus m. — Acetabulum

Heart — Pericardial fat — Diaphragm — Stomach — Splenic v. — Pancreas, body — Small intestine — Transverse colon — Mesenteric vessel — Small intestine — Abdominal mm. — Psoas m. — Iliacus m.

Figure 8.3.3

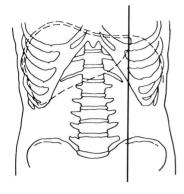

1. The kidneys are oriented obliquely with the lower pole in a more lateral and anterior position than the upper pole.

2. The rectus abdominis muscle is characterized by transversely oriented tendinous intersections.

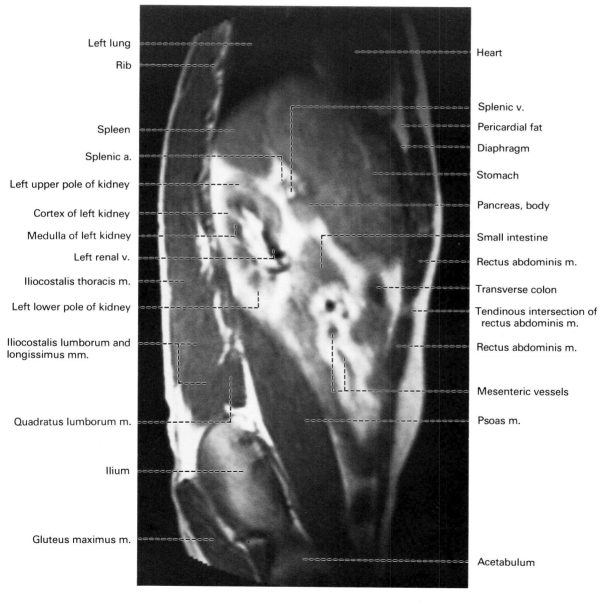

Left lung

Rib

Spleen

Splenic a.

Left upper pole of kidney

Cortex of left kidney

Medulla of left kidney

Left renal v.

Iliocostalis thoracis m.

Left lower pole of kidney

Iliocostalis lumborum and longissimus mm.

Quadratus lumborum m.

Ilium

Gluteus maximus m.

Heart

Splenic v.

Pericardial fat

Diaphragm

Stomach

Pancreas, body

Small intestine

Rectus abdominis m.

Transverse colon

Tendinous intersection of rectus abdominis m.

Rectus abdominis m.

Mesenteric vessels

Psoas m.

Acetabulum

Figure 8.3.4

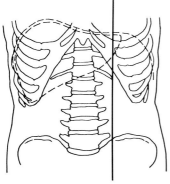

1. Note that the renal pelvis usually lies posterior to renal vessels with the order from front to back being vein, artery, and pelvis.

2. The irregular contour of the sacroiliac joint is appreciated in this section.

3. The psoas muscle proceeds distally to insert along with the iliacus muscle on the lesser trochanter.

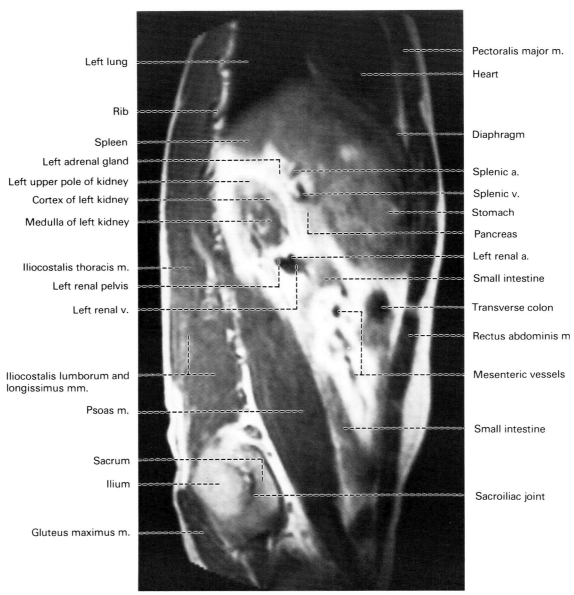

Figure 8.3.5

1. The left ureter can be demonstrated as a linear structure just anterior to the psoas muscle.

2. The left adrenal gland lies anterior and superior to the upper pole of the left kidney.

3. The erector spinae muscles originate from the dorsal aspect of the sacrum.

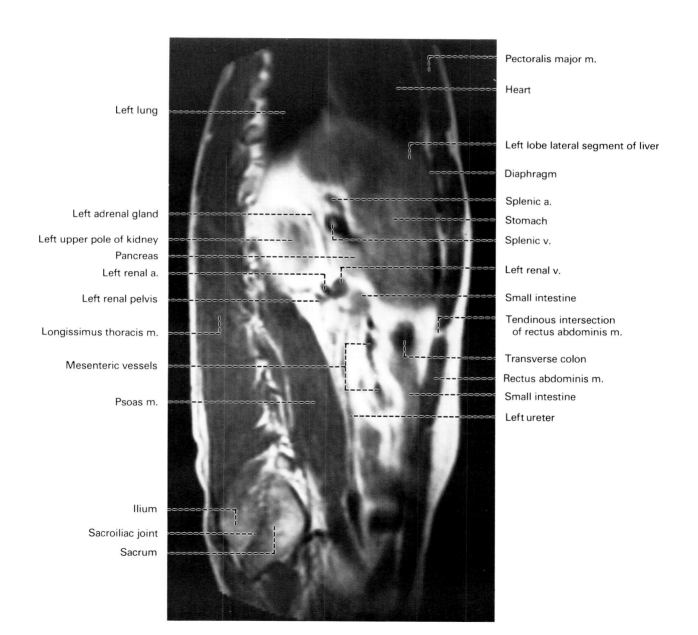

Figure 8.3.6

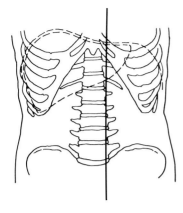

1. The renal artery and vein are seen in cross section; the vein is anterior to the artery.

2. In the pelvis, the common iliac artery is anterior to the common iliac vein.

3. The lumbar arteries supply the back and abdominal musculature. They also give rise to spinal arteries that supply the spinal cord. Lumbar arteries arise from the posterolateral surface of the abdominal aorta.

4. Below the level of the left atrium (not demonstrated) the esophagus moves to the left of midline just anterior to the aorta and traverses the diaphragm at the T10 level.

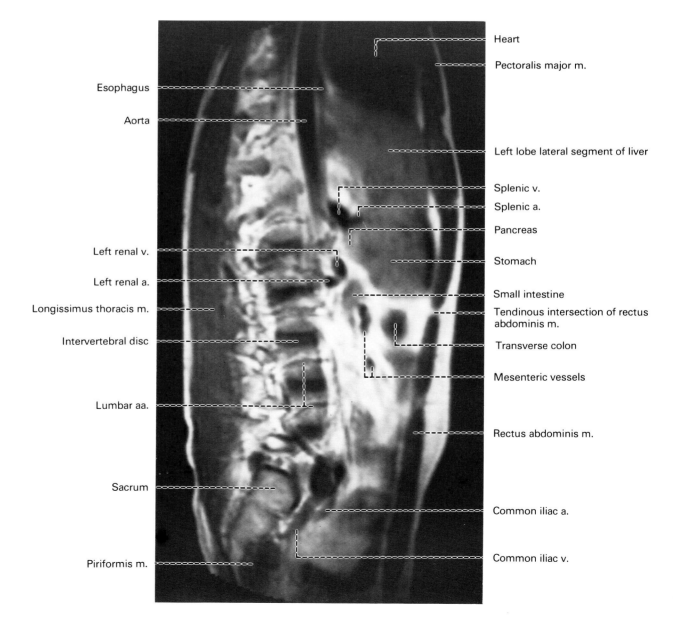

Figure 8.3.7

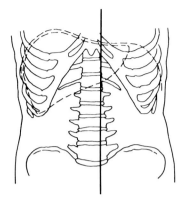

1. Note the origin of the celiac and superior mesenteric arteries from the anterior surface of the abdominal aorta. The celiac artery usually leaves the aorta at the level of T12-L1. The superior mesenteric artery branches off 0.5 – 2 cm distal to the celiac artery.

2. The pedicle and neural foramina are clearly depicted. Nerve roots are seen in the upper portion of the foramina.

3. Note the origin of the lumbar arteries from the posterolateral aspect of the abdominal aorta.

4. The left gastric artery originates from the celiac axis and runs on the surface of the lesser curvature of the stomach.

5. The potential space between the pancreas and the stomach represents the lesser sac. The anterior boundary of the lesser sac is formed by the posterior wall of the stomach, the lesser omentum, and the anterior reflection of the greater omentum. Posteriorly, the lesser sac is bounded by the peritoneal reflection over the pancreas.

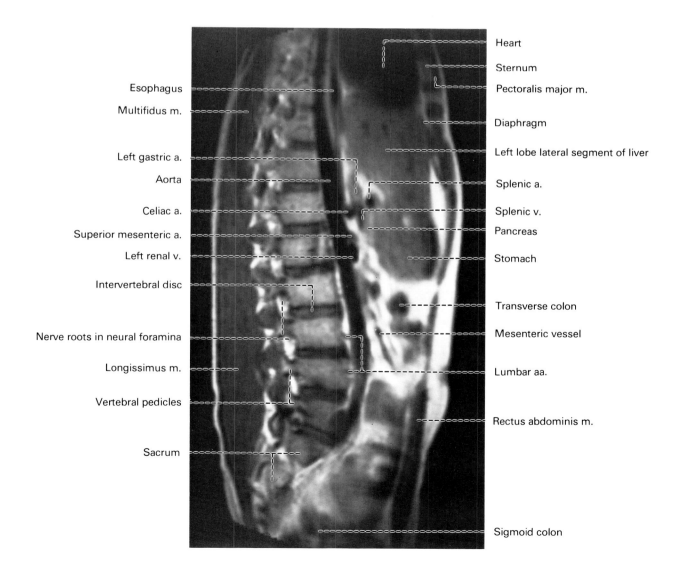

Figure 8.3.8

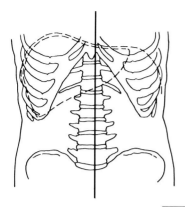

1. This is a midsagittal section that passes through the linea alba.

2. The linea alba is a median raphe formed by the anterior and posterior walls of the rectus sheath from both sides that come together and fuse.

3. Note the thick fibrous ligament, the supraspinous ligament, connecting the tips of the spinous processes.

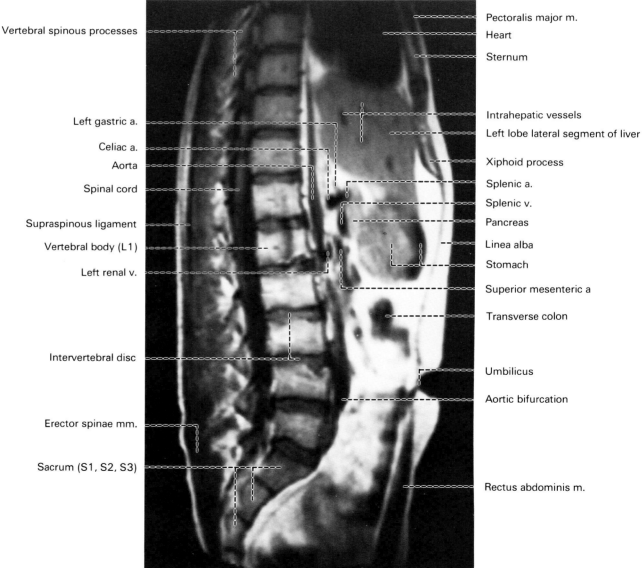

Vertebral spinous processes

Left gastric a.

Celiac a.

Aorta

Spinal cord

Supraspinous ligament

Vertebral body (L1)

Left renal v.

Intervertebral disc

Erector spinae mm.

Sacrum (S1, S2, S3)

Pectoralis major m.

Heart

Sternum

Intrahepatic vessels

Left lobe lateral segment of liver

Xiphoid process

Splenic a.

Splenic v.

Pancreas

Linea alba

Stomach

Superior mesenteric a

Transverse colon

Umbilicus

Aortic bifurcation

Rectus abdominis m.

Figure 8.3.9

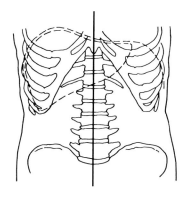

1. The left hepatic vein is seen draining into the inferior vena cava.

2. At the T12-L1 level the spinal cord enlarges and forms the conus. Below L1 only nerve roots will be identified within the thecal sac.

3. At this level the portal vein is surrounded by the pancreatic head.

4. The right renal artery courses between the inferior vena cava and anterior margin of the vertebral body.

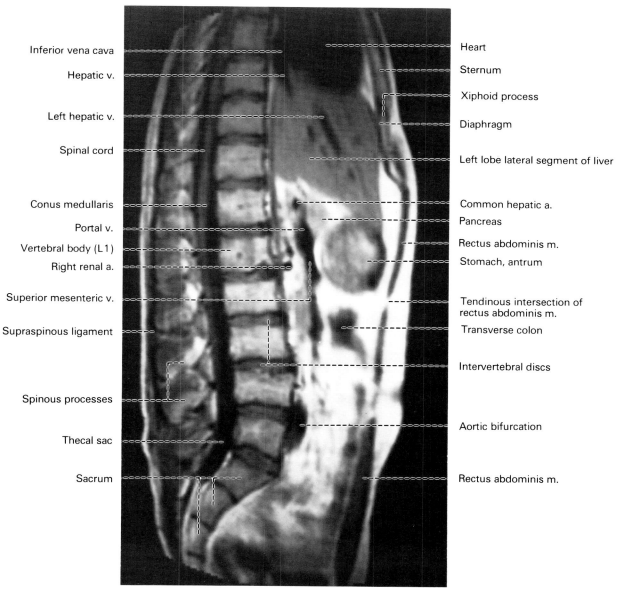

Left column labels: Inferior vena cava, Hepatic v., Left hepatic v., Spinal cord, Conus medullaris, Portal v., Vertebral body (L1), Right renal a., Superior mesenteric v., Supraspinous ligament, Spinous processes, Thecal sac, Sacrum

Right column labels: Heart, Sternum, Xiphoid process, Diaphragm, Left lobe lateral segment of liver, Common hepatic a., Pancreas, Rectus abdominis m., Stomach, antrum, Tendinous intersection of rectus abdominis m., Transverse colon, Intervertebral discs, Aortic bifurcation, Rectus abdominis m.

Figure 8.3.10

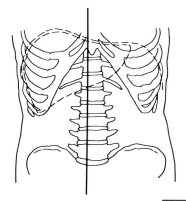

1. The superior mesenteric and splenic veins merge to form the portal vein.

2. Portions of the inferior vena cava are demonstrated in this section.

3. Note the segmented rectus abdominis muscle. Three tendinous intersections are present in this muscle.

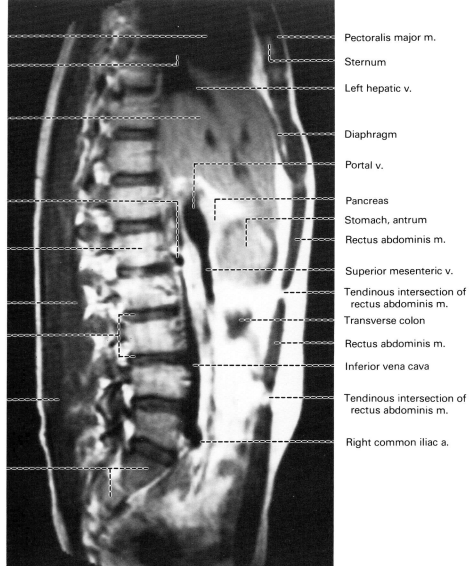

Heart

Inferior vena cava

Left lobe lateral segment of liver

Right renal a.

Vertebral body (L1)

Multifidus m.

Intervertebral disc

Erector spinae m.

Sacrum

Pectoralis major m.

Sternum

Left hepatic v.

Diaphragm

Portal v.

Pancreas

Stomach, antrum

Rectus abdominis m.

Superior mesenteric v.

Tendinous intersection of rectus abdominis m.

Transverse colon

Rectus abdominis m.

Inferior vena cava

Tendinous intersection of rectus abdominis m.

Right common iliac a.

Figure 8.3.11

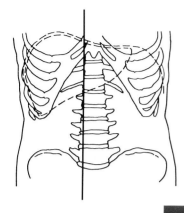

1. Note that the renal artery courses posterior to the inferior vena cava.

2. The internal iliac artery is seen dividing just superior to the piriformis muscle.

3. The superior gluteal artery originates from the internal iliac artery.

4. The fissure of ligamentum venosum lies between the left lobe and the caudate lobe.

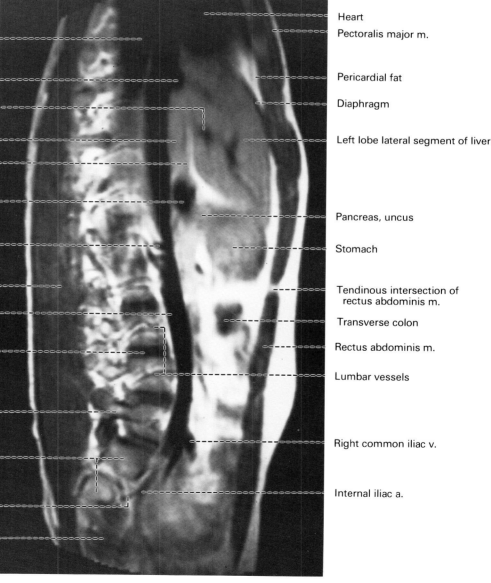

Right lung

Hepatic v.

Left portal v.

Caudate lobe of liver

Fissure of ligamentum venosum

Portal v.

Right renal a.

Longissimus thoracis m.

Inferior vena cava

Intervertebral disc

Vertebral pedicle

Sacrum

Superior gluteal a.

Piriformis m.

Heart
Pectoralis major m.

Pericardial fat

Diaphragm

Left lobe lateral segment of liver

Pancreas, uncus

Stomach

Tendinous intersection of rectus abdominis m.

Transverse colon

Rectus abdominis m.

Lumbar vessels

Right common iliac v.

Internal iliac a.

Figure 8.3.12

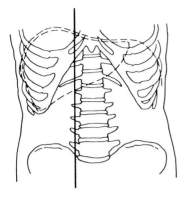

1. Extrahepatic and intrahepatic portions of the portal vein are well demonstrated.

2. The common iliac artery courses anterior to the common iliac vein.

3. The piriformis muscle is a significant anatomic landmark in the pelvis because the sacral plexus forms on its anterior surface.

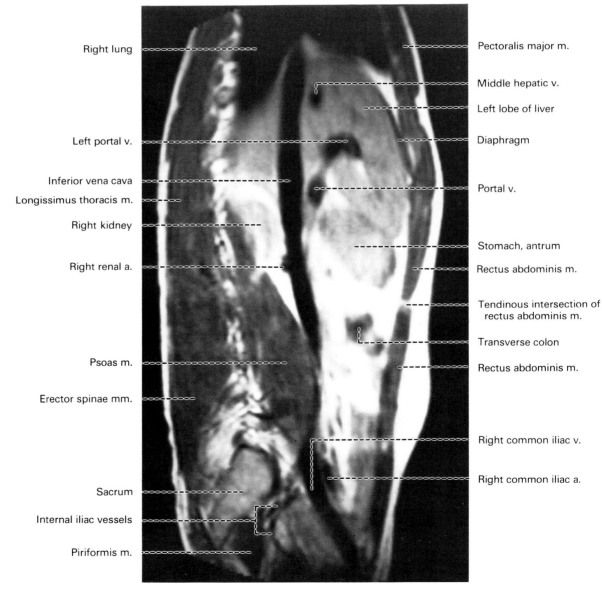

Figure 8.3.13

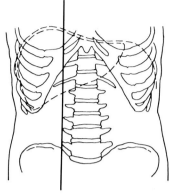

1. The renal vein is seen draining into the inferior vena cava.

2. The liver vasculature is well represented in this section with portions of the portal and right and middle hepatic veins demonstrated.

3. The psoas muscle exits the pelvis beneath the inguinal ligament and proceeds to its insertion on the lesser trochanter along with the iliacus muscle.

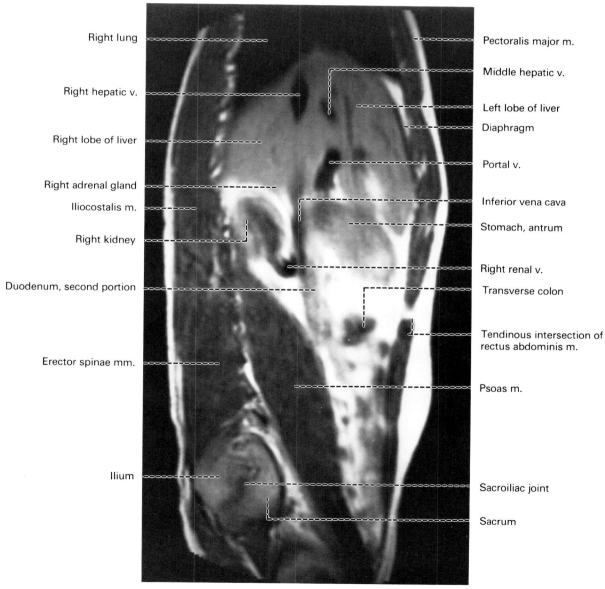

Right lung

Right hepatic v.

Right lobe of liver

Right adrenal gland

Iliocostalis m.

Right kidney

Duodenum, second portion

Erector spinae mm.

Ilium

Pectoralis major m.

Middle hepatic v.

Left lobe of liver

Diaphragm

Portal v.

Inferior vena cava

Stomach, antrum

Right renal v.

Transverse colon

Tendinous intersection of rectus abdominis m.

Psoas m.

Sacroiliac joint

Sacrum

Figure 8.3.14

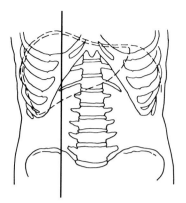

1. The portal vein can be seen within the fissure of ligamentum venosum.

2. Note the relation of the right kidney to the liver and duodenum.

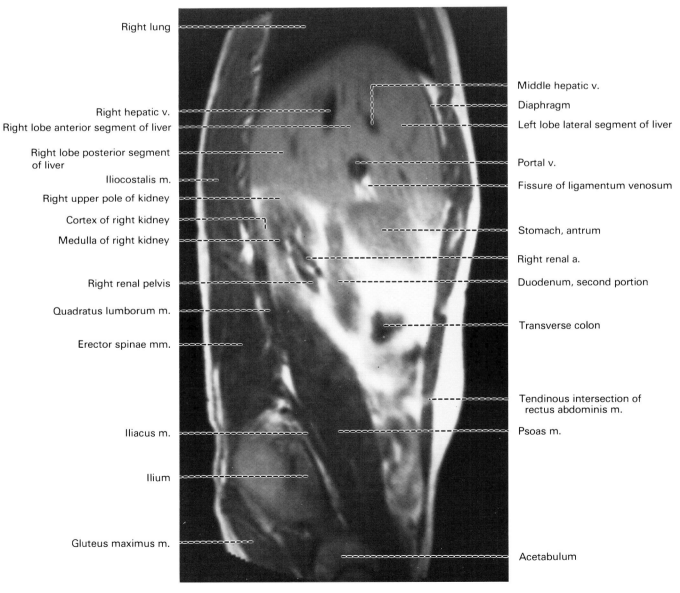

Right lung

Right hepatic v.
Right lobe anterior segment of liver

Right lobe posterior segment of liver

Iliocostalis m.
Right upper pole of kidney

Cortex of right kidney

Medulla of right kidney

Right renal pelvis

Quadratus lumborum m.

Erector spinae mm.

Iliacus m.

Ilium

Gluteus maximus m.

Middle hepatic v.
Diaphragm
Left lobe lateral segment of liver

Portal v.
Fissure of ligamentum venosum

Stomach, antrum

Right renal a.
Duodenum, second portion

Transverse colon

Tendinous intersection of rectus abdominis m.
Psoas m.

Acetabulum

Figure 8.3.15

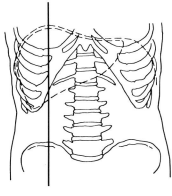

1. Between the diaphragm and the surface of the liver there is a potential space called the right subphrenic space.

2. The potential space formed between the inferior surface of the liver, right kidney, and right adrenal gland is called the hepatorenal recess or Morison's pouch.

3. The psoas and iliacus muscles merge to form one muscle, the iliopsoas.

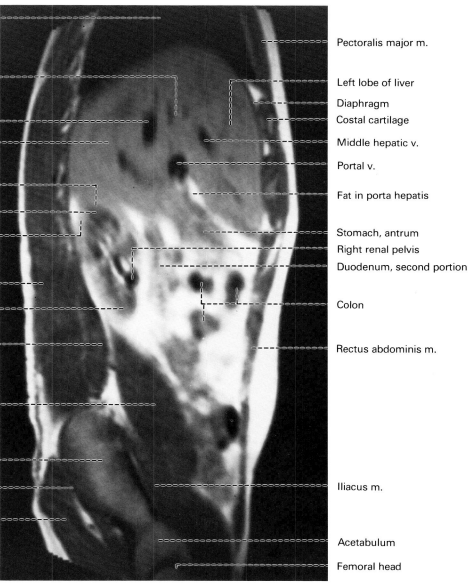

Right lung

Right lobe anterior segment of liver

Right hepatic v.

Right lobe posterior segment of liver

Right upper pole of kidney

Medulla of right kidney

Cortex of right kidney

Iliocostalis lumborum m.

Right lower pole of kidney

Quadratus lumborum m.

Psoas m.

Ilium

Gluteus medius m.

Gluteus maximus m.

Pectoralis major m.

Left lobe of liver

Diaphragm

Costal cartilage

Middle hepatic v.

Portal v.

Fat in porta hepatis

Stomach, antrum

Right renal pelvis

Duodenum, second portion

Colon

Rectus abdominis m.

Iliacus m.

Acetabulum

Femoral head

Figure 8.3.16

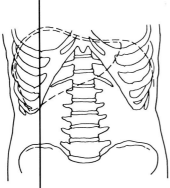

1. Note the relationship of the hepatic flexure to the right kidney and inferior surface of the liver.

2. At the hepatic flexure, the colon becomes intraperitoneal. The entire transverse colon is intraperitoneal.

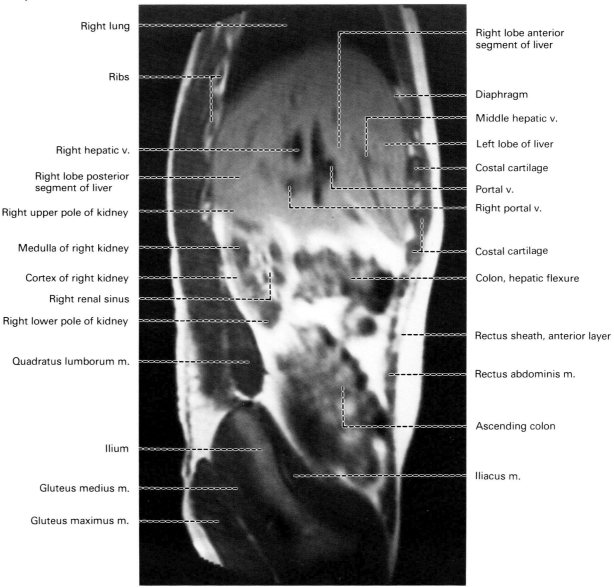

Right lung

Ribs

Right hepatic v.

Right lobe posterior segment of liver

Right upper pole of kidney

Medulla of right kidney

Cortex of right kidney

Right renal sinus

Right lower pole of kidney

Quadratus lumborum m.

Ilium

Gluteus medius m.

Gluteus maximus m.

Right lobe anterior segment of liver

Diaphragm

Middle hepatic v.

Left lobe of liver

Costal cartilage

Portal v.

Right portal v.

Costal cartilage

Colon, hepatic flexure

Rectus sheath, anterior layer

Rectus abdominis m.

Ascending colon

Iliacus m.

Chapter 9

CT OF THE ABDOMEN

AXIAL

Figure 9.1.1

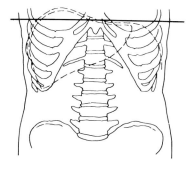

1. Just above the left diaphragm the esophagus moves slightly to the left of midline and descends anterior to the aorta.

2. The intrahepatic portion of the inferior vena cava is located at the posterior medial margin of the liver. The three major hepatic veins (right, middle, and left) drain into it at about this level.

3. The azygos vein is seen anterior to the vertebral body and the hemiazygos vein posterior to the aorta.

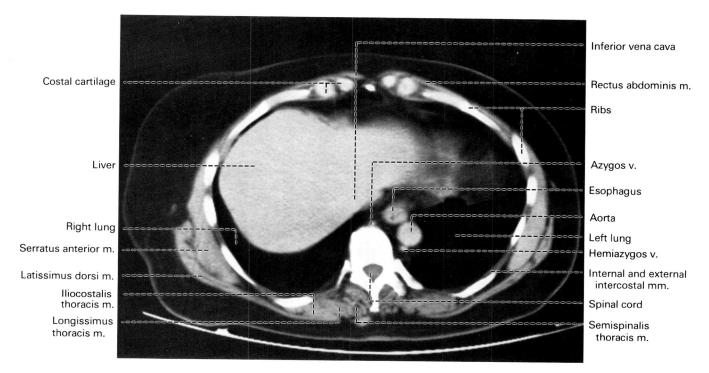

Figure 9.1.2

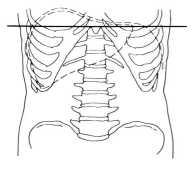

1. There are three openings in the diaphragm; one for each of the following structures: aorta, esophagus, and inferior vena cava.

2. After the esophagus crosses the diaphragm, it turns left to enter the gastric fundus.

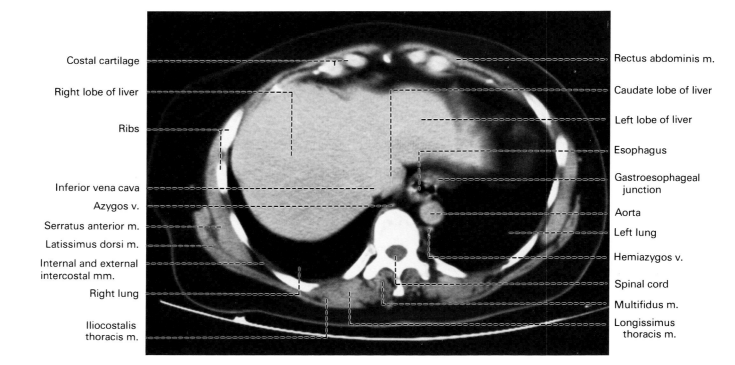

Costal cartilage

Right lobe of liver

Ribs

Inferior vena cava

Azygos v.

Serratus anterior m.

Latissimus dorsi m.

Internal and external
intercostal mm.

Right lung

Iliocostalis
thoracis m.

Rectus abdominis m.

Caudate lobe of liver

Left lobe of liver

Esophagus

Gastroesophageal
junction

Aorta

Left lung

Hemiazygos v.

Spinal cord

Multifidus m.

Longissimus
thoracis m.

Figure 9.1.3

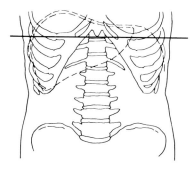

1. This section passes through the upper part of the spleen.

2. The diaphragm is demonstrated as a wavy structure inside of the abdominal wall.

3. The gastroesophageal junction is seen along the medial aspect of the fundus of the stomach.

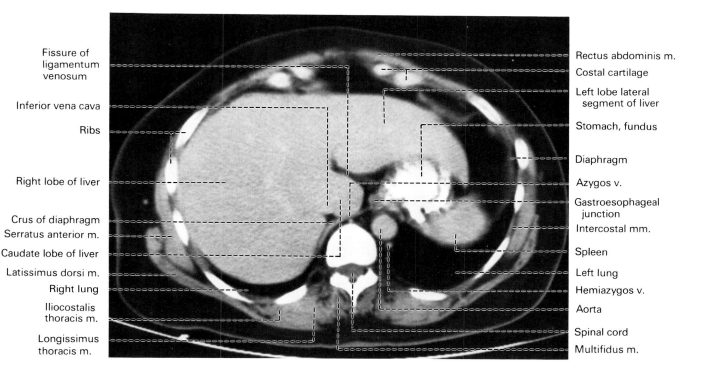

Fissure of ligamentum venosum

Inferior vena cava

Ribs

Right lobe of liver

Crus of diaphragm
Serratus anterior m.
Caudate lobe of liver
Latissimus dorsi m.
Right lung
Iliocostalis thoracis m.
Longissimus thoracis m.

Rectus abdominis m.
Costal cartilage
Left lobe lateral segment of liver
Stomach, fundus
Diaphragm
Azygos v.
Gastroesophageal junction
Intercostal mm.
Spleen
Left lung
Hemiazygos v.
Aorta
Spinal cord
Multifidus m.

Figure 9.1.4

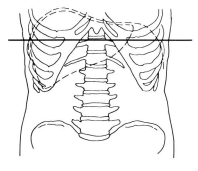

1. The diaphragmatic crura ascend along the anterior aspect of the spine, on each side of the aorta, merging anterior to the aorta to form the aortic hiatus.

2. The right crus arises from the front and side of the bodies of the upper three or four lumbar vertebrae and intervening discs, and is stouter and longer than the left crus, which arises from the upper two or three vertebrae and intervening discs.

3. The hemiazygos vein is demonstrated posterior to the aorta.

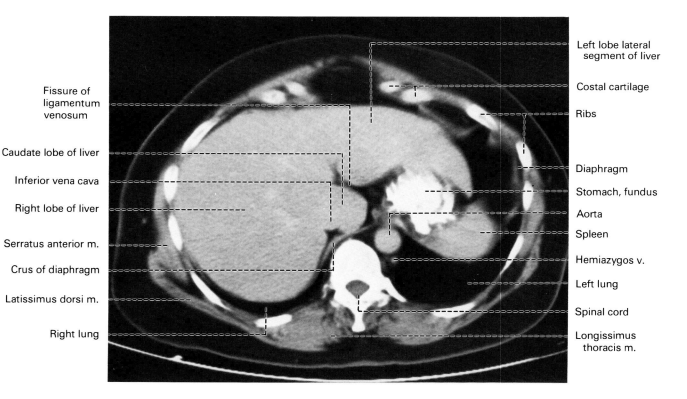

Left lobe lateral segment of liver

Costal cartilage

Ribs

Diaphragm

Stomach, fundus

Aorta

Spleen

Hemiazygos v.

Left lung

Spinal cord

Longissimus thoracis m.

Fissure of ligamentum venosum

Caudate lobe of liver

Inferior vena cava

Right lobe of liver

Serratus anterior m.

Crus of diaphragm

Latissimus dorsi m.

Right lung

Figure 9.1.5

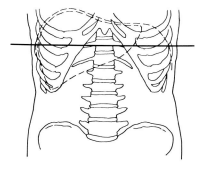

1. The caudate lobe of the liver is located between the fossa of the inferior vena cava and ligamentum venosum.

2. The medial and lateral segments of the left lobe are separated by ligamentum teres.

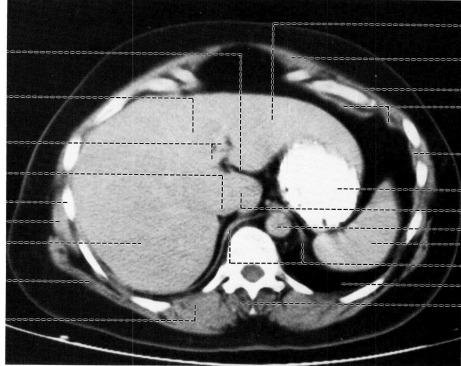

Fissure of ligamentum venosum

Left lobe medial segment of liver

Right and left branches of portal v.

Inferior vena cava

Rib

Serratus anterior m.

Right lobe of liver

Latissimus dorsi m.

Iliocostalis thoracis m.

Left lobe lateral segment of liver

Rectus abdominis m.

External oblique m.

Diaphragm

Internal and external intercostal mm.

Stomach, fundus

Caudate lobe of liver

Aorta

Spleen

Crura of diaphragm

Left lung

Multifidus m.

Figure 9.1.6

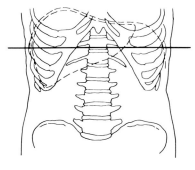

1. The stomach is surrounded by the diaphragm, spleen, lateral segment of the left lobe of the liver, jejunum, tail of the pancreas, and the splenic flexure of the colon.

2. The hepatic triad, seen in the porta hepatis, consists of the common bile duct, portal vein, and hepatic artery.

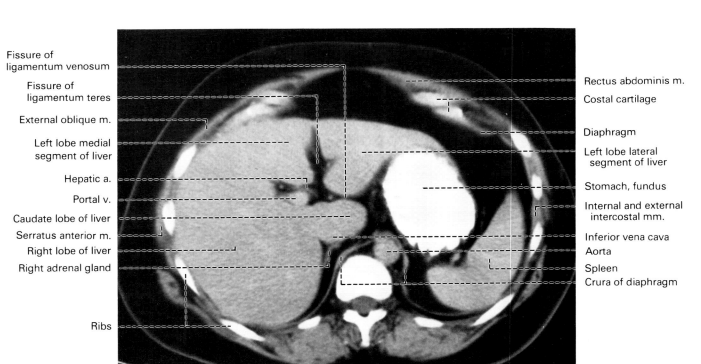

Fissure of ligamentum venosum
Fissure of ligamentum teres
External oblique m.
Left lobe medial segment of liver
Hepatic a.
Portal v.
Caudate lobe of liver
Serratus anterior m.
Right lobe of liver
Right adrenal gland
Ribs

Rectus abdominis m.
Costal cartilage
Diaphragm
Left lobe lateral segment of liver
Stomach, fundus
Internal and external intercostal mm.
Inferior vena cava
Aorta
Spleen
Crura of diaphragm

Figure 9.1.7

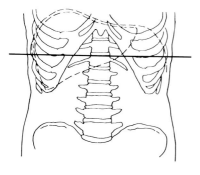

1. The hepatic artery arises from the celiac axis; it runs anterior to the portal vein and divides into the right and left hepatic arteries in the porta hepatis.

2. The medial segment of the left lobe of the liver lies between the fossa of the gallbladder and ligamentum teres.

3. The right adrenal gland is located posterior to the inferior vena cava.

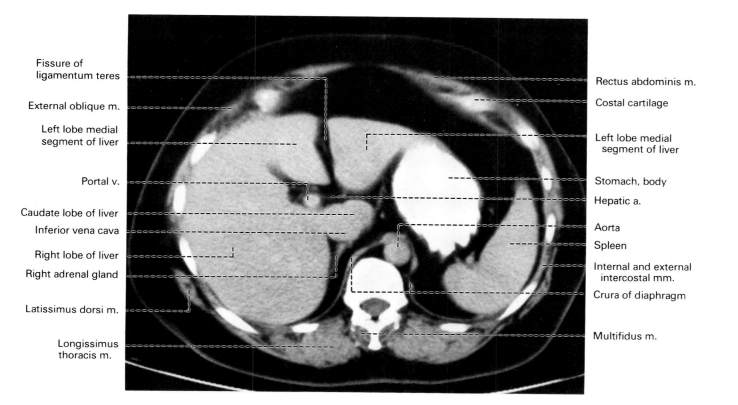

Fissure of ligamentum teres

External oblique m.

Left lobe medial segment of liver

Portal v.

Caudate lobe of liver

Inferior vena cava

Right lobe of liver

Right adrenal gland

Latissimus dorsi m.

Longissimus thoracis m.

Rectus abdominis m.

Costal cartilage

Left lobe medial segment of liver

Stomach, body

Hepatic a.

Aorta

Spleen

Internal and external intercostal mm.

Crura of diaphragm

Multifidus m.

Figure 9.1.8

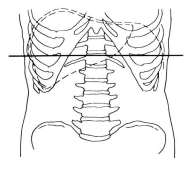

1. The main portal vein courses within the gastrohepatic (hepatoduodenal) ligament anterior to the inferior vena cava and into the porta hepatis, where it bifurcates into the right and left portal veins.

2. The main portal vein always lies posterior to the main hepatic artery and common bile duct.

3. The papillary process of the caudate lobe of the liver is seen between the portal vein and inferior vena cava.

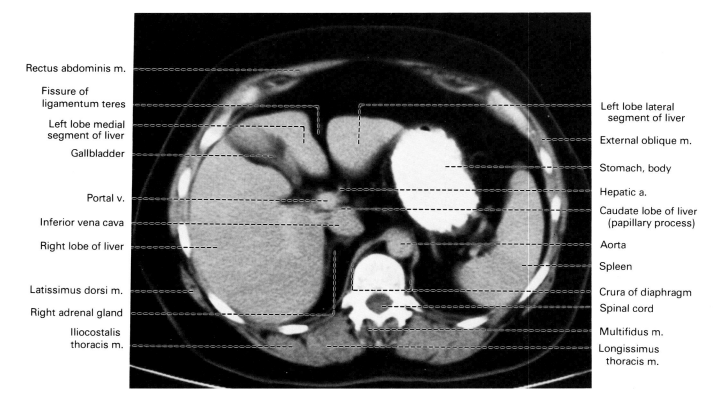

Figure 9.1.9

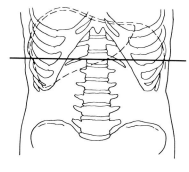

1. The celiac axis is the first unpaired branch of the abdominal aorta; it divides into the common hepatic, splenic, and left gastric arteries.

2. The gallbladder is well seen when distended as an oval sac of water density lying in a fossa on the inferior hepatic surface.

3. The left adrenal gland is located lateral to the crus of the left diaphragm.

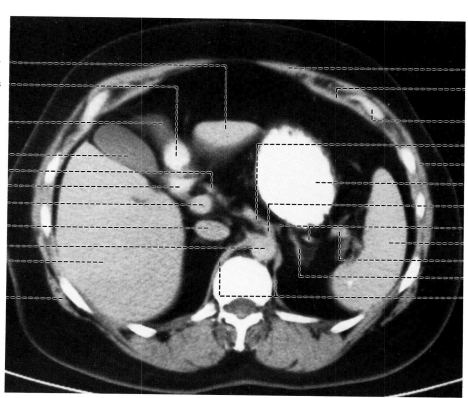

Left lobe lateral segment of liver
Stomach, pylorus
Left lobe medial segment of liver
Gallbladder
Hepatic a.
Duodenal bulb
Portal v.
Inferior vena cava
Aorta
Right lobe of liver
Latissimus dorsi m.

Rectus abdominis m.
Transversus abdominis m.
Costal cartilage
Common hepatic a.
External oblique m.
Stomach, body
Celiac a.
Splenic a.
Spleen
Splenic v.
Left adrenal gland
Crura of diaphragm

Figure 9.1.10

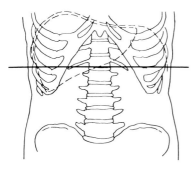

1. The tail of the pancreas reaches the hilus of the spleen and is located in the splenorenal ligament.

2. The duodenal bulb and the second and third portions of the duodenum surround the head and uncinate process of the pancreas; this is called the C-loop.

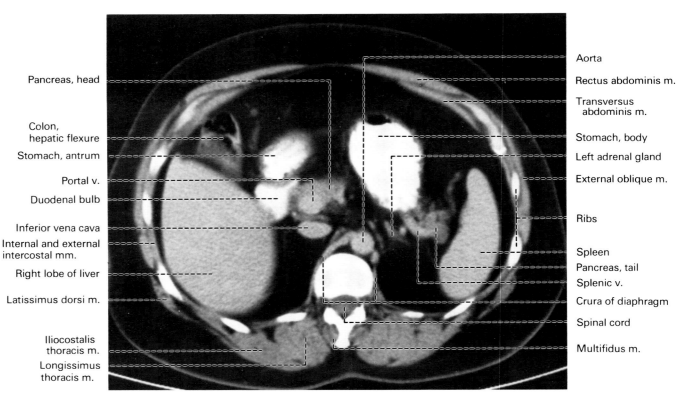

Labels, left side:
Pancreas, head
Colon, hepatic flexure
Stomach, antrum
Portal v.
Duodenal bulb
Inferior vena cava
Internal and external intercostal mm.
Right lobe of liver
Latissimus dorsi m.
Iliocostalis thoracis m.
Longissimus thoracis m.

Labels, right side:
Aorta
Rectus abdominis m.
Transversus abdominis m.
Stomach, body
Left adrenal gland
External oblique m.
Ribs
Spleen
Pancreas, tail
Splenic v.
Crura of diaphragm
Spinal cord
Multifidus m.

Figure 9.1.11

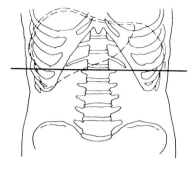

1. The body of the pancreas lies immediately posterior to the antrum of the stomach and the head lies just medial to the duodenum.

2. The superior mesenteric artery is seen as it originates from the aorta.

3. The potential space between the stomach and pancreas is called the lesser sac. Normally this potential space is not demonstrated by CT.

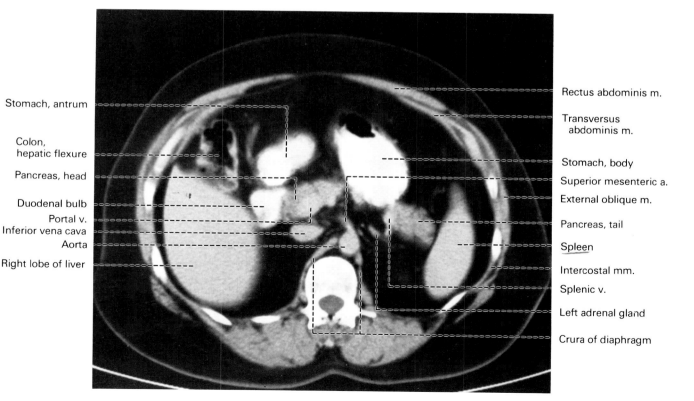

Stomach, antrum

Colon, hepatic flexure

Pancreas, head

Duodenal bulb

Portal v.
Inferior vena cava

Aorta

Right lobe of liver

Rectus abdominis m.

Transversus abdominis m.

Stomach, body

Superior mesenteric a.

External oblique m.

Pancreas, tail

Spleen

Intercostal mm.

Splenic v.

Left adrenal gland

Crura of diaphragm

Figure 9.1.12

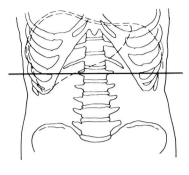

1. The right crus of the diaphragm is longer and larger than the left crus, and it extends approximately to the third or fourth lumbar vertebra. The left crus extends to the second or third lumbar vertebra.

2. The splenic vein courses posterior to the pancreas.

3. Usually the left kidney is somewhat higher than the right kidney. In this subject the superior poles of both kidneys are at the same level.

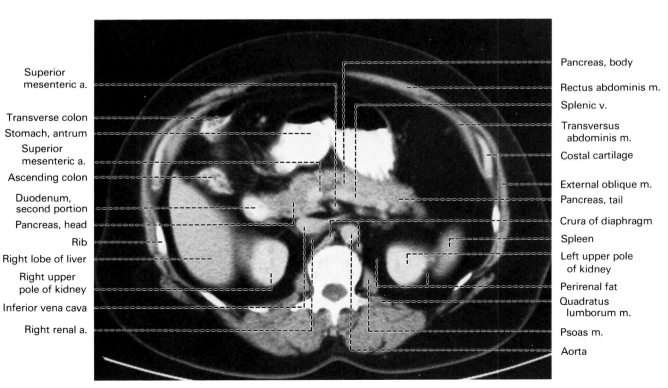

Superior mesenteric a.

Transverse colon
Stomach, antrum
Superior mesenteric a.

Ascending colon

Duodenum, second portion
Pancreas, head
Rib
Right lobe of liver

Right upper pole of kidney

Inferior vena cava

Right renal a.

Pancreas, body

Rectus abdominis m.
Splenic v.
Transversus abdominis m.
Costal cartilage

External oblique m.
Pancreas, tail

Crura of diaphragm
Spleen
Left upper pole of kidney

Perirenal fat
Quadratus lumborum m.

Psoas m.

Aorta

Figure 9.1.13

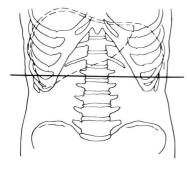

1. The renal arteries course posterior to the renal veins. The right renal artery crosses behind the inferior vena cava.

2. The renal veins are usually larger than the arteries. The left renal vein crosses the midline anterior to the aorta and drains into the inferior vena cava at the level of the uncinate process of the pancreas.

3. The pancreas lies anterior to the portal vein, splenic vein, and superior mesenteric artery and vein.

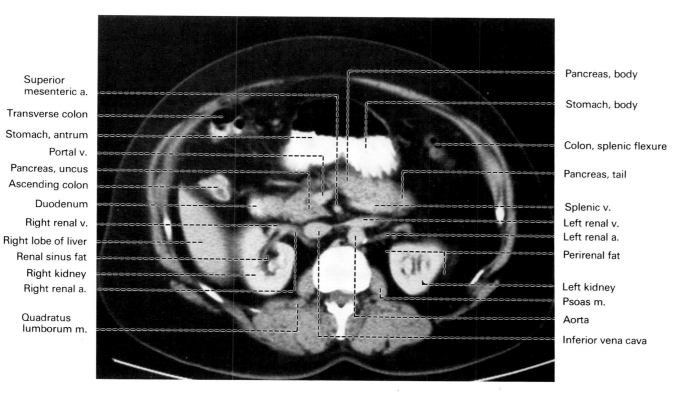

Superior mesenteric a.
Transverse colon
Stomach, antrum
Portal v.
Pancreas, uncus
Ascending colon
Duodenum
Right renal v.
Right lobe of liver
Renal sinus fat
Right kidney
Right renal a.
Quadratus lumborum m.

Pancreas, body
Stomach, body
Colon, splenic flexure
Pancreas, tail
Splenic v.
Left renal v.
Left renal a.
Perirenal fat
Left kidney
Psoas m.
Aorta
Inferior vena cava

Figure 9.1.14

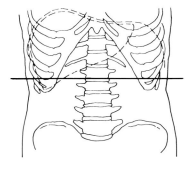

1. The wall thickness of the colon is 3 to 5 mm. The outer colonic margin is outlined by pericolic fat.

2. The inferior mesenteric vein drains into either the splenic or superior mesenteric vein.

3. The head and uncinate process of the pancreas lie posterolateral to the superior mesenteric vein.

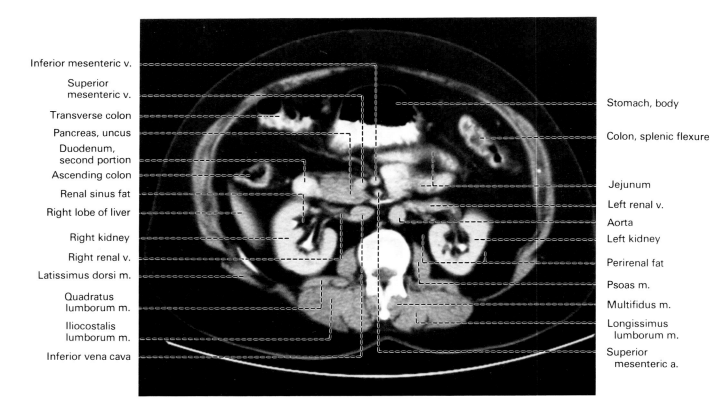

Figure 9.1.15

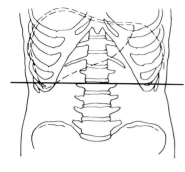

1. The transverse (third) portion of the duodenum runs between the superior mesenteric artery and aorta.

2. The superior mesenteric vein courses to the right of the superior mesenteric artery.

3. The hilum of the kidney faces anteromedially.

4. The left gonadal vein (testicular vein in males and ovarian vein in females) usually drains into the left renal vein.

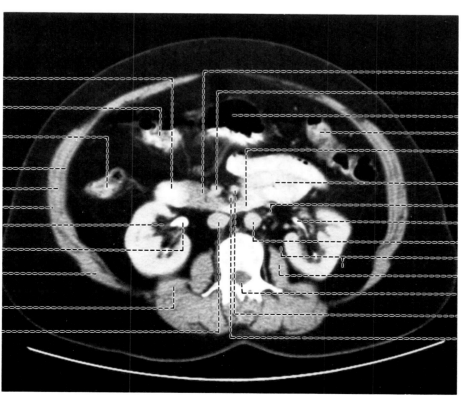

Duodenum, second portion
Transverse colon
Ascending colon
Transversus abdominus m.
Internal oblique m.
External oblique m.
Renal sinus fat
Right renal pelvis
Latissimus dorsi m.
Quadratus lumborum m.
Inferior vena cava

Pancreas, uncus
Superior mesenteric v.
Stomach
Colon, splenic flexure
Duodenum, fourth portion
Jejunum
Left gonadal v.
Left renal pelvis
Aorta
Perirenal fat
Psoas m.
Thecal sac
Inferior mesenteric v.
Superior mesenteric a.

Figure 9.1.16

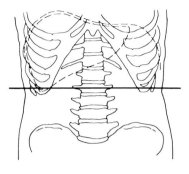

1. The right gonadal vein drains into the inferior vena cava.

2. All three muscles forming the anterolateral aspect of the abdominal wall are depicted in this section: external oblique, internal oblique, and transversus abdominis muscles.

3. The quadratus lumborum muscle originates from the iliac crest and transverse process of the lower three lumbar vertebrae and inserts on the transverse processes of the upper three lumbar vertebrae and proximal part of the twelfth rib.

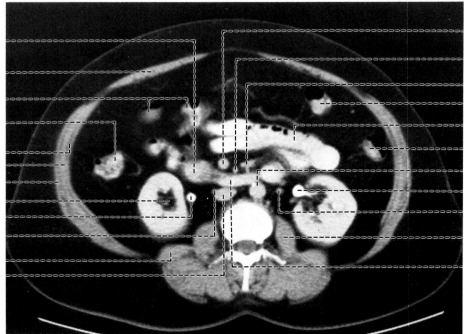

Duodenum, second portion
Rectus abdominis m.
Transverse colon
Ascending colon
Transversus abdominis m.
Internal oblique m.
External oblique m.
Renal sinus fat
Right renal pelvis
Right gonadal v.
Quadratus lumborum m.
Inferior vena cava

Superior mesenteric v.
Superior mesenteric a.
Inferior mesenteric v.
Transverse colon
Small intestine
Descending colon
Aorta
Left renal pelvis
Left gonadal v.
Psoas m.
Duodenum, third portion

Figure 9.1.17

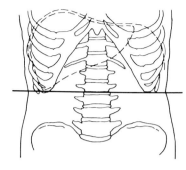

1. Perirenal fat completely invests the kidneys and proximal ureters.

2. The ureter begins at the renal pelvis. It is approximately 25 cm long and is divided into abdominal and pelvic portions.

3. The third portion of the duodenum crosses between the superior mesenteric artery and vein anteriorly and the inferior vena cava posteriorly.

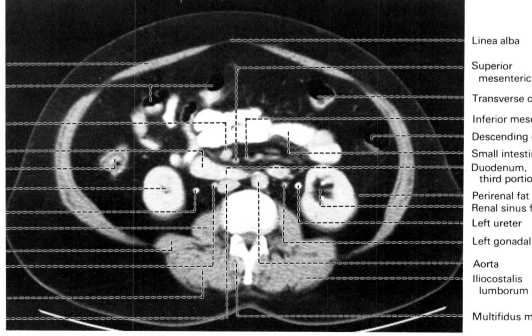

Figure 9.1.18

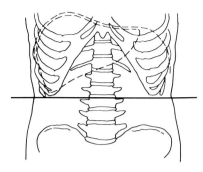

1. This section is through the lower poles of the kidneys.

2. The proximal part of the gonadal veins runs medial to the ureters.

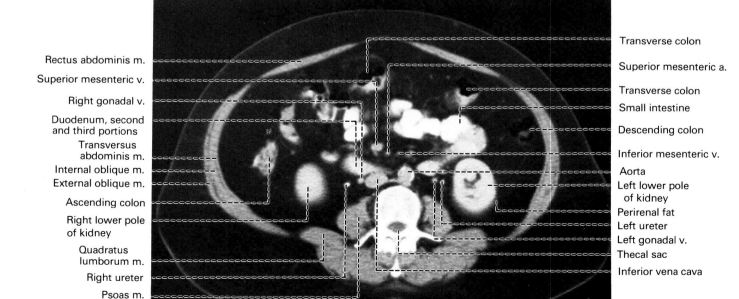

Rectus abdominis m.
Superior mesenteric v.
Right gonadal v.
Duodenum, second and third portions
Transversus abdominis m.
Internal oblique m.
External oblique m.
Ascending colon
Right lower pole of kidney
Quadratus lumborum m.
Right ureter
Psoas m.

Transverse colon
Superior mesenteric a.
Transverse colon
Small intestine
Descending colon
Inferior mesenteric v.
Aorta
Left lower pole of kidney
Perirenal fat
Left ureter
Left gonadal v.
Thecal sac
Inferior vena cava

Figure 9.1.19

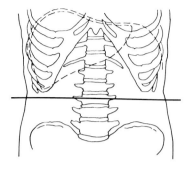

1. The transverse colon is intraperitoneal but the ascending and descending colon are retroperitoneal.

2. The lumbar plexus forms within the psoas muscle.

3. A persistent left inferior vena cava is seen in this subject.

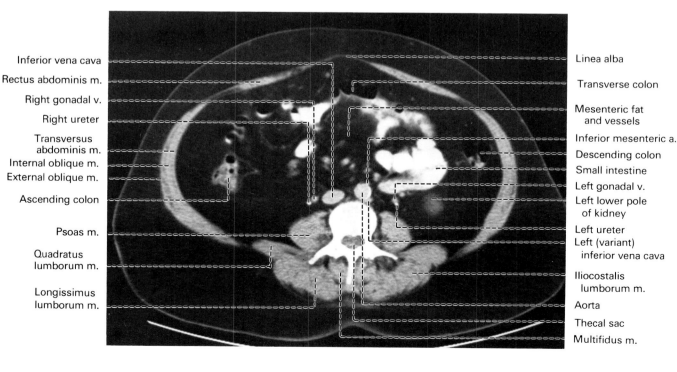

Inferior vena cava
Rectus abdominis m.
Right gonadal v.
Right ureter
Transversus abdominis m.
Internal oblique m.
External oblique m.
Ascending colon
Psoas m.
Quadratus lumborum m.
Longissimus lumborum m.

Linea alba
Transverse colon
Mesenteric fat and vessels
Inferior mesenteric a.
Descending colon
Small intestine
Left gonadal v.
Left lower pole of kidney
Left ureter
Left (variant) inferior vena cava
Iliocostalis lumborum m.
Aorta
Thecal sac
Multifidus m.

Figure 9.1.20

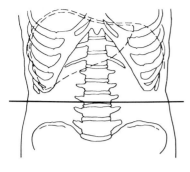

1. The inferior mesenteric artery is the last of the unpaired visceral arteries originating from the aorta. It usually arises at the level of the third lumbar vertebra or at the intervertebral disc between L3 and L4.

2. Note the gonadal veins as they cross anterior to the ureters.

3. In the lumbar spine, three muscles are grouped under the term erector spinae muscles: multifidus, longissimus lumborum, and iliocostalis lumborum.

Linea alba
Inferior vena cava
Small intestine
Right gonadal v.
Ascending colon
Transversus abdominis m.
Internal oblique m.
External oblique m.
Right ureter
Psoas m.
Quadratus lumborum m.
Iliocostalis lumborum m.
Multifidus m.

Rectus abdominis m.
Mesenteric fat and vessels
Small intestine
Descending colon
Inferior mesenteric a.
Left gonadal v.
Left ureter
Left (variant) inferior vena cava
Aorta
Longissimus lumborum m.
Thecal sac

Figure 9.1.21

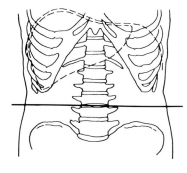

1. The gonadal veins have crossed over the ureters, and in more caudal sections they run lateral to the ureters.

2. This section is just cephalad to the umbilicus.

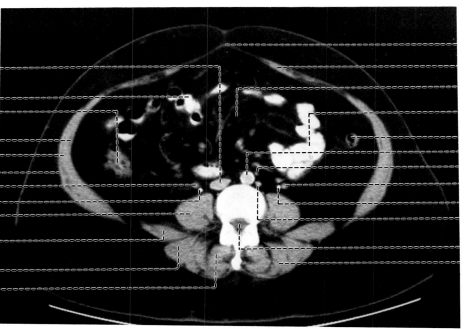

Inferior vena cava

Small intestine
Ascending colon
Transversus abdominis m.
Internal oblique m.
External oblique m.
Right gonadal v.
Right ureter
Psoas m.
Quadratus lumborum m.
Iliocostalis lumborum m.
Multifidus m.

Linea alba
Rectus abdominis m.
Mesenteric fat and vessels
Small intestine
Descending colon
Aorta
Inferior mesenteric a.
Left gonadal v.
Left ureter
Left (variant) inferior vena cava
Thecal sac
Longissimus lumborum m.

Figure 9.1.22

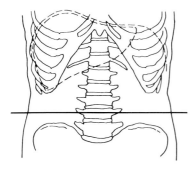

1. This section is at the level of the umbilicus.

2. The small intestine is outlined by oral contrast.

3. The inferior mesenteric artery is seen to the left of the aorta.

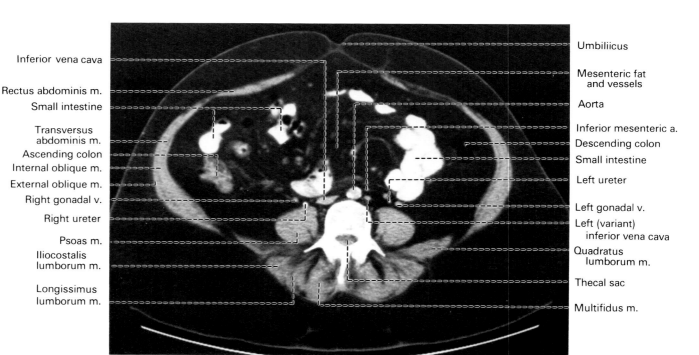

Inferior vena cava

Rectus abdominis m.

Small intestine

Transversus
abdominis m.

Ascending colon

Internal oblique m.

External oblique m.

Right gonadal v.

Right ureter

Psoas m.

Iliocostalis
lumborum m.

Longissimus
lumborum m.

Umbiliicus

Mesenteric fat
and vessels

Aorta

Inferior mesenteric a.

Descending colon

Small intestine

Left ureter

Left gonadal v.

Left (variant)
inferior vena cava

Quadratus
lumborum m.

Thecal sac

Multifidus m.

Figure 9.1.23

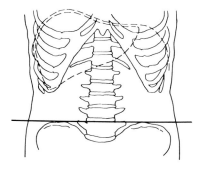

1. The umbilicus serves as an approximate reference point for the bifurcation of the aorta.

2. The aorta bifurcates into the common iliac arteries at about L3-L4 level.

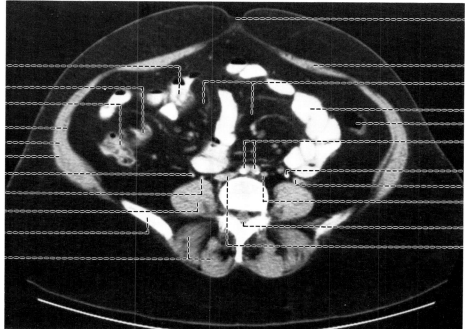

Small intestine

Terminal ileum

Ascending colon

Transversus abdominis m.

Internal oblique m.

External oblique m.

Right gonadal v.

Right ureter

Psoas m.

Iliac crest

Sacrospinalis mm.

Umbilicus

Rectus abdominis m.

Mesenteric fat and vessels

Small intestine

Descending colon

Right and left common iliac aa.

Left ureter

Left gonadal v.

Left (variant) inferior vena cava

Thecal sac

Inferior vena cava

Figure 9.1.24

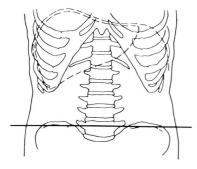

1. The terminal ileum empties into the cecum.

2. The ileocecal valve is usually seen as a fatty mass and should not be mistaken for cecal cancer or lipoma.

3. The gonadal veins are seen just anterior to the psoas muscles.

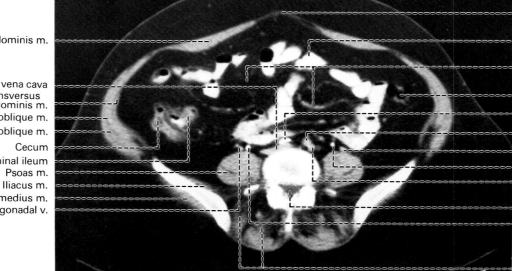

Rectus abdominis m.

Inferior vena cava
Transversus abdominis m.
Internal oblique m.
External oblique m.
Cecum
Terminal ileum
Psoas m.
Iliacus m.
Gluteus medius m.
Right gonadal v.

Linea alba

Small intestine

Mesenteric fat and vessels
Descending colon
Right common iliac a.
Left common iliac a.
Left gonadal v.
Left ureter
Left (variant) inferior vena cava
Thecal sac
Right ureter

Sacrospinalis mm.

Figure 9.1.25

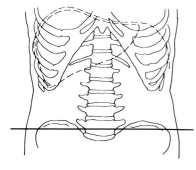

1. The appendix usually arises from the posteromedial surface of the cecum several centimeters below the ileocecal valve.

2. The common iliac veins join to form the inferior vena cava about 1 to 3 cm below the aortic bifurcation.

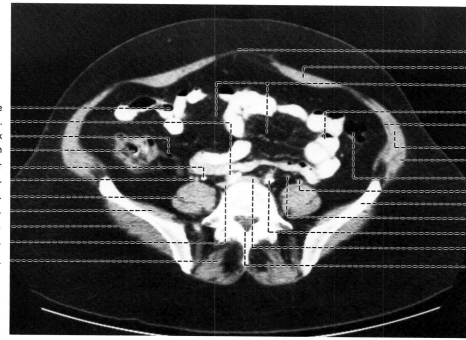

Small intestine
Right common iliac a.
Appendix
Cecum
Right ureter
Right gonadal v.
Psoas m.
Iliacus m.
Gluteus medius m.
Right common iliac v.
Sacrospinalis mm.

Linea alba
Rectus abdominis m.
Mesenteric fat
  and vessels
Small intestine
Transversus
  abdominis m.
Internal oblique m.
External oblique m.
Descending colon
Left gonadal v.
Ilium
Left ureter
Left common iliac a.
Left common iliac v.

Thecal sac

Figure 9.1.26

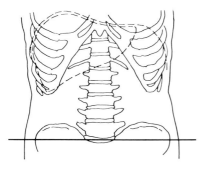

1. The psoas muscle approximates the iliacus muscle before they merge to form the iliopsoas muscle.

2. The common iliac veins run posterior to the common iliac arteries as they course more distally in the pelvis.

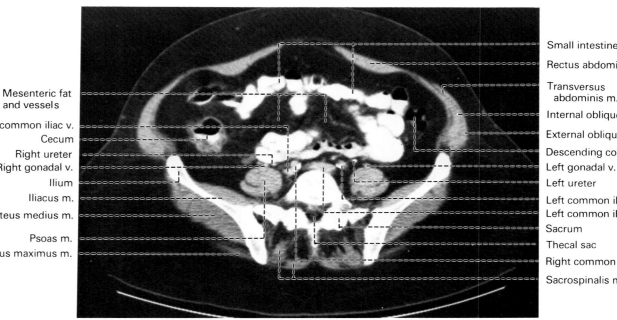

Mesenteric fat and vessels
Right common iliac v.
Cecum
Right ureter
Right gonadal v.
Ilium
Iliacus m.
Gluteus medius m.
Psoas m.
Gluteus maximus m.

Small intestine
Rectus abdominis m.
Transversus abdominis m.
Internal oblique m.
External oblique m.
Descending colon
Left gonadal v.
Left ureter
Left common iliac a.
Left common iliac v.
Sacrum
Thecal sac
Right common iliac a.
Sacrospinalis mm.

Figure 9.1.27

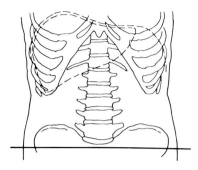

1. This section is through the upper part of the sacrum.

2. All three gluteal muscles are demonstrated in this section.

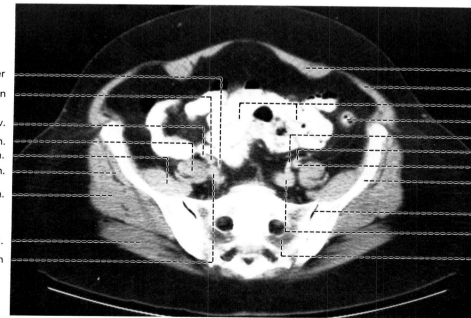

Right ureter

Right common
iliac a.

Right gonadal v.

Psoas m.

Iliacus m.

Gluteus minimus m.

Gluteus medius m.

Gluteus maximus m.

Right common
iliac v.

Rectus abdominis m.

Abdominal mm.

Ileum

Descending colon

Left ureter

Left gonadal v.

Left common iliac a.

Ilium

Sacroiliac joint

Left common iliac v.

Sacrum

IV
PELVIS AND HIP

Chapter 10

MALE PELVIS

Figure 10.1.1

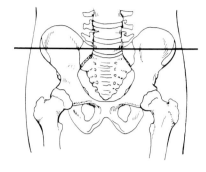

1. At this level, the rectus abdominis is a major component of the anterior abdominal wall muscles.

2. Note the linea alba forming a midline aponeurosis between the right and left rectus abdominis muscles.

3. The external oblique, internal oblique, and transversus abdominis muscles make up the anterolateral portion of the abdominal wall at this level.

4. The iliacus and psoas muscles are fusing.

5. At this level, sacral plexus elements course over the anterior surface of the sacrum.

6. Note the irregular configuration of the sacroiliac joint.

7. At this level, two large pelvic (anterior) foramina are imaged, and within them are ventral rami of the sacral nerves.

8. Note also that there are dorsal sacral foramina that transmit the dorsal rami of the sacral nerves.

9. Note that the thecal sac extends to the sacrum, usually to the level of S2.

10. The three gluteal muscles are distinguished.

11. Note the common iliac vessels medial to the iliopsoas.

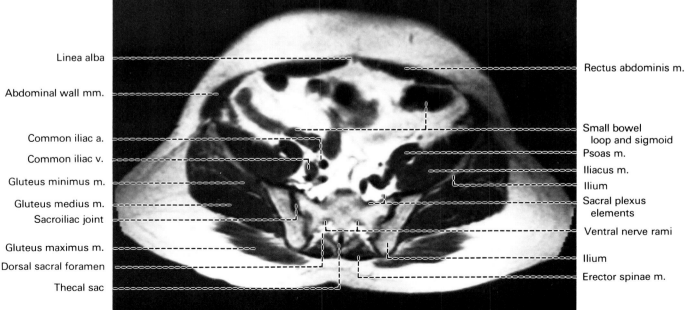

Figure 10.1.2

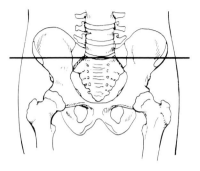

1. Note that the common iliac vessels have divided into the paired external and internal iliac vessels.

2. At its origin on the sacrum, the erector spinae muscle is small and tendinous.

3. The external oblique, internal oblique, and transversus abdominis muscles (lateral abdominal wall muscles) cannot be individually distinguished at this level.

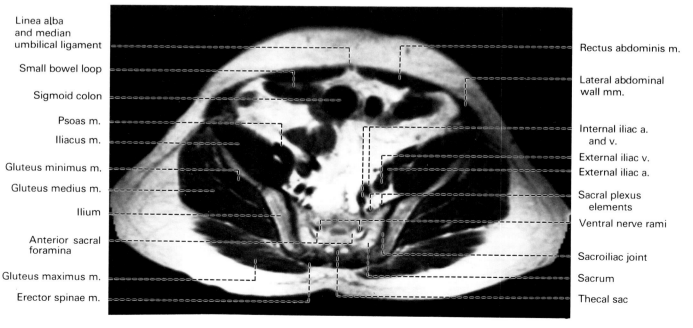

Linea alba and median umbilical ligament

Small bowel loop

Sigmoid colon

Psoas m.

Iliacus m.

Gluteus minimus m.

Gluteus medius m.

Ilium

Anterior sacral foramina

Gluteus maximus m.

Erector spinae m.

Rectus abdominis m.

Lateral abdominal wall mm.

Internal iliac a. and v.

External iliac v.
External iliac a.

Sacral plexus elements

Ventral nerve rami

Sacroiliac joint

Sacrum

Thecal sac

Figure 10.1.3

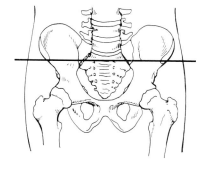

1. The rounded structure within the linea alba is the median umbilical ligament.

2. Observe that the internal iliac vessels remain in the posterior portion of the pelvis while the external iliac vessels begin to course more anteriorly.

3. In the more inferior portion of the ilium, the iliac wing becomes shorter in its anteroposterior dimension and broader in its lateral dimension.

4. The sigmoid colon courses posteriorly and inferiorly to become the rectum.

5. On the right, note the anterior superior iliac spine from which the sartorius originates.

6. The psoas and iliacus have become the iliopsoas.

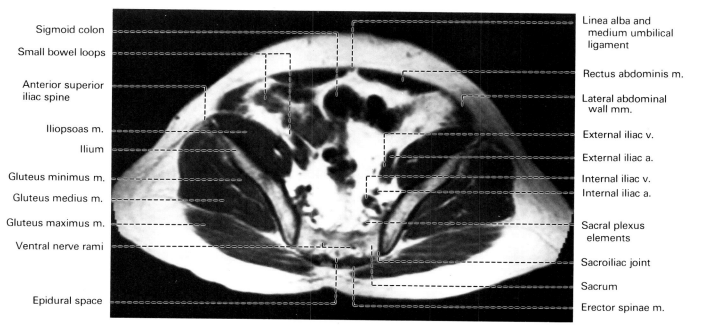

Figure 10.1.4

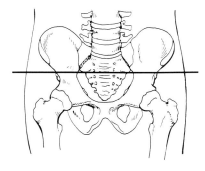

1. The sartorius originates from the anterior superior iliac spine.

2. On the left the tensor fasciae latae is noted anterior to the gluteus medius and minimus.

3. This image is at the level of the greater sciatic notch. Through this notch pass the sciatic nerve and the superior and inferior gluteal vessels and nerves.

4. The piriformis muscle, which also passes through the greater sciatic notch, originates from the anterior surface of the sacrum.

5. The sciatic nerve forms on the anterior surface of the piriformis.

6. The superior gluteal vessels have branched from their internal iliac origins and exit through the greater sciatic notch immediately under the ilium.

7. The femoral nerve is noted anterior to the iliopsoas and anterolateral to the external iliac vessels.

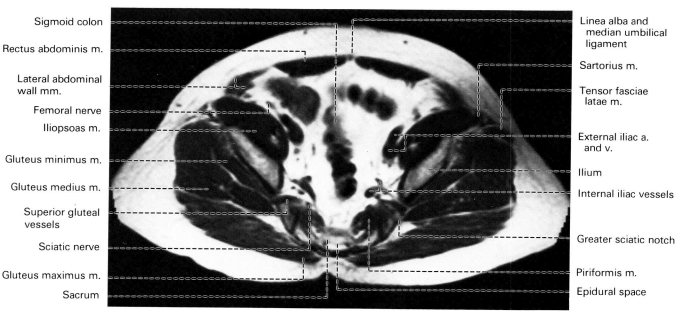

Figure 10.1.5

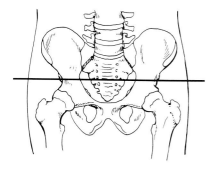

1. The sciatic nerve at this level lies immediately lateral to the internal iliac vessels, all of which course on the anterior surface of the piriformis.

2. At this section the dome of the bladder can be seen.

3. Note the arrangement of the external iliac vessels and the femoral nerve; from medial to lateral: vein, artery, nerve.

4. Observe the origin of the gluteus maximus from the dorsum of the sacrum. It courses laterally and inferiorly inserting into the iliotibial tract.

5. This portion of the ilium constitutes the weight-bearing portion of the acetabulum (acetabular roof).

6. Note the tendon of the psoas minor as it inserts on the iliopubic eminence. It is an inconsistent structure, present in only 60 percent of individuals.

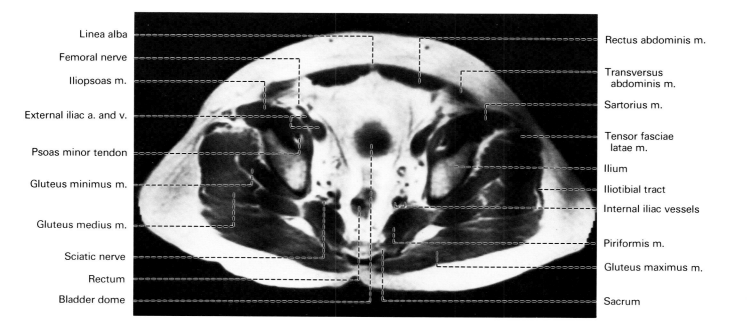

Figure 10.1.6

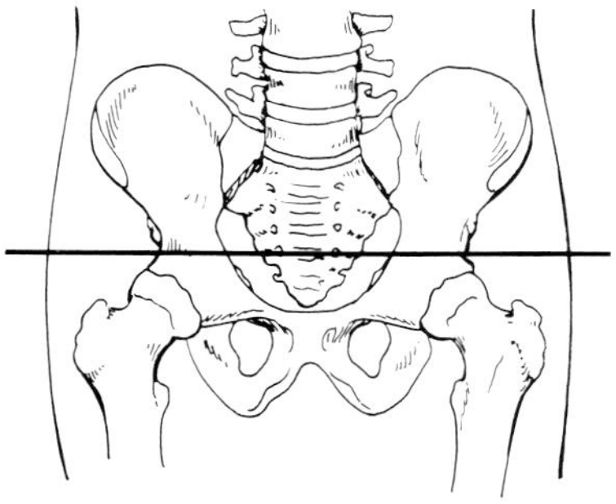

1. Note that the urinary bladder is surrounded by the perivesical fat.
2. The obturator nerve lies on the medial surface of the obturator internus.
3. The inferior gluteal vessels branch from the internal iliac vessels adjacent to the piriformis. These vessels will exit beneath the piriformis.
4. Note the tendinous portion of the piriformis that courses laterally and inferiorly to insert on the upper border of the greater trochanter.
5. Observe the presacral space filled with fat posterior to the rectum.

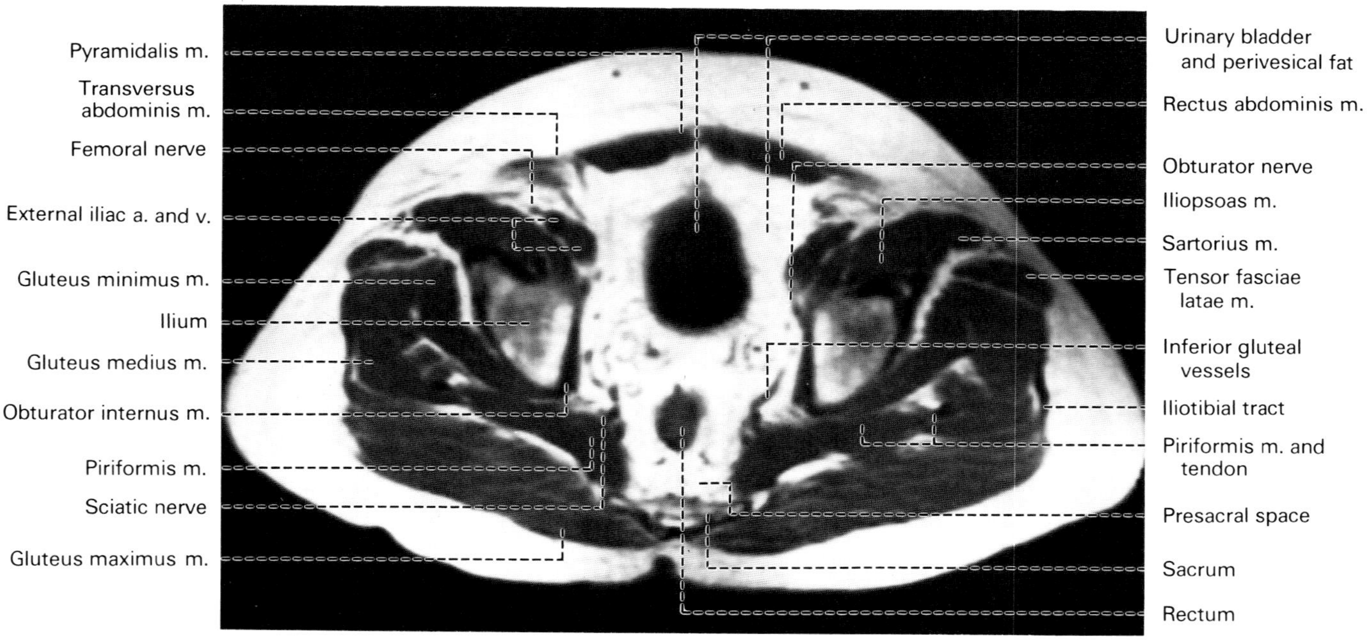
Pyramidalis m.
Transversus abdominis m.
Femoral nerve
External iliac a. and v.
Gluteus minimus m.
Ilium
Gluteus medius m.
Obturator internus m.
Piriformis m.
Sciatic nerve
Gluteus maximus m.
Urinary bladder and perivesical fat
Rectus abdominis m.
Obturator nerve
Iliopsoas m.
Sartorius m.
Tensor fasciae latae m.
Inferior gluteal vessels
Iliotibial tract
Piriformis m. and tendon
Presacral space
Sacrum
Rectum

Figure 10.1.7

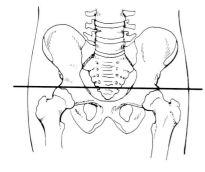

1. This image is at the level of the acetabulum. The superior portion of the femoral head is imaged.

2. The proximal portion of the rectus femoris originates from the anterior-inferior iliac spine (straight head) and the groove above the acetabulum (reflected head).

3. The gemelli and obturator internus converge to insert on the medial surface of the greater trochanter.

4. Observe the paired seminal vesicles posterior to the bladder.

5. The pyramidalis is clearly distinguished from the rectus abdominis.

6. At this level the external iliac vessels have crossed the inguinal ligament and are renamed femoral vessels.

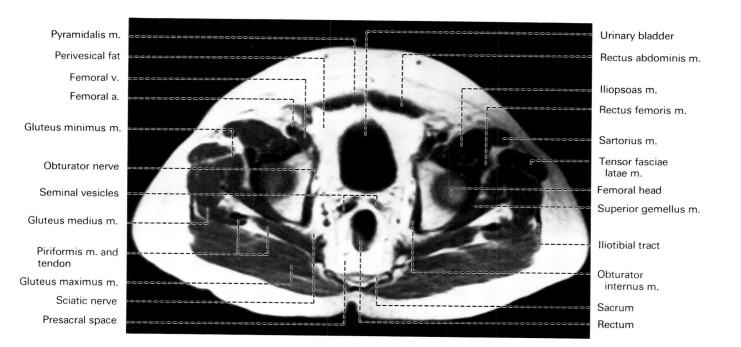

Figure 10.1.8

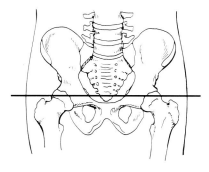

1. The seminal vesicles posterior to the bladder converge medially. Just lateral to them the ductus deferens can be seen.

2. Note the sacrospinous ligament. It courses from the sacrum toward the ischial spine.

3. Note that the sciatic nerve is posterior to the ischial spine.

4. The acetabulum is now separated into its anterior and posterior columns, the latter ending in the ischial spine.

5. The central depression in the acetabulum is a nonarticular surface to which the ligamentum teres is attached.

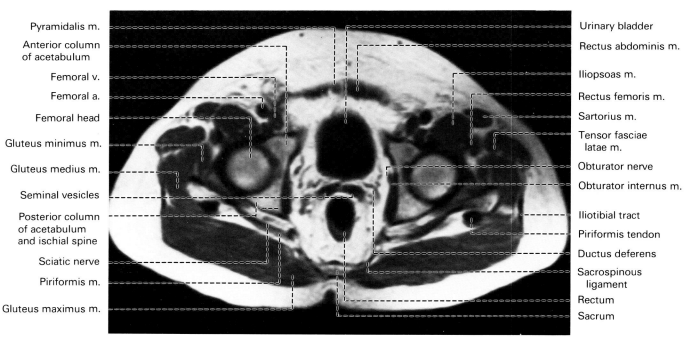

Pyramidalis m.
Anterior column of acetabulum
Femoral v.
Femoral a.
Femoral head
Gluteus minimus m.
Gluteus medius m.
Seminal vesicles
Posterior column of acetabulum and ischial spine
Sciatic nerve
Piriformis m.
Gluteus maximus m.

Urinary bladder
Rectus abdominis m.
Iliopsoas m.
Rectus femoris m.
Sartorius m.
Tensor fasciae latae m.
Obturator nerve
Obturator internus m.
Iliotibial tract
Piriformis tendon
Ductus deferens
Sacrospinous ligament
Rectum
Sacrum

Figure 10.1.9

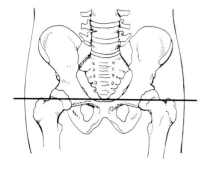

1. Note that the superior pubic ramus contributes to the anterior column of the acetabulum.

2. The pectineus arises from the crest (pectin) of the pubis.

3. This section passes through the ischial spine.

4. Note the gluteus medius insertion on the greater trochanter.

5. Note the obturator vessels and nerve as they course inferiorly toward the obturator foramen.

6. The inferior gluteal vessels are depicted on the anterior surface of gluteus maximus, the muscle they supply.

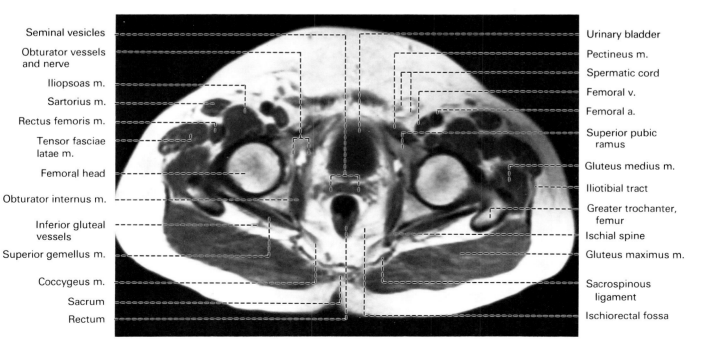

Seminal vesicles
Obturator vessels and nerve
Iliopsoas m.
Sartorius m.
Rectus femoris m.
Tensor fasciae latae m.
Femoral head
Obturator internus m.
Inferior gluteal vessels
Superior gemellus m.
Coccygeus m.
Sacrum
Rectum

Urinary bladder
Pectineus m.
Spermatic cord
Femoral v.
Femoral a.
Superior pubic ramus
Gluteus medius m.
Iliotibial tract
Greater trochanter, femur
Ischial spine
Gluteus maximus m.
Sacrospinous ligament
Ischiorectal fossa

Figure 10.1.10

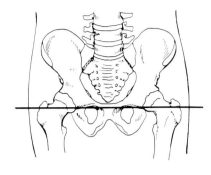

1. The perivesical space adjacent to the bladder floor should be noted.

2. The prostate gland at the base of the bladder is seen at this level. Its proximity to the rectum should be noted.

3. At this level, the obturator internus has a large muscle belly that courses around the ischium and then toward its insertion with the gemelli in the trochanteric fossa.

4. The sciatic nerve descends posterior to the obturator internus and is covered by the gluteus maximus at the level of the greater trochanter.

5. A portion of the sacrotuberous ligament is identified in this image.

6. The spermatic cord courses superficially and is medial to the femoral vessels at this level.

7. The levator ani and the coccygeal muscles form the floor of the pelvis.

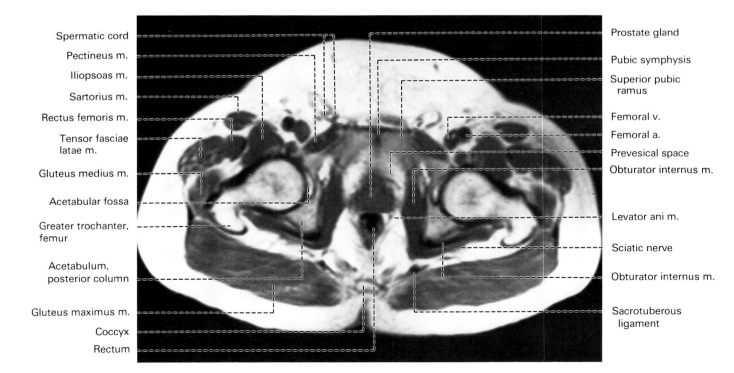

Spermatic cord
Pectineus m.
Iliopsoas m.
Sartorius m.
Rectus femoris m.
Tensor fasciae latae m.
Gluteus medius m.
Acetabular fossa
Greater trochanter, femur
Acetabulum, posterior column
Gluteus maximus m.
Coccyx
Rectum

Prostate gland
Pubic symphysis
Superior pubic ramus
Femoral v.
Femoral a.
Prevesical space
Obturator internus m.
Levator ani m.
Sciatic nerve
Obturator internus m.
Sacrotuberous ligament

Figure 10.1.11

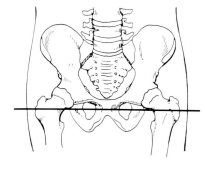

1. The obturator externus and internus are noted on either side of the obturator foramen.

2. The vascular structures anterior to the prostate represent the prostatic venous plexus.

3. Note that the femoral neck courses posterolaterally creating what is known as the anteversion angle.

4. The levator ani is seen on both sides of the rectum.

5. The inferior gemellus arises from the ischium.

6. The tensor fasciae latae is distinguished by its marbled appearance due to the abundance of interfascicular fat.

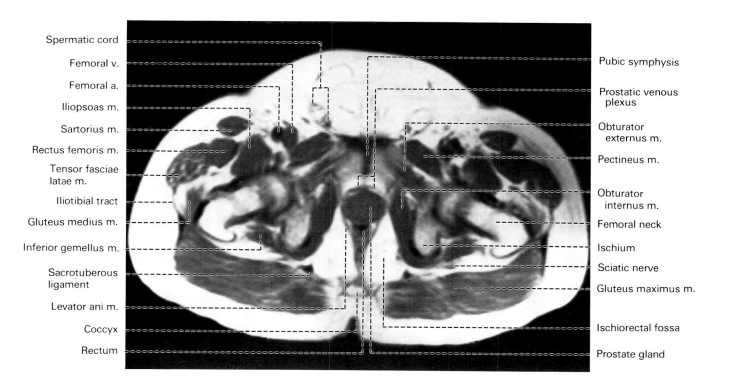

Spermatic cord
Femoral v.
Femoral a.
Iliopsoas m.
Sartorius m.
Rectus femoris m.
Tensor fasciae latae m.
Iliotibial tract
Gluteus medius m.
Inferior gemellus m.
Sacrotuberous ligament
Levator ani m.
Coccyx
Rectum

Pubic symphysis
Prostatic venous plexus
Obturator externus m.
Pectineus m.
Obturator internus m.
Femoral neck
Ischium
Sciatic nerve
Gluteus maximus m.
Ischiorectal fossa
Prostate gland

Figure 10.1.12

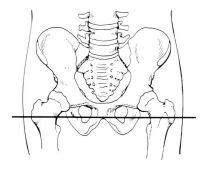

1. The adductor brevis arises from the inferior pubic ramus and body of the pubis adjacent to the symphysis.

2. The intertrochanteric ridge, a bony prominence connecting the greater and lesser trochanters, is identified in this image.

3. Note the well-defined, fat-filled ischiorectal fossa.

4. Note that the iliotibial tract is a distinct entity composed of fascial contributions from gluteus maximus and tensor fasciae latae.

5. Note the origin of the vastus lateralis from the anterolateral aspect of the proximal femur.

6. The great saphenous vein drains into the femoral vein.

7. The spermatic cord is seen in the anterior subcutaneous tissues.

8. The medial femoral circumflex vessels course toward the femoral neck. They are an important vascular supply of the femoral head.

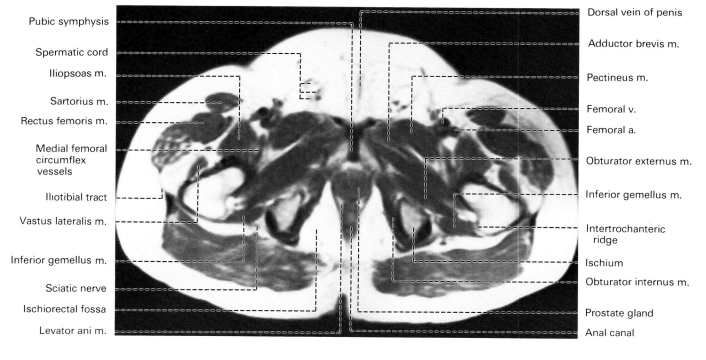

Pubic symphysis
Spermatic cord
Iliopsoas m.
Sartorius m.
Rectus femoris m.
Medial femoral circumflex vessels
Iliotibial tract
Vastus lateralis m.
Inferior gemellus m.
Sciatic nerve
Ischiorectal fossa
Levator ani m.

Dorsal vein of penis
Adductor brevis m.
Pectineus m.
Femoral v.
Femoral a.
Obturator externus m.
Inferior gemellus m.
Intertrochanteric ridge
Ischium
Obturator internus m.
Prostate gland
Anal canal

Figure 10.1.13

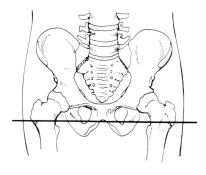

1. Note the paired corpora cavernosa.

2. The adductor longus arises from the body of the pubis adjacent to the symphysis.

3. Note that the iliopsoas inserts onto the lesser trochanter.

4. Observe the origin of the hamstring muscles from the ischium.

5. Note the entire course of quadratus femoris; it originates from the lateral aspect of the ischial tuberosity and inserts into the inferior aspect of the intertrochanteric ridge.

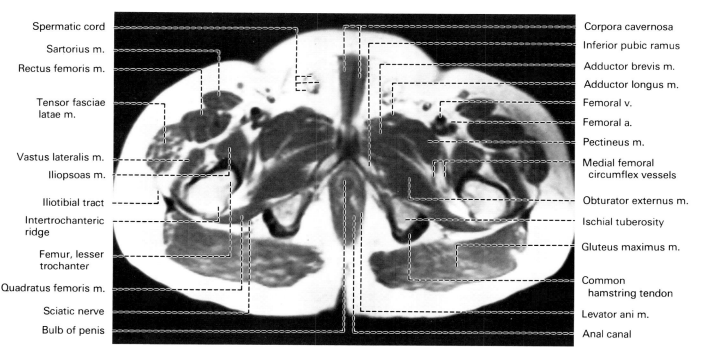

Spermatic cord
Sartorius m.
Rectus femoris m.
Tensor fasciae latae m.
Vastus lateralis m.
Iliopsoas m.
Iliotibial tract
Intertrochanteric ridge
Femur, lesser trochanter
Quadratus femoris m.
Sciatic nerve
Bulb of penis

Corpora cavernosa
Inferior pubic ramus
Adductor brevis m.
Adductor longus m.
Femoral v.
Femoral a.
Pectineus m.
Medial femoral circumflex vessels
Obturator externus m.
Ischial tuberosity
Gluteus maximus m.
Common hamstring tendon
Levator ani m.
Anal canal

Figure 10.1.14

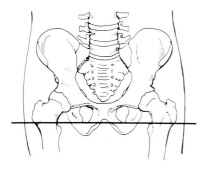

1. The adductor group is composed of the adductor longus, brevis, and magnus muscles. This order as seen from anterior to posterior is preserved as the adductors course inferiorly until the adductor brevis inserts into the linea aspera.

2. Note that the common tendon of origin of the hamstring muscles has divided into the more anterior tendon of the semimembranosus and the more posterior conjoint tendon of biceps femoris and semitendinosus.

3. The sciatic nerve courses on the posterior surface of quadratus femoris and is still covered primarily by the gluteus maximus.

4. The vastus intermedius originates from the anterolateral portion of the proximal femur deep to vastus lateralis.

5. Note the origin of vastus lateralis from the lateral lip of the linea aspera at this level.

6. The lateral femoral circumflex vessels course toward the femoral neck between the iliopsoas and rectus femoris muscles. The lateral femoral circumflex artery arises from the deep femoral artery.

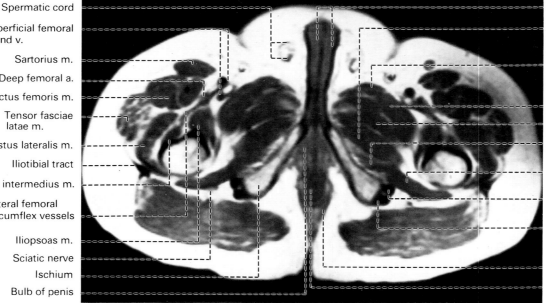

Spermatic cord
Superficial femoral a. and v.
Sartorius m.
Deep femoral a.
Rectus femoris m.
Tensor fasciae latae m.
Vastus lateralis m.
Iliotibial tract
Vastus intermedius m.
Lateral femoral circumflex vessels
Iliopsoas m.
Sciatic nerve
Ischium
Bulb of penis

Corpora cavernosa
Adductor magnus m.
Adductor longus m.
Pectineus m.
Adductor brevis m.
Obturator externus m.
Quadratus femoris m.
Semimembranosus tendon
Biceps femoris and semitendinosus tendons
Levator ani m.
Anal canal

Figure 10.1.15

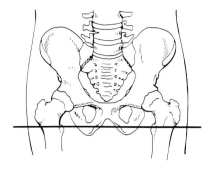

1. Note the position of the urethra.

2. A portion of gluteus maximus inserts into the iliotibial tract.

3. Note the insertion of iliopsoas.

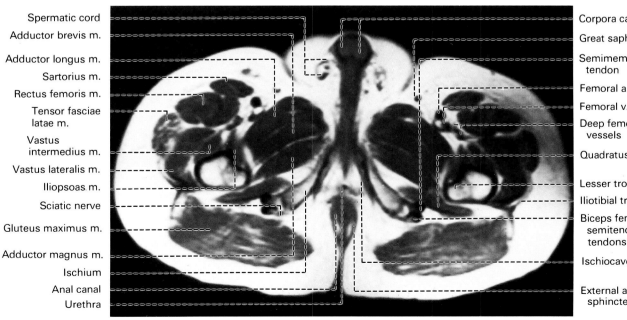

Spermatic cord
Adductor brevis m.
Adductor longus m.
Sartorius m.
Rectus femoris m.
Tensor fasciae latae m.
Vastus intermedius m.
Vastus lateralis m.
Iliopsoas m.
Sciatic nerve
Gluteus maximus m.
Adductor magnus m.
Ischium
Anal canal
Urethra

Corpora cavernosa
Great saphenous v.
Semimembranosus tendon
Femoral a.
Femoral v.
Deep femoral vessels
Quadratus femoris m.
Lesser trochanter
Iliotibial tract
Biceps femoris and semitendinosus tendons
Ischiocavernosus m.
External anal sphincter m.

Figure 10.1.16

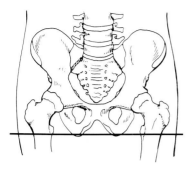

1. Note the spermatic cord ascending from the scrotum.

2. Semitendinosus is becoming muscular at this level. The other two hamstrings remain tendinous.

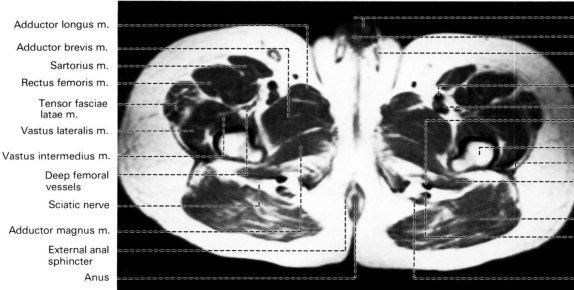

Adductor longus m.

Adductor brevis m.

Sartorius m.

Rectus femoris m.

Tensor fasciae latae m.

Vastus lateralis m.

Vastus intermedius m.

Deep femoral vessels

Sciatic nerve

Adductor magnus m.

External anal sphincter

Anus

Corpora cavernosa

Corpus spongiosum

Spermatic cord

Femoral a.

Femoral v.

Semimembranosus tendon

Femur

Iliotibial tract

Quadratus femoris m.

Gluteus maximus m.

Biceps femoris (long head) tendon

Semitendinosus m.

Figure 10.1.17

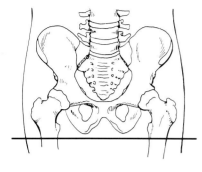

1. Note that the penile urethra courses through corpus spongiosum.

2. The head of the epididymis on the right is identified.

3. At this level the sciatic nerve courses on the posterior surface of adductor magnus.

4. The most medial muscle of the thigh is gracilis.

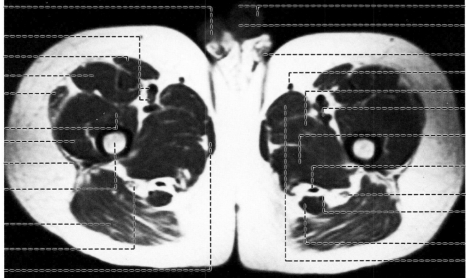

Epididymis, head — Corpora cavernosa

Femoral a. and v. — Corpus spongiosum and urethra

Sartorius m. — Spermatic cord

Rectus femoris m. — Great saphenous v.

Tensor fasciae latae m. — Adductor brevis m.

Vastus intermedius m. — Deep femoral vessels

Vastus lateralis m. — Adductor magnus m.

Iliotibial tract — Semimembranosus tendon

Femur — Sciatic nerve

Gluteus maximus m. — Biceps femoris (long head) tendon

Sciatic nerve — Semitendinosus m.

Gracilis m. — Adductor longus m.

Figure 10.2.1

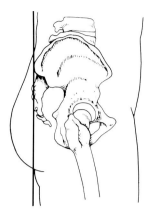

1. The gluteus maximus fibers originate from the ilium and the sacrum.

2. The posterior sacral foramina can be identified.

3. The longissimus portion of erector spinae is noted.

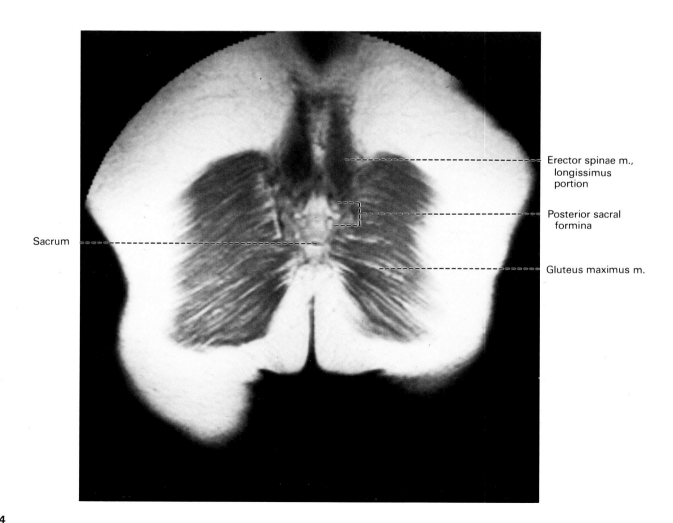

Erector spinae m., longissimus portion

Posterior sacral formina

Gluteus maximus m.

Sacrum

Figure 10.2.2

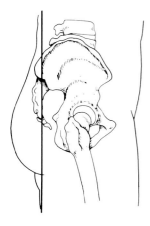

1. The sacroiliac joint can be visualized at this posterior level. Note that the ilium is superior and lateral to the sacrum.

2. The origin of piriformis is identifiable as it courses laterally and inferiorly.

3. Gluteus maximus originates from the ilium, sacrum, sacrotuberous ligament, and coccyx.

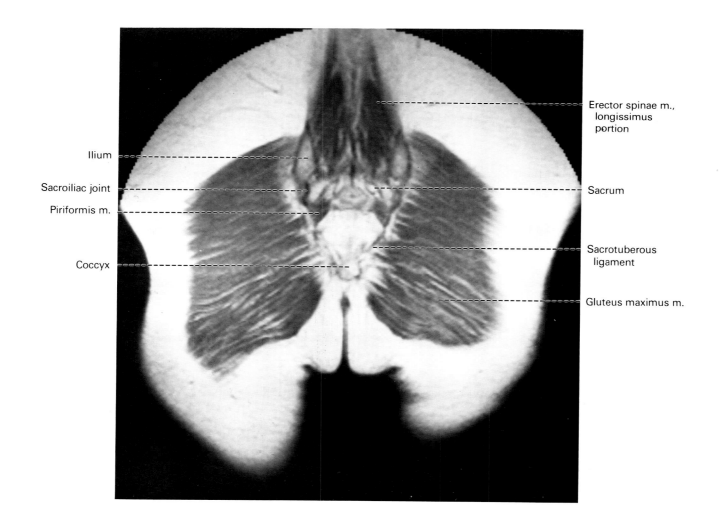

Figure 10.2.3

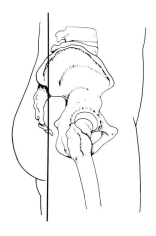

1. Gluteus medius should be appreciated in its position slightly superior to gluteus maximus.

2. Semitendinosus and the long head of biceps femoris are seen.

3. Levator ani is shown.

4. The third member of the hamstring group, semimembranosus, will be seen medial to semitendinosus in more anterior sections.

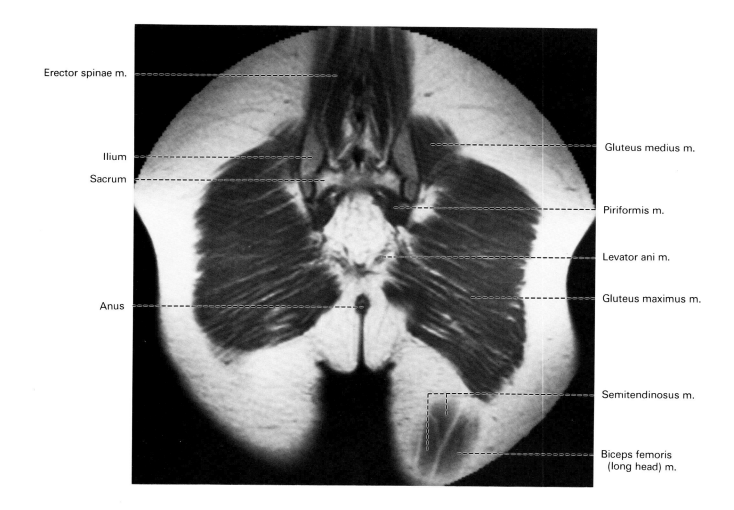

Figure 10.2.4

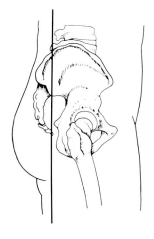

1. The increased complexity of the erector spinae muscle should be appreciated.

2. The posterior portion of the iliotibial tract is seen laterally over the lower half of gluteus maximus.

3. All three muscles of the hamstring group (semitendinosus, semimembranosus, and long head of biceps femoris) are identified on the left.

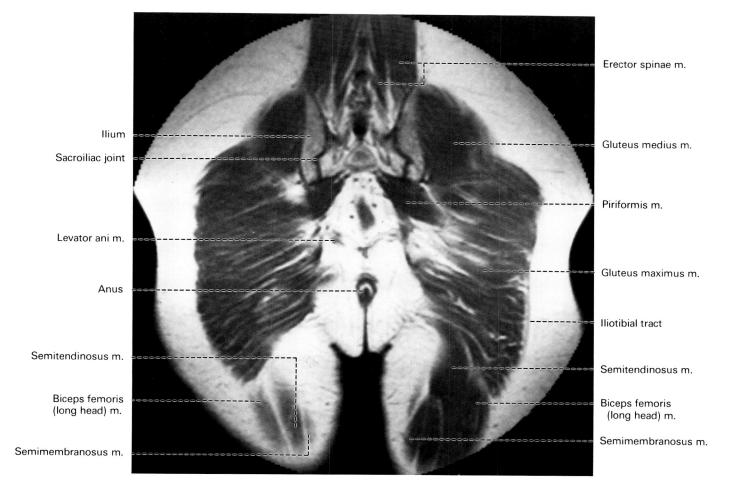

Ilium
Sacroiliac joint
Levator ani m.
Anus
Semitendinosus m.
Biceps femoris (long head) m.
Semimembranosus m.

Erector spinae m.
Gluteus medius m.
Piriformis m.
Gluteus maximus m.
Iliotibial tract
Semitendinosus m.
Biceps femoris (long head) m.
Semimembranosus m.

Figure 10.2.5

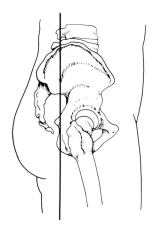

1. The caudal portion of the thecal sac is visualized.

2. The ischiorectal fossa is clearly demonstrated. Note the pudendal artery on the right entering the fossa posterior to the sacrotuberous ligament. The pudendal artery in this subject arises as a branch of the inferior gluteal. It may arise from a common trunk with the inferior gluteal or as a separate branch from the internal iliac.

3. Note that piriformis is exiting through the greater sciatic foramen. The inferior gluteal artery is situated below piriformis. The superior gluteal artery is above piriformis.

4. In this section levator ani courses from the ischial spine and can be seen inserting above the anus.

5. The common tendon of semitendinosus and long head of biceps femoris is identifiable.

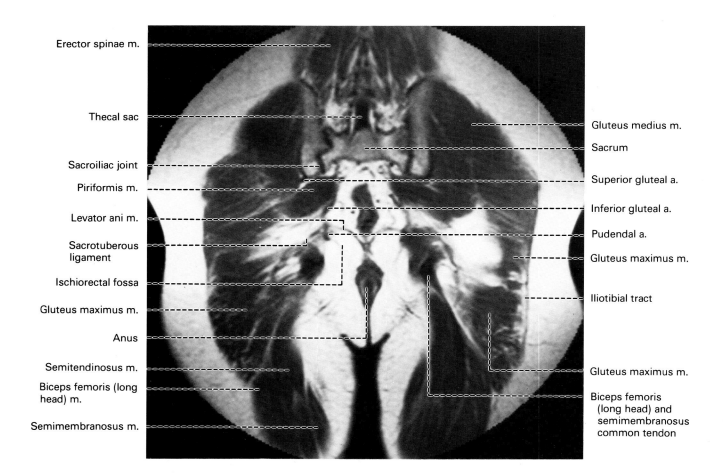

Figure 10.2.6

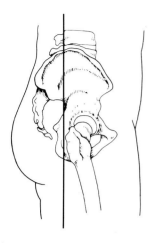

1. Two sacral nerve roots are seen exiting from their anterior sacral foramina.

2. The hamstring muscles arise from the ischial tuberosity.

3. The laterally positioned tendinous origin of the long head of biceps femoris can be seen on the right. Inferior to their common tendinous origin semitendinosus becomes muscular but the long head of biceps femoris remains tendinous for several more centimeters.

4. The superior and inferior gluteal arteries are seen in their respective superior and inferior relations to piriformis.

5. Obturator internus abuts the medial aspect of the ischium.

6. The medially located adductor magnus is noted. This portion is functionally included with the hamstring muscles.

7. The fleshy quadratus femoris courses from the ischium to the posterior aspect of the proximal femur.

8. The sciatic nerve on the right is seen just below piriformis, exiting through the greater sciatic foramen. On the left it is imaged inferior to quadratus femoris.

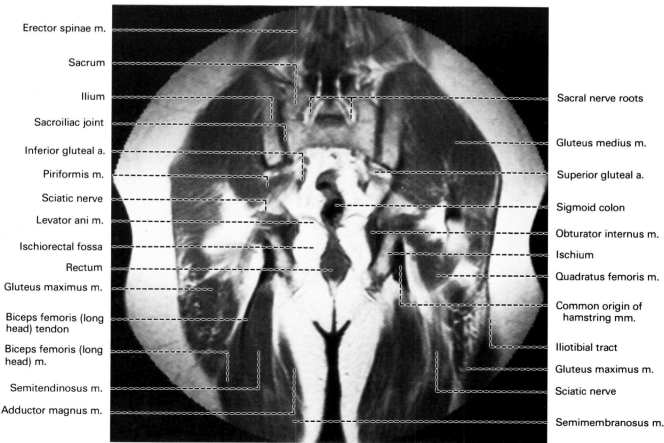

Figure 10.2.7

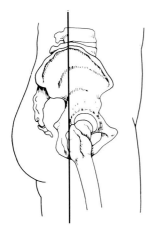

1. The piriformis tendon is seen on the left coursing to its insertion on the greater trochanter.

2. On the left, just below the piriformis tendon, obturator internus is situated between the superior and inferior gemelli.

3. Below the gemelli muscles a flat muscle, quadratus femoris, is seen extending from the ischial tuberosity to the inferior aspect of the intertrochanteric ridge.

4. Sacral plexus elements can be seen in their position just anterior to the sacrum.

5. The thecal sac and several nerve roots in the lumbar region are demonstrated.

6. Note the posterior portion of adductor magnus, originating from the ischial tuberosity. This portion functions as a hamstring muscle and is innervated by the sciatic. The more medial and anterior fibers of adductor magnus (seen on more anterior images) function as a powerful adductor and are innervated by the obturator nerve.

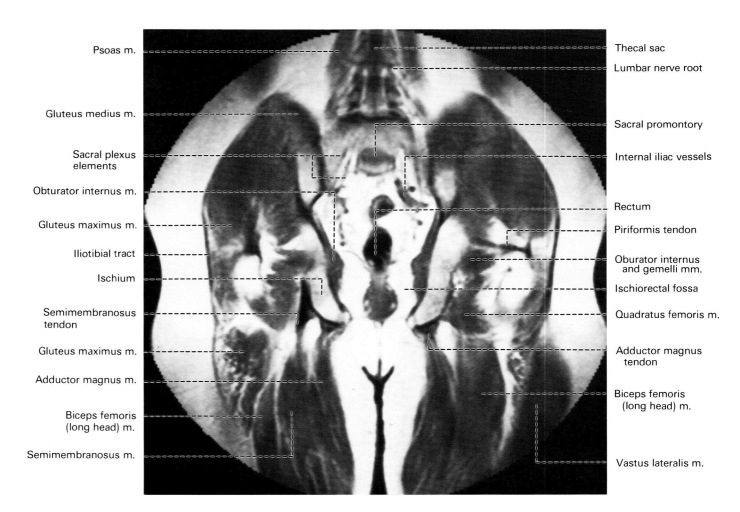

Psoas m.

Gluteus medius m.

Sacral plexus elements

Obturator internus m.

Gluteus maximus m.

Iliotibial tract

Ischium

Semimembranosus tendon

Gluteus maximus m.

Adductor magnus m.

Biceps femoris (long head) m.

Semimembranosus m.

Thecal sac

Lumbar nerve root

Sacral promontory

Internal iliac vessels

Rectum

Piriformis tendon

Oburator internus and gemelli mm.

Ischiorectal fossa

Quadratus femoris m.

Adductor magnus tendon

Biceps femoris (long head) m.

Vastus lateralis m.

Figure 10.2.8

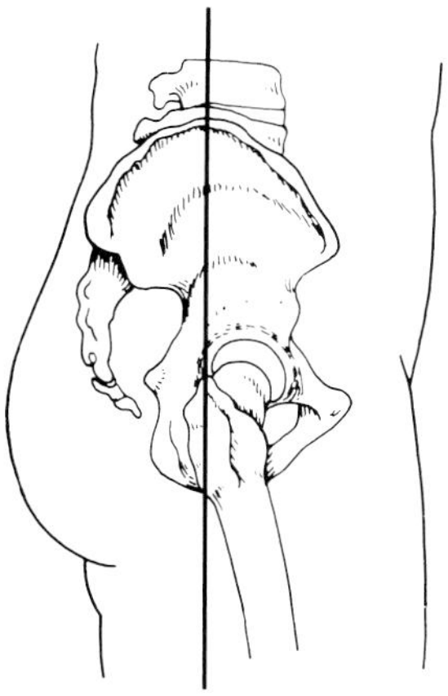

1. This coronal image is at the level of the ischial tuberosities.
2. At this level obturator externus on the right can be seen coursing toward the trochanteric fossa.
3. The gluteus medius and minimus muscles can be easily distinguished with the latter lying deep to the former.
4. The vastus lateralis is seen on the right but is better visualized on the left.
5. The vas deferens can be seen coming into the posterior portion of the prostate joining the seminal vesicles.

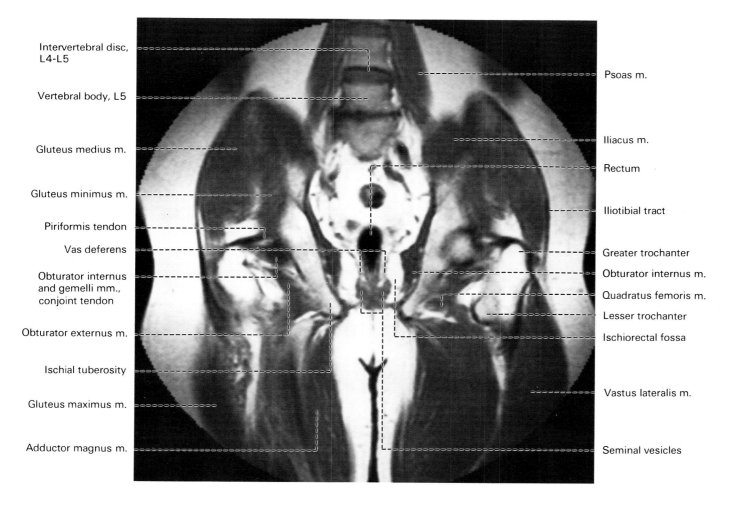

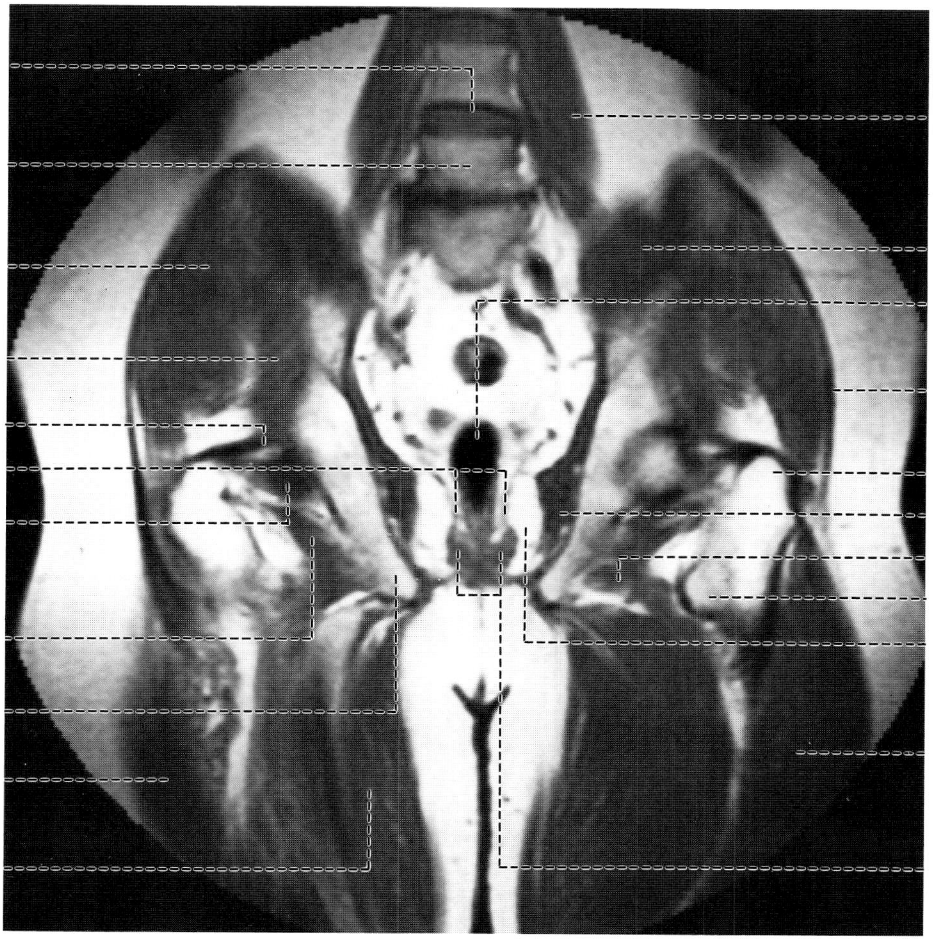
Intervertebral disc, L4-L5
Vertebral body, L5
Gluteus medius m.
Gluteus minimus m.
Piriformis tendon
Vas deferens
Obturator internus and gemelli mm., conjoint tendon
Obturator externus m.
Ischial tuberosity
Gluteus maximus m.
Adductor magnus m.
Psoas m.
Iliacus m.
Rectum
Iliotibial tract
Greater trochanter
Obturator internus m.
Quadratus femoris m.
Lesser trochanter
Ischiorectal fossa
Vastus lateralis m.
Seminal vesicles

Figure 10.2.9

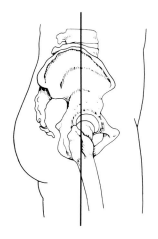

1. The iliacus muscle defines the medial wall of the ilium while gluteus medius and minimus define the lateral wall of the ilium on the left.

2. The prostate gland and a small portion of the seminal vesicles are visualized.

3. The iliotibial tract is seen distinctly because it is surrounded by fat.

4. The obturator externus is seen coursing to the trochanteric fossa.

5. The obturator internus and externus muscles define the obturator foramen.

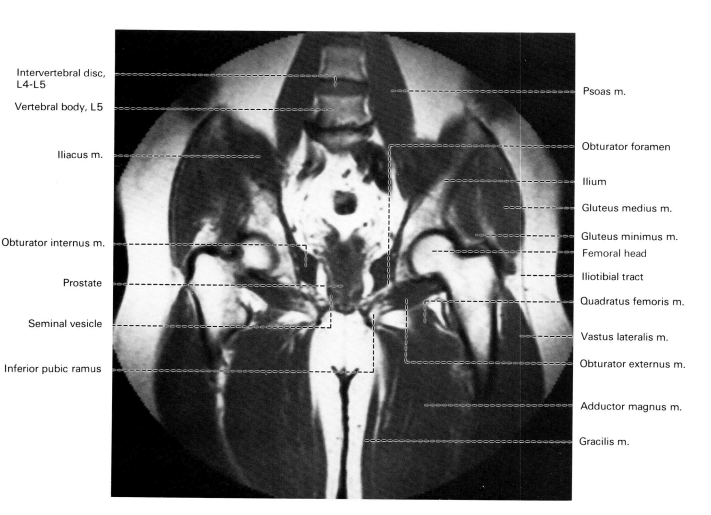

Intervertebral disc, L4-L5
Vertebral body, L5
Iliacus m.
Obturator internus m.
Prostate
Seminal vesicle
Inferior pubic ramus

Psoas m.
Obturator foramen
Ilium
Gluteus medius m.
Gluteus minimus m.
Femoral head
Iliotibial tract
Quadratus femoris m.
Vastus lateralis m.
Obturator externus m.
Adductor magnus m.
Gracilis m.

Figure 10.2.10

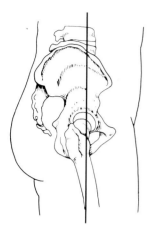

1. This image is at the level of the membranous urethra and penile root.

2. Adductor longus and adductor brevis are superior and lateral to adductor magnus at this level.

3. The iliopsoas tendon is noted as it approaches the lesser trochanter.

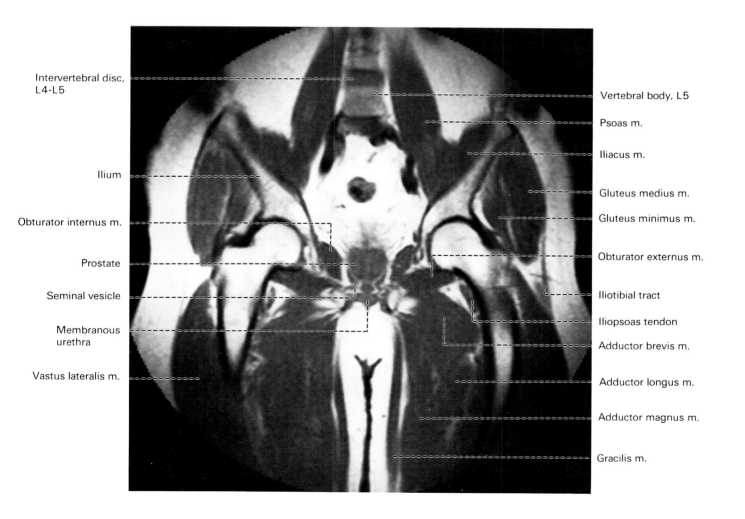

Intervertebral disc, L4-L5

Vertebral body, L5

Psoas m.

Iliacus m.

Ilium

Gluteus medius m.

Obturator internus m.

Gluteus minimus m.

Prostate

Obturator externus m.

Seminal vesicle

Iliotibial tract

Membranous urethra

Iliopsoas tendon

Adductor brevis m.

Vastus lateralis m.

Adductor longus m.

Adductor magnus m.

Gracilis m.

Figure 10.2.11

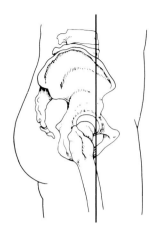

1. At this level the posterior portion of the urinary bladder is imaged.

2. The aorta, inferior vena cava, and iliac vessels are noted.

3. Tensor fasciae latae is well visualized on the left and to a lesser extent on the right.

4. Gracilis is the most medial thigh muscle originating from the inferior pubic rami.

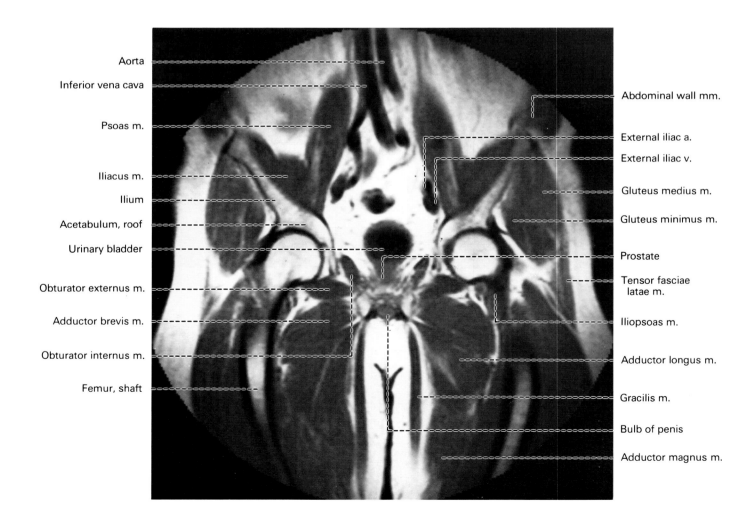

Aorta
Inferior vena cava
Psoas m.
Iliacus m.
Ilium
Acetabulum, roof
Urinary bladder
Obturator externus m.
Adductor brevis m.
Obturator internus m.
Femur, shaft

Abdominal wall mm.
External iliac a.
External iliac v.
Gluteus medius m.
Gluteus minimus m.
Prostate
Tensor fasciae latae m.
Iliopsoas m.
Adductor longus m.
Gracilis m.
Bulb of penis
Adductor magnus m.

Figure 10.2.12

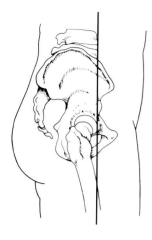

1. Pectineus is the most anterior muscle arising from the superior pubic ramus.

2. The iliacus and psoas muscles are imaged before they fuse.

3. On this image branches of the right femoral circumflex artery are seen. The medial femoral circumflex is seen between psoas and adductor brevis. A branch of the lateral femoral circumflex is seen between iliopsoas and vastus lateralis.

4. The low signal area superior and lateral to the femoral head represents the reflected head of rectus femoris. The straight head is not imaged because of its more anterior origin at the anterior inferior iliac spine.

5. Note the perivesical fat and its relationship to the bladder.

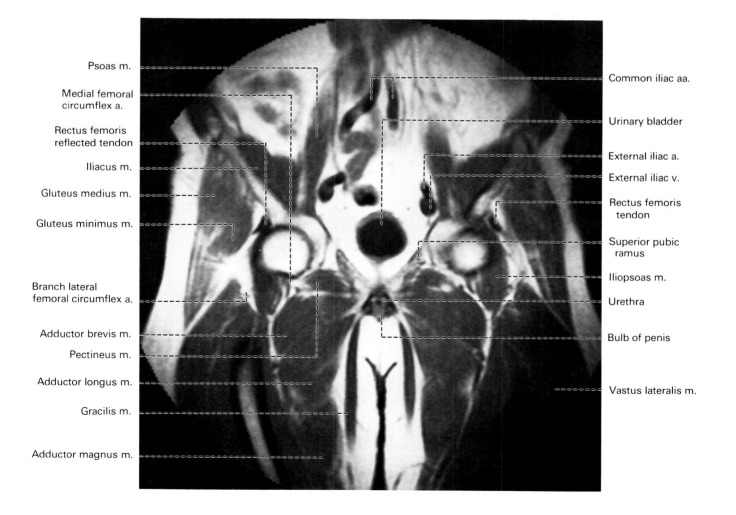

Psoas m.

Medial femoral circumflex a.

Rectus femoris reflected tendon

Iliacus m.

Gluteus medius m.

Gluteus minimus m.

Branch lateral femoral circumflex a.

Adductor brevis m.

Pectineus m.

Adductor longus m.

Gracilis m.

Adductor magnus m.

Common iliac aa.

Urinary bladder

External iliac a.

External iliac v.

Rectus femoris tendon

Superior pubic ramus

Iliopsoas m.

Urethra

Bulb of penis

Vastus lateralis m.

Figure 10.2.13

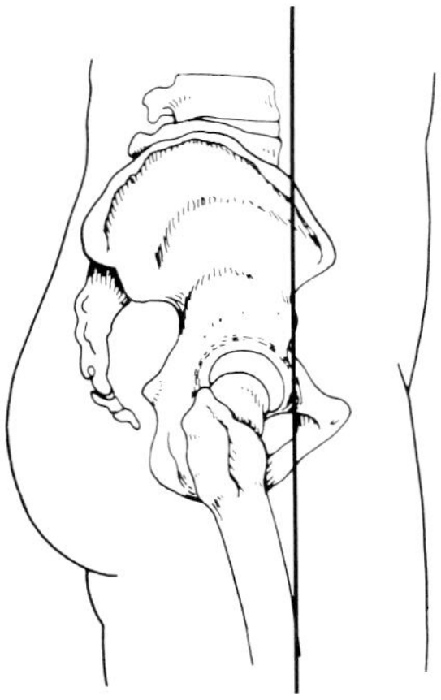

1. On the left, the straight head of rectus femoris originates from the anterior inferior iliac spine.

2. Note the erectile components of the penis (the paired corpora cavernosa and the corpus spongiosum).

3. Iliopsoas is covering the anterior portion of the femoral head on the left and is inferior to the femoral head on the right.

4. The superficial femoral artery is noted in the medial intermuscular septum, separating the adductors from the anterior compartment muscles.

5. The medial portion of the pectineus muscle is visualized at this level.

6. Tensor fasciae latae is seen on both sides. Its normal fatty infiltration is better demonstrated on the right. In cross section the fatty infiltration gives it a characteristic marbled appearance.

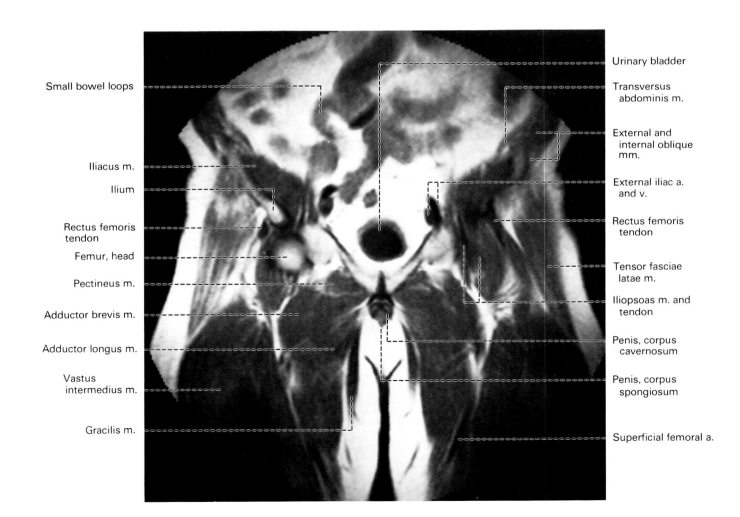

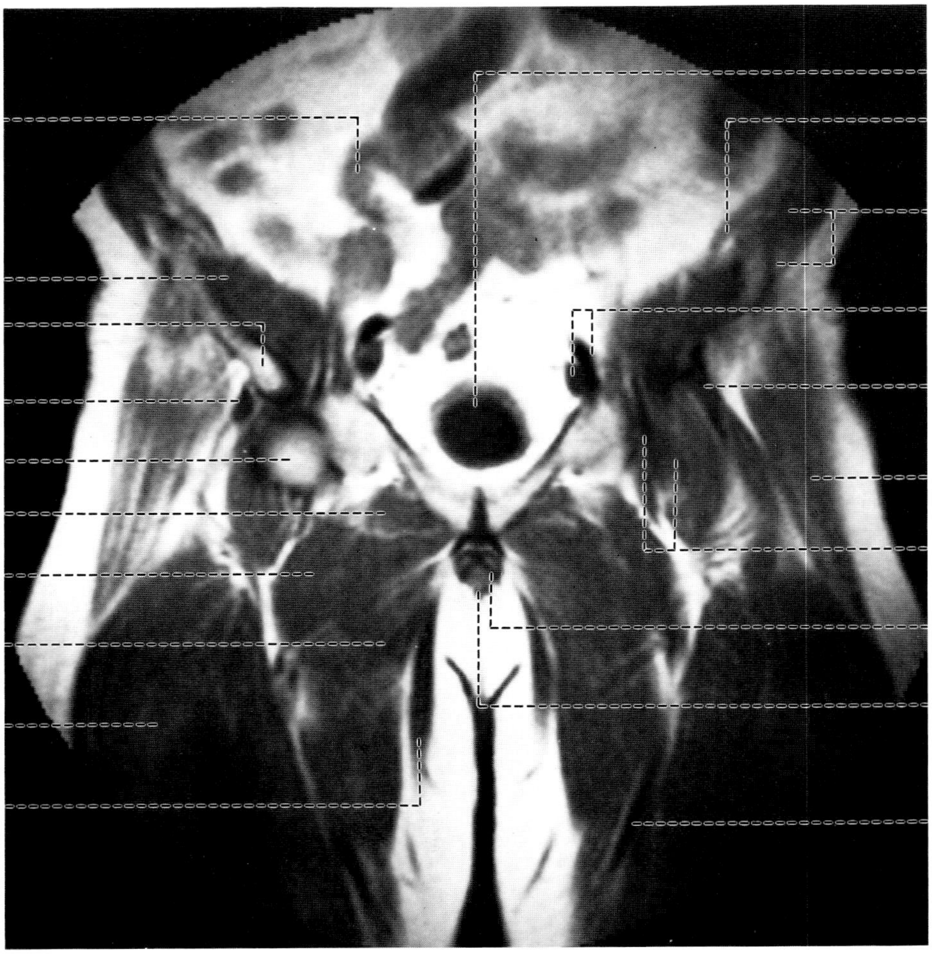
Small bowel loops
Iliacus m.
Ilium
Rectus femoris tendon
Femur, head
Pectineus m.
Adductor brevis m.
Adductor longus m.
Vastus intermedius m.
Gracilis m.
Urinary bladder
Transversus abdominis m.
External and internal oblique mm.
External iliac a. and v.
Rectus femoris tendon
Tensor fasciae latae m.
Iliopsoas m. and tendon
Penis, corpus cavernosum
Penis, corpus spongiosum
Superficial femoral a.

Figure 10.2.14

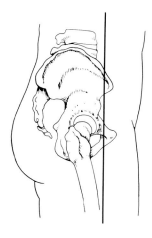

1. The abdominal muscles are broadly attached to the iliac crest.

2. Iliopsoas is broad as it exits the pelvis and crosses anterior to the femoral head.

3. The femoral artery and femoral vein are seen coursing anterior to the superior pubic ramus, with the artery lateral to the vein.

4. Note the origins of the three adductor muscles and their relationships.

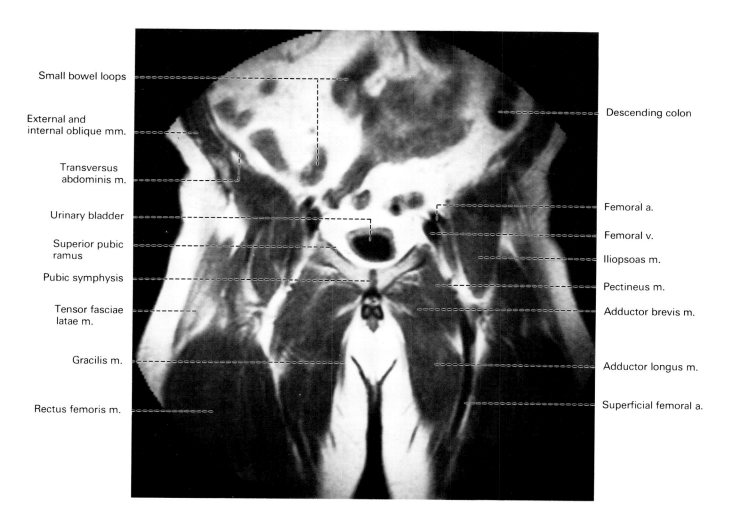

Small bowel loops

External and internal oblique mm.

Transversus abdominis m.

Urinary bladder

Superior pubic ramus

Pubic symphysis

Tensor fasciae latae m.

Gracilis m.

Rectus femoris m.

Descending colon

Femoral a.

Femoral v.

Iliopsoas m.

Pectineus m.

Adductor brevis m.

Adductor longus m.

Superficial femoral a.

Figure 10.2.15

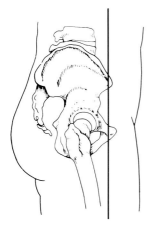

1. Sartorius is situated directly anterior to the femoral artery and vein in the inferior aspect of this image.

2. Rectus femoris is prominent, reflecting its anterior position within quadriceps femoris.

3. Transversus abdominis is distinguished from the internal and external oblique abdominal muscles.

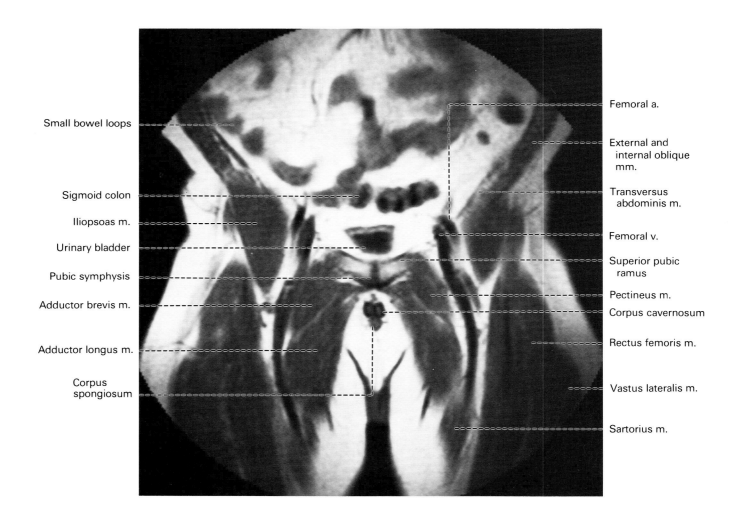

Small bowel loops

Sigmoid colon

Iliopsoas m.

Urinary bladder

Pubic symphysis

Adductor brevis m.

Adductor longus m.

Corpus spongiosum

Femoral a.

External and internal oblique mm.

Transversus abdominis m.

Femoral v.

Superior pubic ramus

Pectineus m.

Corpus cavernosum

Rectus femoris m.

Vastus lateralis m.

Sartorius m.

Figure 10.2.16

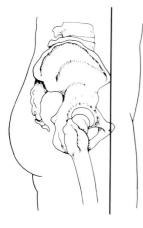

1. Adductor longus and pectineus are the most anterior of the medial compartment muscles.

2. Transversus abdominis can be differentiated from the internal and external oblique muscles on this image.

3. The greater saphenous vein is noted traversing superficial to adductor longus.

4. The femoral vessels exit the pelvis under the inguinal ligament.

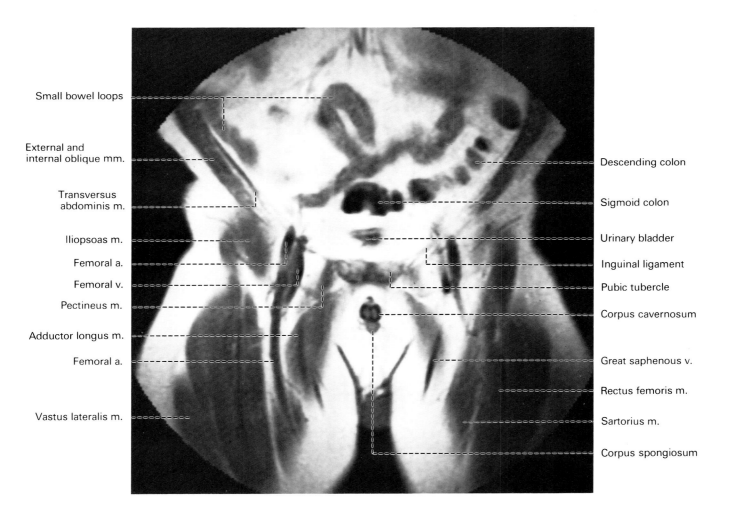

Small bowel loops

External and internal oblique mm.

Transversus abdominis m.

Iliopsoas m.

Femoral a.

Femoral v.

Pectineus m.

Adductor longus m.

Femoral a.

Vastus lateralis m.

Descending colon

Sigmoid colon

Urinary bladder

Inguinal ligament

Pubic tubercle

Corpus cavernosum

Great saphenous v.

Rectus femoris m.

Sartorius m.

Corpus spongiosum

Figure 10.2.17

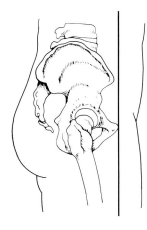

1. The paired corpora cavernosa and the corpus spongiosum are easily identifiable.

2. The greater saphenous vein courses superiorly to join the femoral vein.

3. The testis is identifiable.

4. Sartorius courses obliquely medial to rectus femoris on this image.

5. Note the haustrations in the descending colon in contradistinction to the smooth appearance of the small intestine.

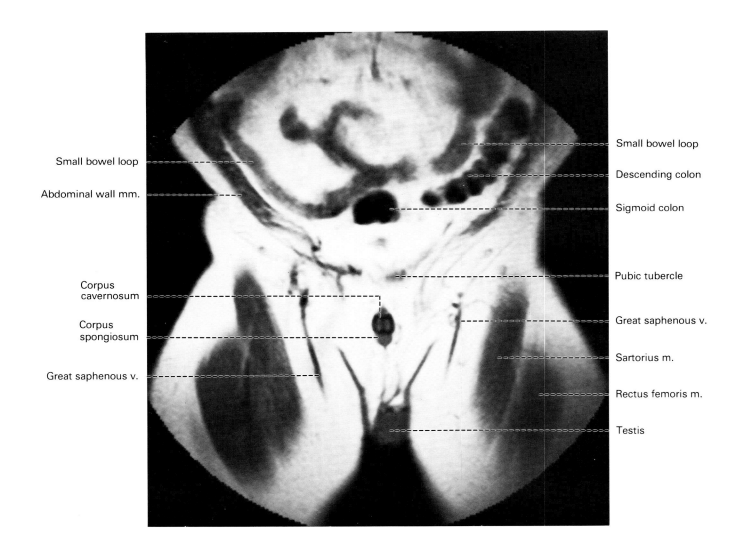

Figure 10.2.18

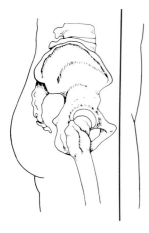

1. The spermatic cord on the left courses superior to the inguinal canal.

2. Note the tubular structures of the head of the epididymis.

3. Superficial inguinal lymph nodes can often be identified in this region.

4. Note the insertion of rectus abdominis onto the crest and symphysis pubis.

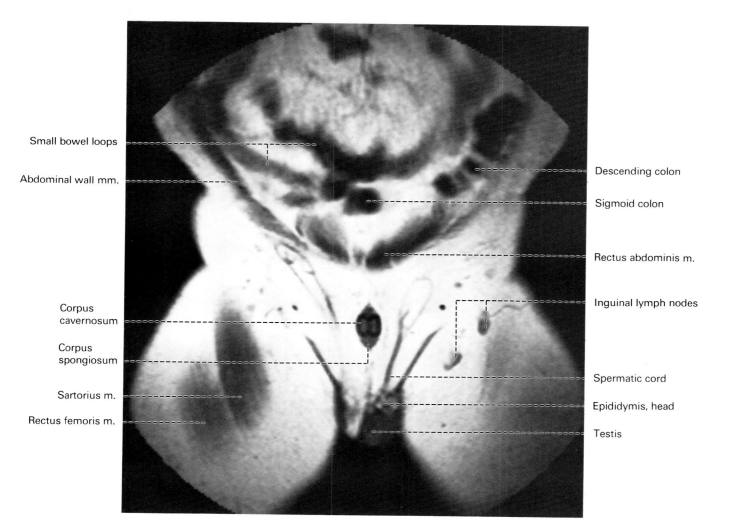

Small bowel loops

Abdominal wall mm.

Descending colon

Sigmoid colon

Rectus abdominis m.

Corpus cavernosum

Inguinal lymph nodes

Corpus spongiosum

Sartorius m.

Spermatic cord

Epididymis, head

Rectus femoris m.

Testis

Figure 10.2.19

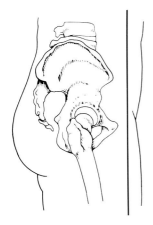

1. The dorsal vein of the penis can be identified.

2. The spermatic cord (vas deferens, vessels) courses toward the inguinal ligament.

3. Note that the external oblique muscle is better demonstrated on the left.

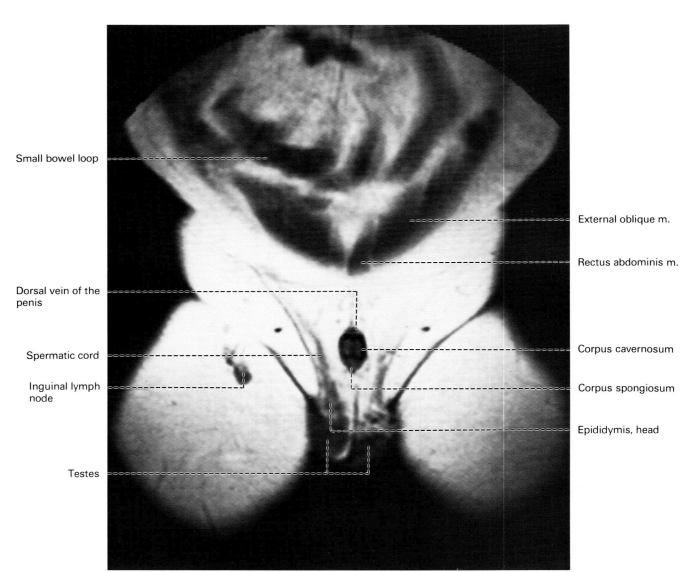

Figure 10.2.20

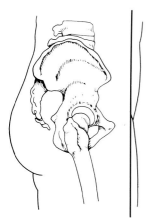

1. In this anterior image, the abdominal muscles are partly visualized.

2. The paired corpora cavernosa and single corpus spongiosum are demonstrated in cross section.

3. The epididymis on the left and testis on the right are well seen.

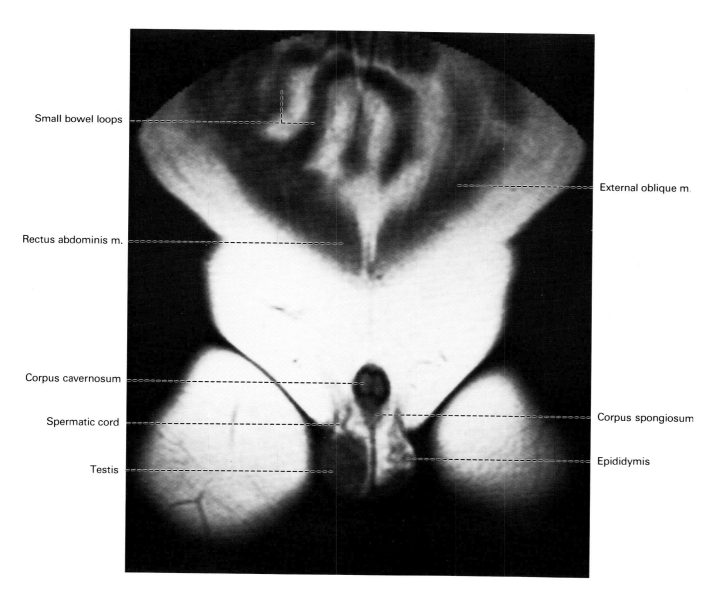

SAGITTAL

Figure 10.3.1

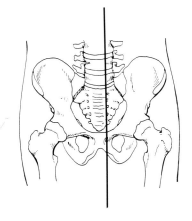

1. This image is just to the left of midline and some midline structures are seen, such as the prostate.

2. The urogenital diaphragm is located anterior and inferior to the prostate, attaching to the pubic bone.

3. The aorta is partly imaged on this section.

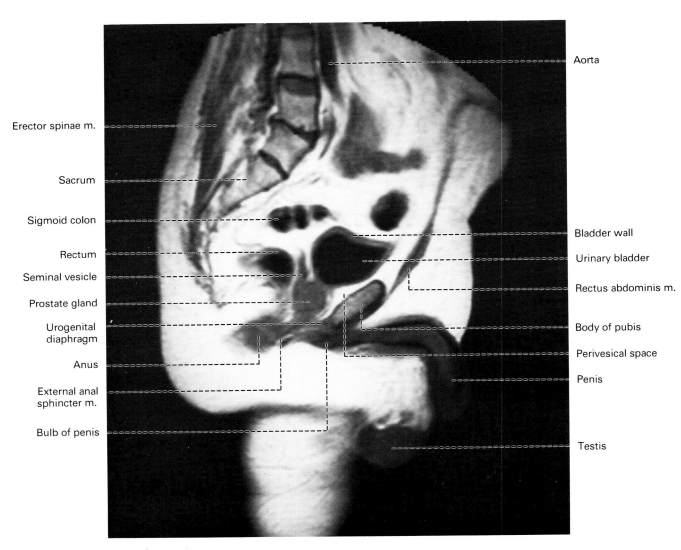

Erector spinae m.

Sacrum

Sigmoid colon

Rectum

Seminal vesicle

Prostate gland

Urogenital diaphragm

Anus

External anal sphincter m.

Bulb of penis

Aorta

Bladder wall

Urinary bladder

Rectus abdominis m.

Body of pubis

Perivesical space

Penis

Testis

Figure 10.3.2

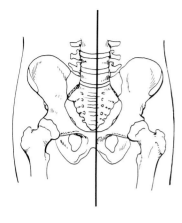

1. This is a midline image.

2. The perivesical space is well visualized.

3. The median umbilical ligament attaches to the anterosuperior aspect of the bladder.

4. The presacral space is clearly seen showing high signal intensity because of its fat content.

5. Levator ani is visualized.

6. The aorta is now clearly visible with aortic bifurcation noted anterior to the lower lumbar spine.

7. The thecal sac ends at the level of the S1-S2 junction.

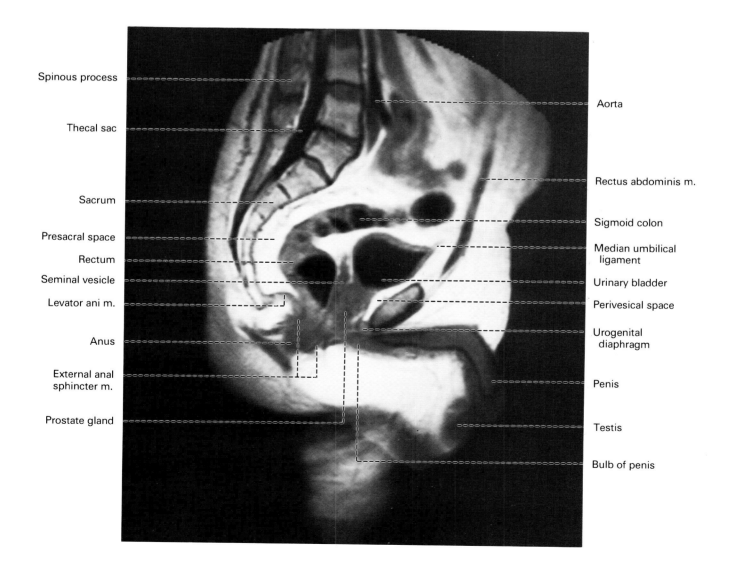

Left labels (top to bottom): Spinous process, Thecal sac, Sacrum, Presacral space, Rectum, Seminal vesicle, Levator ani m., Anus, External anal sphincter m., Prostate gland

Right labels (top to bottom): Aorta, Rectus abdominis m., Sigmoid colon, Median umbilical ligament, Urinary bladder, Perivesical space, Urogenital diaphragm, Penis, Testis, Bulb of penis

Figure 10.3.3

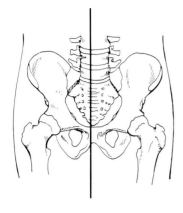

1. The inferior vena cava is well demonstrated in this section.

2. The right common iliac artery is anterior to the distal portion of the inferior vena cava.

3. The right seminal vesical is directed posterior and superior to the prostate gland.

4. The perivesical space is seen between the pubis and urinary bladder.

5. The testis, vas deferens, body of epididymis, and efferent ductules are all clearly depicted.

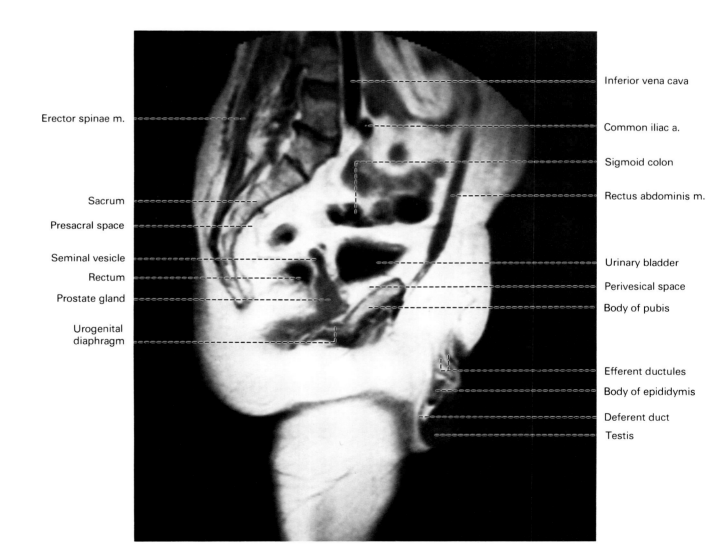

Figure 10.3.4

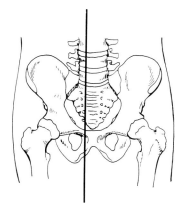

1. The gracilis is demonstrated and is the most medial muscle of the thigh. It originates from the body and inferior pubic ramus and descends to insert on the tibia as part of the pes anserine complex.

2. The right common iliac artery is seen dividing into the internal iliac artery and the more anterior external iliac artery.

3. The common iliac vein is posterior to the iliac artery.

4. The spermatic cord courses superiorly from the testis.

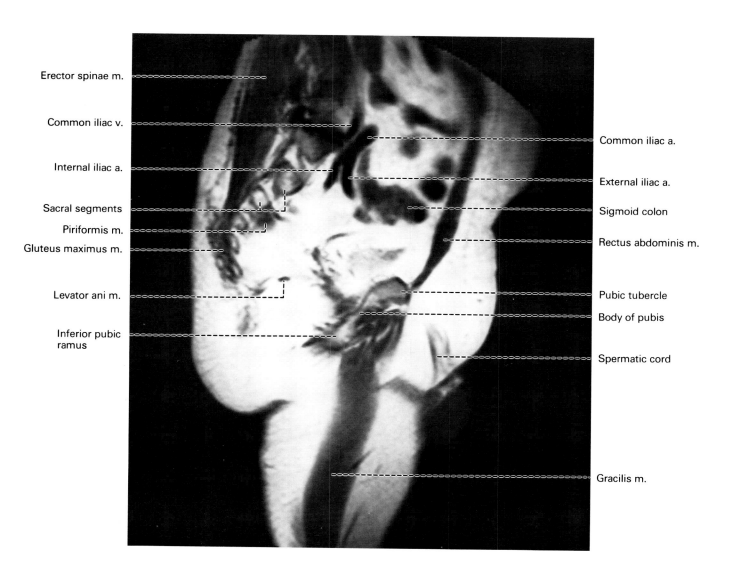

Figure 10.3.5

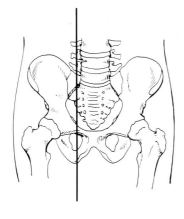

1. Adductor magnus has two heads at its origin. One is more posterior and functions as a hamstring muscle, being innervated from the sciatic. The other head is more anterior, grouped with the other adductors, and innervated by the obturator nerve.

2. The internal iliac artery is seen posteriorly as it gives rise to the superior and inferior gluteal arteries. The external iliac artery projects anterior to the common iliac vein in this image.

3. Piriformis originates as a broad muscle from the anterior aspect of the sacrum.

4. Obturator internus and externus are seen on each side of the obturator foramen.

5. Gluteus maximus is shown. It originates in part from the posterior aspect of the sacrum.

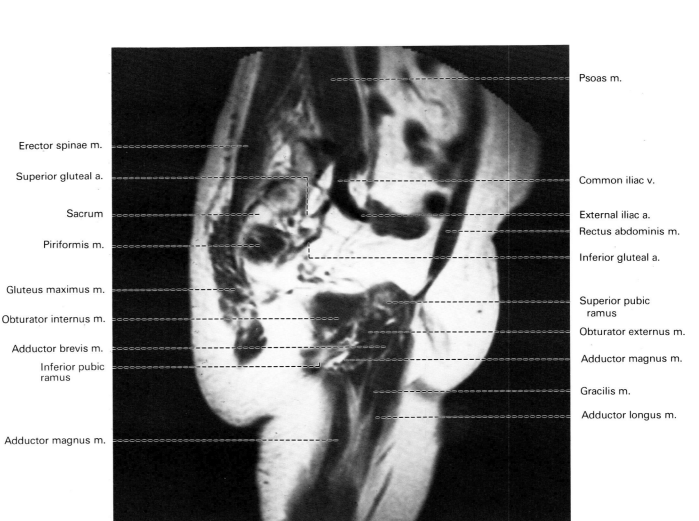

Figure 10.3.6

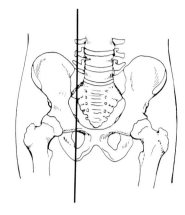

1. Note the two heads of adductor magnus that are now muscular.

2. The external iliac vein is posterior to the internal iliac artery.

3. This parasagittal section gives a new perspective on the sacroiliac joint.

4. Special attention should be paid to piriformis. The sacral plexus forms on its surface.

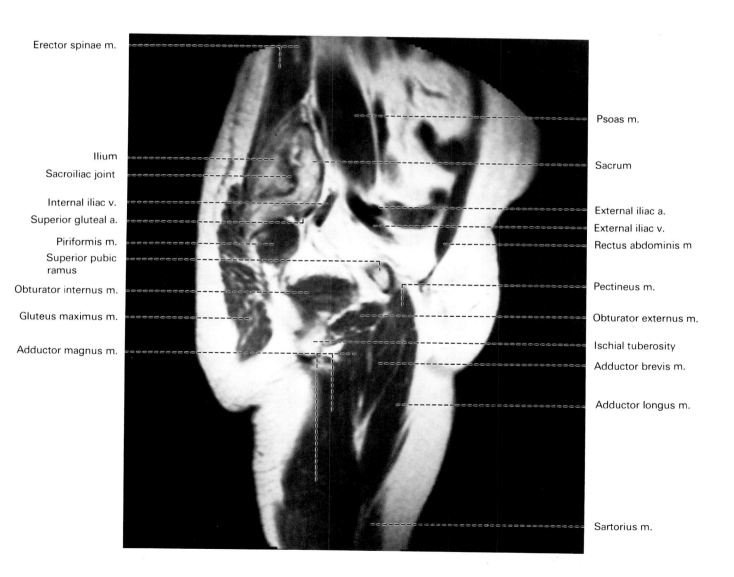

Erector spinae m.

Psoas m.

Ilium

Sacrum

Sacroiliac joint

Internal iliac v.

External iliac a.

Superior gluteal a.

External iliac v.

Piriformis m.

Rectus abdominis m

Superior pubic ramus

Obturator internus m.

Pectineus m.

Gluteus maximus m.

Obturator externus m.

Adductor magnus m.

Ischial tuberosity

Adductor brevis m.

Adductor longus m.

Sartorius m.

Figure 10.3.7

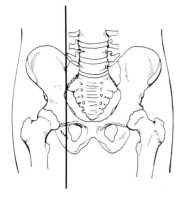

1. At this level the external iliac artery is anterior to the external iliac vein.

2. The sacrotuberous ligament is demonstrated.

3. The curvature of the sacroiliac joint in the sagittal plane should be appreciated.

4. The piriformis exits through the greater sciatic foramen, with the superior gluteal artery and nerve above and the inferior gluteal artery and nerve below. The sciatic nerve courses inferior to piriformis (not seen in this section).

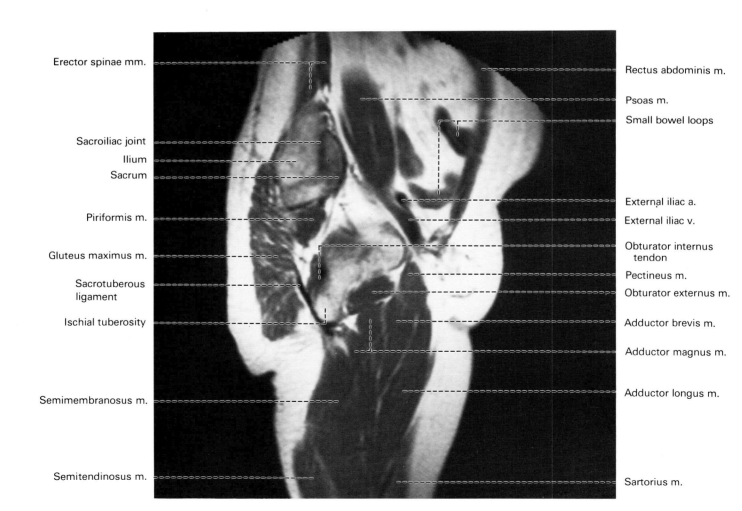

Erector spinae mm.

Sacroiliac joint

Ilium

Sacrum

Piriformis m.

Gluteus maximus m.

Sacrotuberous ligament

Ischial tuberosity

Semimembranosus m.

Semitendinosus m.

Rectus abdominis m.

Psoas m.

Small bowel loops

External iliac a.

External iliac v.

Obturator internus tendon

Pectineus m.

Obturator externus m.

Adductor brevis m.

Adductor magnus m.

Adductor longus m.

Sartorius m.

Figure 10.3.8

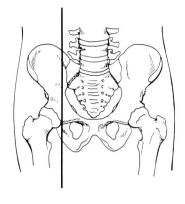

1. Lateral to erector spinae is quadratus lumborum, inserting onto the iliac crest lateral to the sacroiliac joint.

2. Gluteus medius is shown to have fibers more superiorly located than gluteus maximus, thus explaining why, on descending axial images, the gluteus medius fibers are encountered first.

3. The superior gluteal artery can be seen (with its flow void) superior to the piriformis muscle, just below the inferior margin of the ilium.

4. Note the origins of the two gemelli (superior and inferior) with the tendinous portion of obturator internus between them. These, along with piriformis and quadratus femoris, are known as the short external rotators of the hip. They insert onto the greater trochanter.

5. Note the greater saphenous vein and its anastomosis with the femoral vein.

6. Note the spermatic cord entering the pelvis via the external (superficial) inguinal ring.

7. The iliacus and psoas muscles merge together to form iliopsoas.

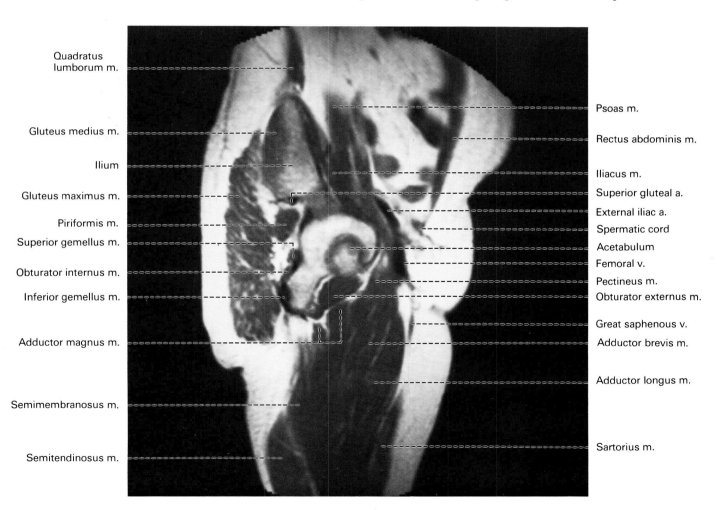

Figure 10.3.9

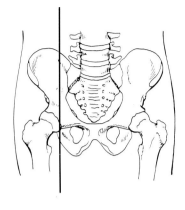

1. The sciatic nerve can be seen exiting beneath the inferior margin of the piriformis. At this level it is coursing obliquely.

2. The tendinous origin of the more anterior semimembranosus is faintly visible on this image. The semitendinosus and long head of the biceps femoris originate here conjointly.

3. Obturator externus courses posterior and inferior to the femoral head.

4. The acetabulum at this level is demonstrated with its anterior and posterior columns. The posterior column is larger than the anterior column.

5. The medial femoral circumflex artery can be seen arising from the common femoral artery and coursing under pectineus.

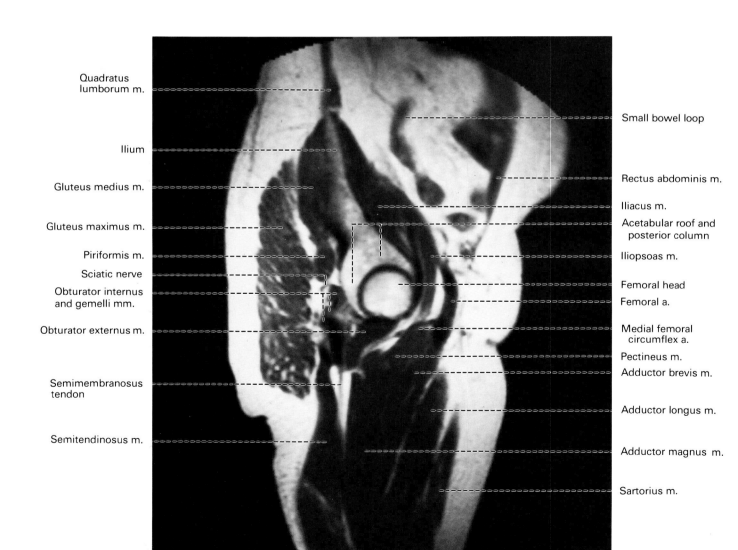

Quadratus lumborum m.

Ilium

Gluteus medius m.

Gluteus maximus m.

Piriformis m.

Sciatic nerve

Obturator internus and gemelli mm.

Obturator externus m.

Semimembranosus tendon

Semitendinosus m.

Small bowel loop

Rectus abdominis m.

Iliacus m.

Acetabular roof and posterior column

Iliopsoas m.

Femoral head

Femoral a.

Medial femoral circumflex a.

Pectineus m.

Adductor brevis m.

Adductor longus m.

Adductor magnus m.

Sartorius m.

Figure 10.3.10

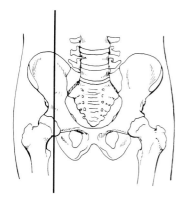

1. The gluteus minimus can now be identified deep to the gluteus medius.

2. The sciatic nerve courses obliquely before descending into the thigh.

3. The tendinous origin of semimembranosus is now clearly visible.

4. The deep femoral artery (profunda femoris) is noted coursing deep to adductor longus.

5. Iliopsoas proceeds anteriorly over the femoral head and then turns sharply posteriorly.

6. This section is lateral to rectus abdominis and through the aponeurosis of the other abdominal wall muscles.

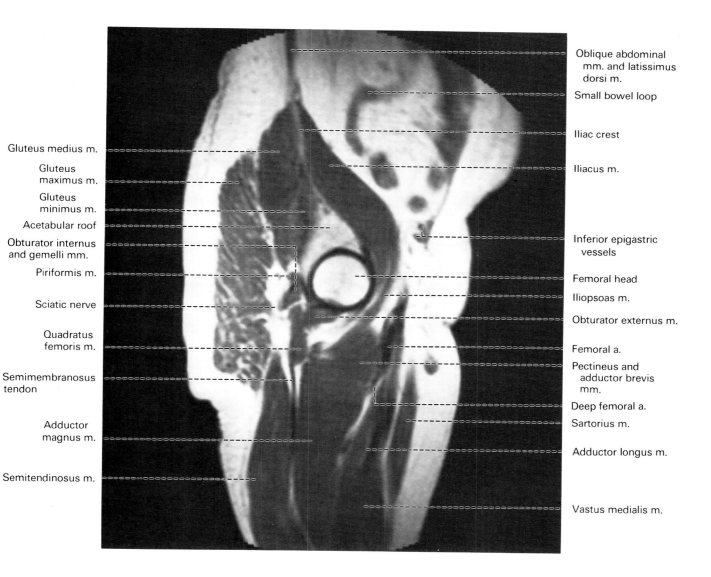

Gluteus medius m.
Gluteus maximus m.
Gluteus minimus m.
Acetabular roof
Obturator internus and gemelli mm.
Piriformis m.
Sciatic nerve
Quadratus femoris m.
Semimembranosus tendon
Adductor magnus m.
Semitendinosus m.

Oblique abdominal mm. and latissimus dorsi m.
Small bowel loop
Iliac crest
Iliacus m.
Inferior epigastric vessels
Femoral head
Iliopsoas m.
Obturator externus m.
Femoral a.
Pectineus and adductor brevis mm.
Deep femoral a.
Sartorius m.
Adductor longus m.
Vastus medialis m.

Figure 10.3.11

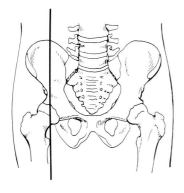

1. Iliopsoas courses inferiorly and posterolaterally to insert onto the lesser trochanter.

2. The deep femoral artery is seen as it gives off its muscular branches.

3. Quadratus femoris is seen as a thick fleshy muscle beneath the short rotators.

4. Obturator externus is seen coursing immediately under the femoral head en route to its insertion in the trochanteric fossa.

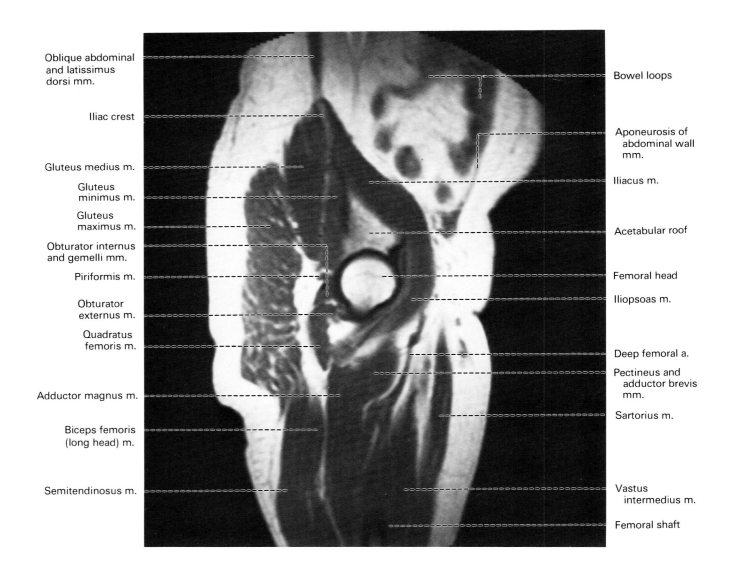

Oblique abdominal and latissimus dorsi mm.

Iliac crest

Gluteus medius m.

Gluteus minimus m.

Gluteus maximus m.

Obturator internus and gemelli mm.

Piriformis m.

Obturator externus m.

Quadratus femoris m.

Adductor magnus m.

Biceps femoris (long head) m.

Semitendinosus m.

Bowel loops

Aponeurosis of abdominal wall mm.

Iliacus m.

Acetabular roof

Femoral head

Iliopsoas m.

Deep femoral a.

Pectineus and adductor brevis mm.

Sartorius m.

Vastus intermedius m.

Femoral shaft

Figure 10.3.12

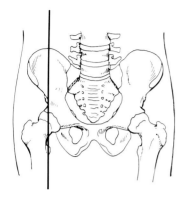

1. The piriformis tendon is seen as it approaches the superior and inferior gemelli and the obturator internus tendon; the piriformis tendon is superior to these other structures.

2. Quadratus femoris is well demonstrated in this section.

3. The sciatic nerve is seen descending posterior to the adductor magnus and anterior to the long head of the biceps femoris.

4. Pectineus and adductor brevis are seen close to their insertions on the proximal femur.

5. The lateral femoral circumflex vessels are coursing under sartorius and rectus femoris.

6. Iliopsoas inserts onto the lesser trochanter.

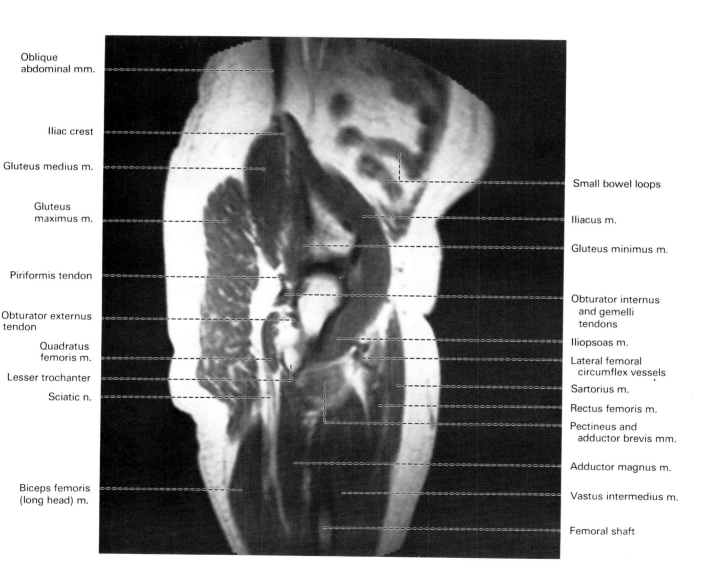

Figure 10.3.13

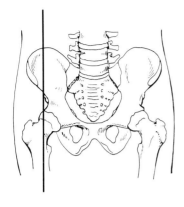

1. There are three small, rounded low intensity structures aligned in the trochanteric fossa. The superior one represents the piriformis tendon; the middle one is a conjoint tendon of obturator internus and gemelli; and the inferior one is the obturator externus tendon.

2. The straight tendon of rectus femoris originates from the anterior inferior iliac spine. The reflected tendon originates from the superior aspect of the acetabulum.

3. Branches from the lateral femoral circumflex vessels are seen between vastus intermedius and rectus femoris.

4. Anastomotic branches of the medial femoral circumflex vessels are seen posterior to the proximal femur between quadratus femoris and adductor magnus.

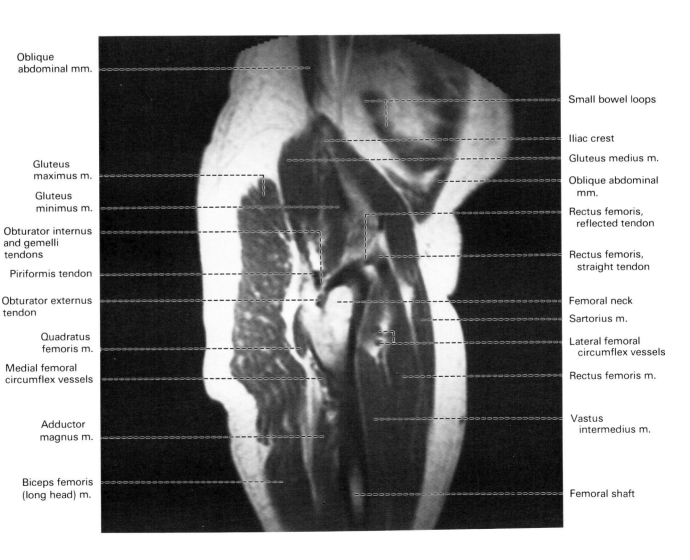

Figure 10.3.14

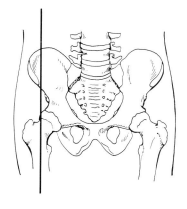

1. The lateral femoral circumflex vessels course toward the femur at the proximal end of vastus intermedius.

2. The posterior position of the greater trochanter should be appreciated. The tendon of gluteus medius attaches to the greater trochanter.

3. Femoral anteversion can be appreciated on this section.

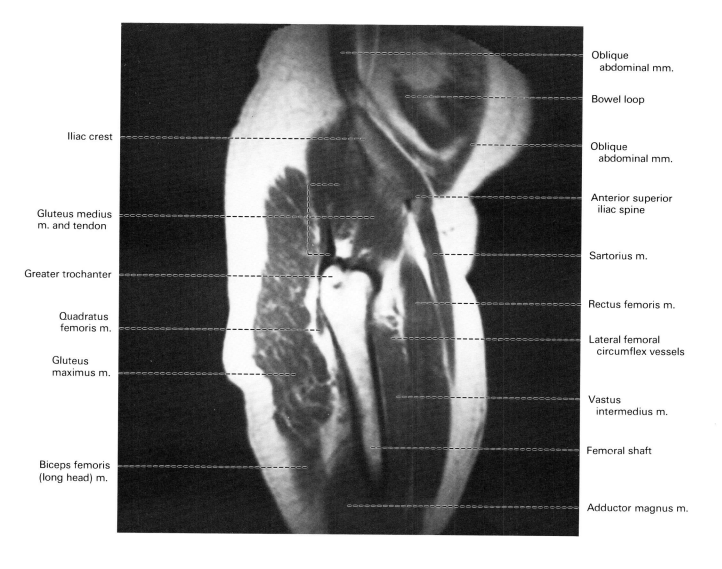

Figure 10.3.15

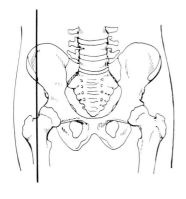

1. The origin of sartorius from the anterior superior iliac spine should be noted.

2. Tensor fasciae latae originates from the anterior superior iliac spine.

3. Note the broad insertion of gluteus medius onto the greater trochanter.

4. Note the posterior extent of vastus lateralis. It originates from the lateral lip of the linea aspera.

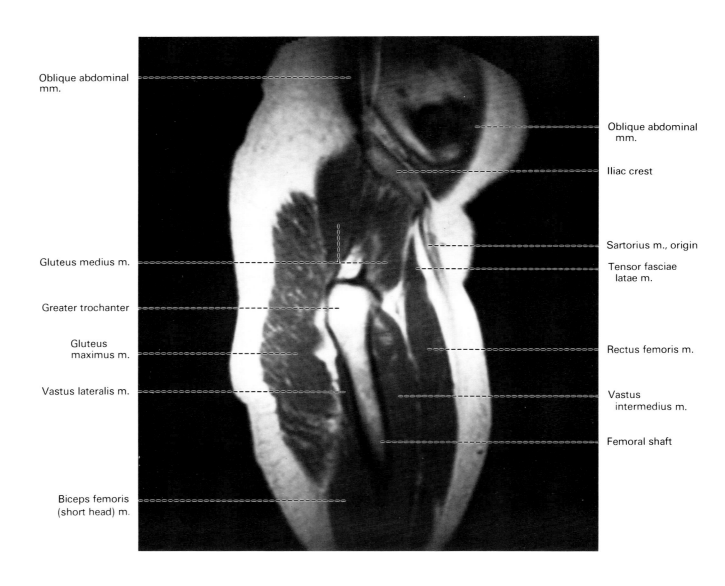

Figure 10.3.16

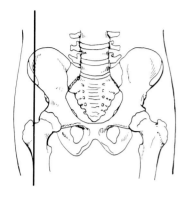

1. Gluteus maximus extends more inferiorly than the other gluteal muscles.

2. Gluteus medius inserts onto the lateral surface of the greater trochanter in this section.

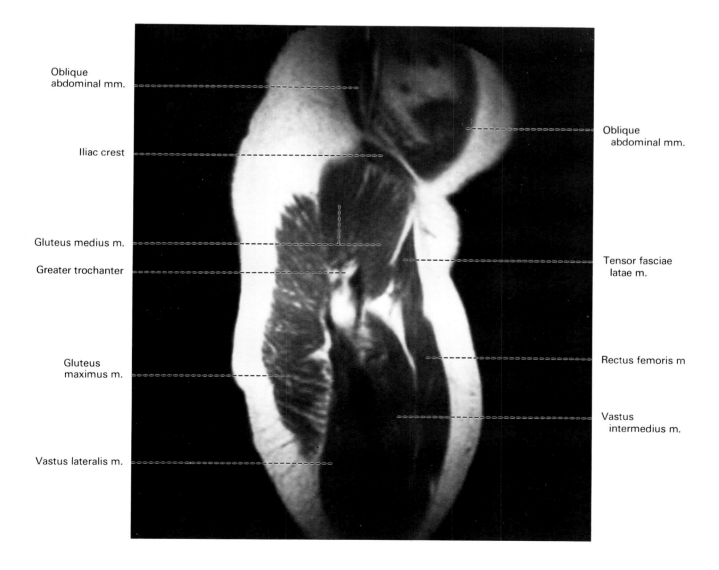

Figure 10.3.17

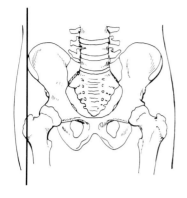

1. The oblique abdominal muscles are seen attaching to the superior margin of the iliac crest.

2. The linear low signal intensity structure between vastus lateralis and gluteus maximus represents the iliotibial tract onto which gluteus maximus inserts.

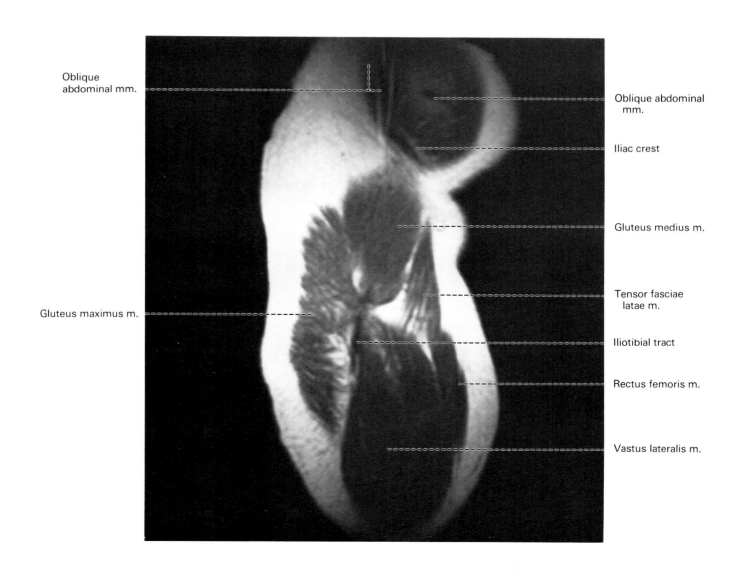

Oblique abdominal mm.

Gluteus maximus m.

Oblique abdominal mm.

Iliac crest

Gluteus medius m.

Tensor fasciae latae m.

Iliotibial tract

Rectus femoris m.

Vastus lateralis m.

Figure 10.3.18

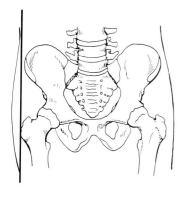

1. The iliotibial tract can be seen at the posterior border of the vastus lateralis muscle.

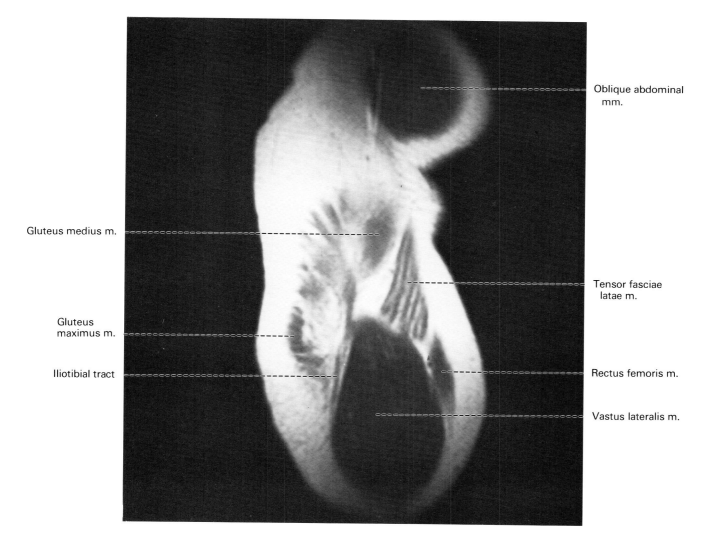

Oblique abdominal mm.

Gluteus medius m.

Gluteus maximus m.

Iliotibial tract

Tensor fasciae latae m.

Rectus femoris m.

Vastus lateralis m.

Figure 10.3.19

1. This most lateral section shows tensor fasciae latae and vastus lateralis.

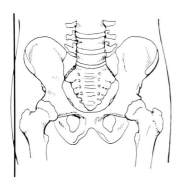

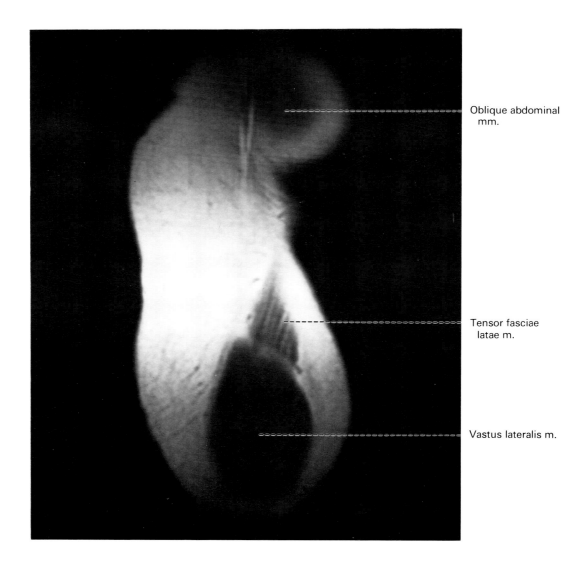

Oblique abdominal mm.

Tensor fasciae latae m.

Vastus lateralis m.

Chapter 11

FEMALE PELVIS

AXIAL

Figure 11.1.1

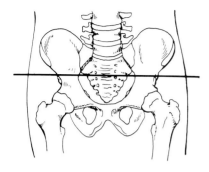

1. This image is obtained at the superior aspect of the uterine fundus.

2. Also noted is the greater sciatic foramen with piriformis exiting through it.

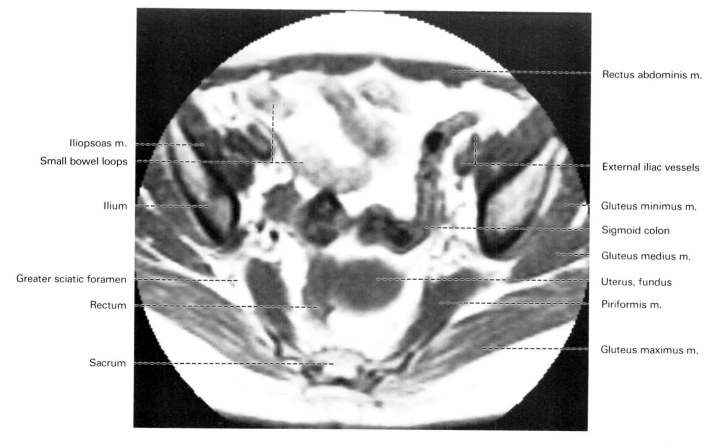

Rectus abdominis m.

Iliopsoas m.

Small bowel loops

External iliac vessels

Ilium

Gluteus minimus m.

Sigmoid colon

Gluteus medius m.

Greater sciatic foramen

Uterus, fundus

Rectum

Piriformis m.

Gluteus maximus m.

Sacrum

Figure 11.1.2

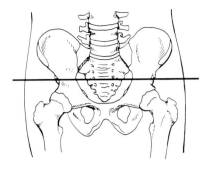

1. This section passes through the dome of the urinary bladder.

2. The broad ligament of the uterus extends laterally and anteriorly.

3. The left ovary is seen near the periphery of the broad ligament.

4. The rectouterine pouch of Douglas represents the lowest peritoneal reflection in the pelvis.

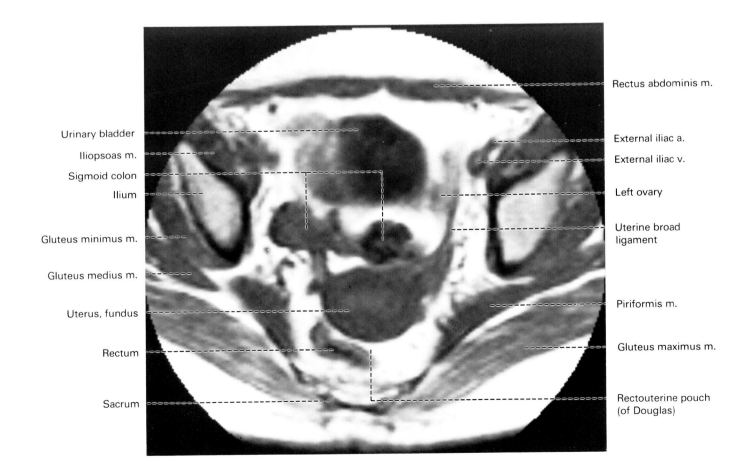

Rectus abdominis m.

Urinary bladder

External iliac a.

Iliopsoas m.

External iliac v.

Sigmoid colon

Left ovary

Ilium

Uterine broad ligament

Gluteus minimus m.

Gluteus medius m.

Uterus, fundus

Piriformis m.

Rectum

Gluteus maximus m.

Sacrum

Rectouterine pouch (of Douglas)

Figure 11.1.3

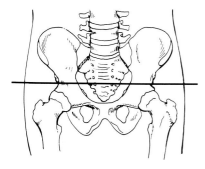

1. Note the relationship of the urinary bladder, uterus, and rectum.

2. Immediately medial to the acetabular margin is the obturator nerve.

3. Immediately lateral to the external iliac artery is the femoral nerve.

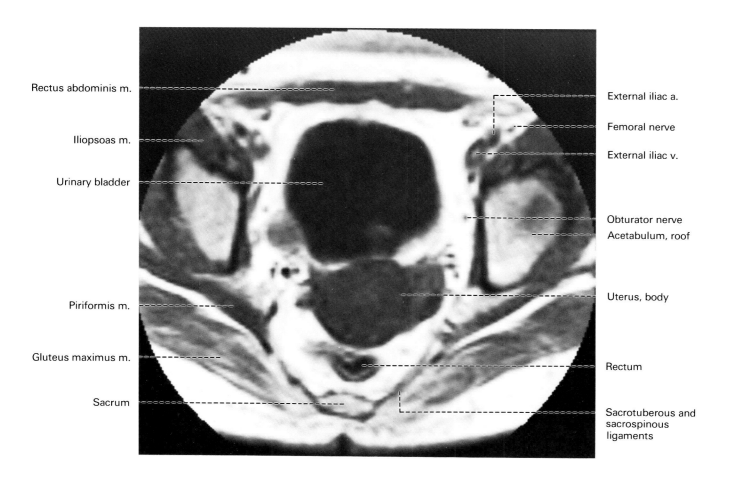

Rectus abdominis m.

Iliopsoas m.

Urinary bladder

Piriformis m.

Gluteus maximus m.

Sacrum

External iliac a.

Femoral nerve

External iliac v.

Obturator nerve
Acetabulum, roof

Uterus, body

Rectum

Sacrotuberous and
sacrospinous
ligaments

Figure 11.1.4

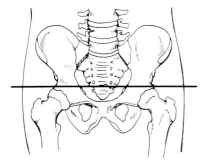

1. Note the uterine vessels that branch from the internal iliac vessels.

2. The rectum, uterus, and urinary bladder are closely apposed.

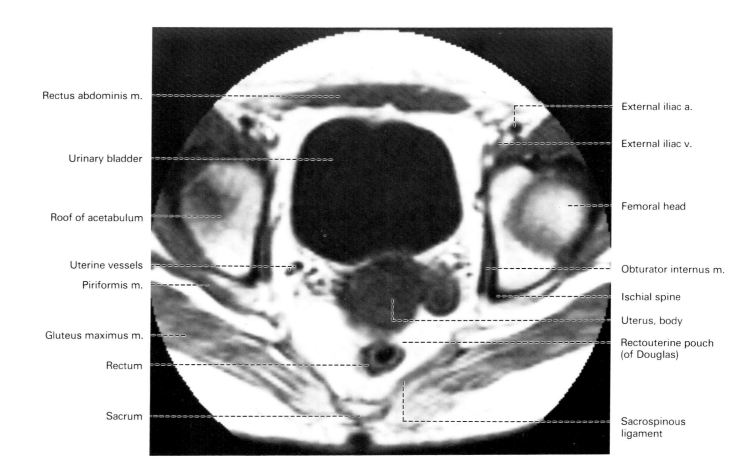

Rectus abdominis m.

Urinary bladder

Roof of acetabulum

Uterine vessels

Piriformis m.

Gluteus maximus m.

Rectum

Sacrum

External iliac a.

External iliac v.

Femoral head

Obturator internus m.

Ischial spine

Uterus, body

Rectouterine pouch (of Douglas)

Sacrospinous ligament

Figure 11.1.5

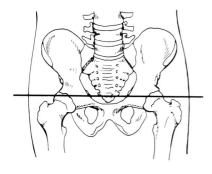

1. Note the uterovaginal vascular plexus. The ureter, at this level, is in the same location but is often difficult to identify.

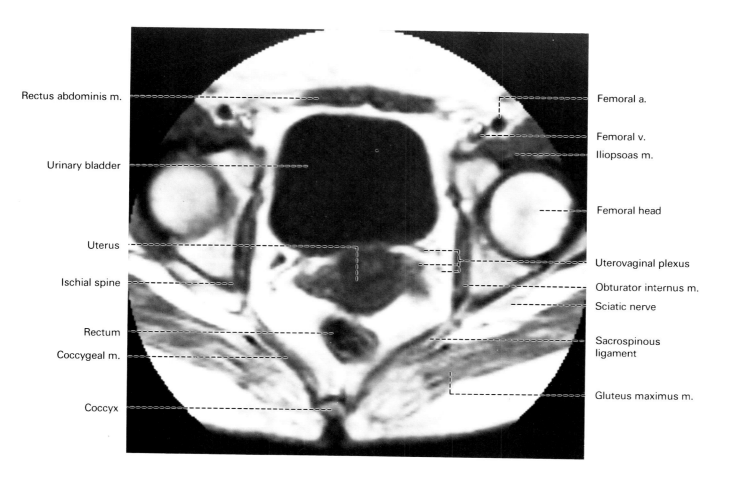

Rectus abdominis m.

Urinary bladder

Uterus

Ischial spine

Rectum

Coccygeal m.

Coccyx

Femoral a.

Femoral v.

Iliopsoas m.

Femoral head

Uterovaginal plexus

Obturator internus m.

Sciatic nerve

Sacrospinous ligament

Gluteus maximus m.

Figure 11.1.6

1. The cervical canal of the uterus can be seen at this level.

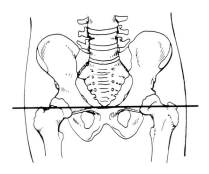

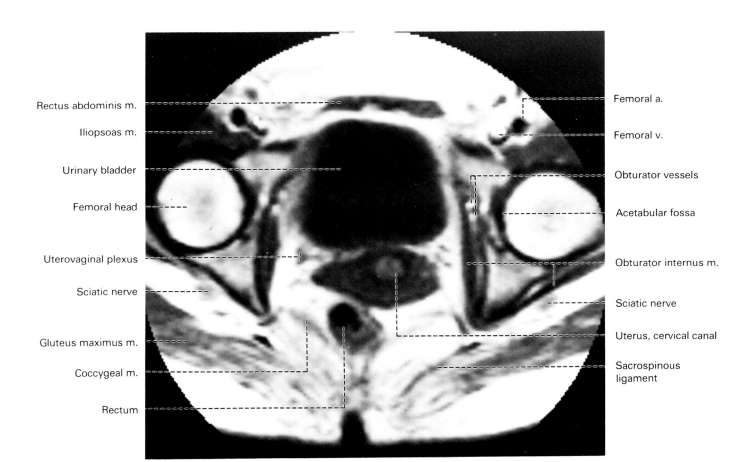

Rectus abdominis m.

Iliopsoas m.

Urinary bladder

Femoral head

Uterovaginal plexus

Sciatic nerve

Gluteus maximus m.

Coccygeal m.

Rectum

Femoral a.

Femoral v.

Obturator vessels

Acetabular fossa

Obturator internus m.

Sciatic nerve

Uterus, cervical canal

Sacrospinous ligament

Figure 11.1.7

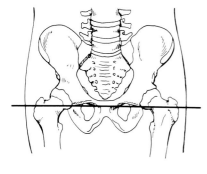

1. The levator ani is identified in this section.

2. The inferior gluteal artery gives rise to the pudendal artery, which courses anteriorly along the medial margin of obturator internus. The pudendal nerve runs with the artery.

3. The cervical canal in the lowest part of the uterus is visualized.

4. The obturator nerve and vessels are seen in the pelvis as they exit anteriorly under the inferior margin of the superior pubic ramus.

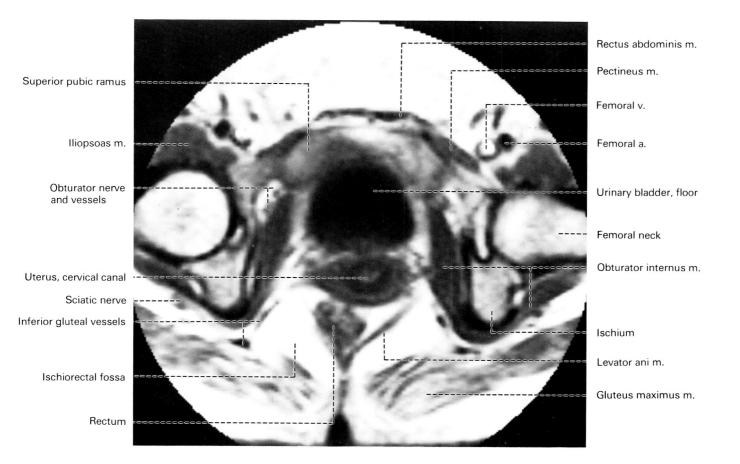

Superior pubic ramus

Iliopsoas m.

Obturator nerve and vessels

Uterus, cervical canal

Sciatic nerve

Inferior gluteal vessels

Ischiorectal fossa

Rectum

Rectus abdominis m.

Pectineus m.

Femoral v.

Femoral a.

Urinary bladder, floor

Femoral neck

Obturator internus m.

Ischium

Levator ani m.

Gluteus maximus m.

Figure 11.1.8

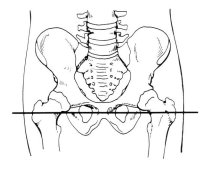

1. Note the urethra and vagina posterior to the symphysis pubis.

2. The flattened shape of the vagina in cross section should be noted.

3. The pudendal vessels and nerve are adjacent to obturator internus.

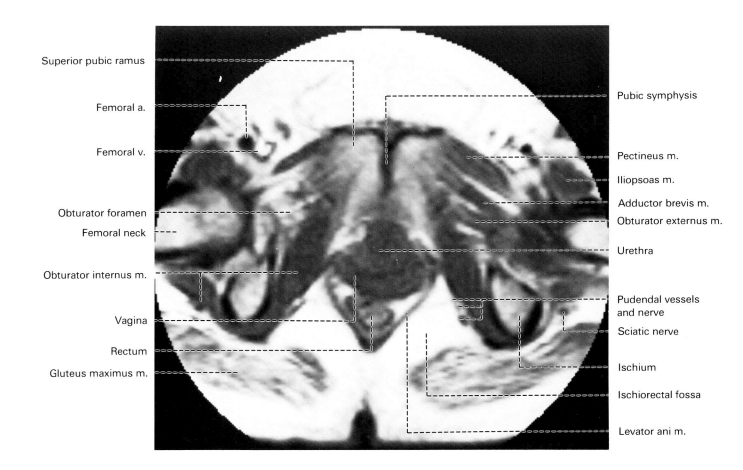

Superior pubic ramus
Femoral a.
Femoral v.
Obturator foramen
Femoral neck
Obturator internus m.
Vagina
Rectum
Gluteus maximus m.

Pubic symphysis
Pectineus m.
Iliopsoas m.
Adductor brevis m.
Obturator externus m.
Urethra
Pudendal vessels and nerve
Sciatic nerve
Ischium
Ischiorectal fossa
Levator ani m.

Figure 11.2.1

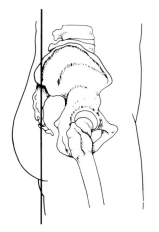

1. This section passes through the posterior aspect of the levator ani muscle as it inserts into the coccyx.

2. The erector spinae muscles are clearly demonstrated in this image.

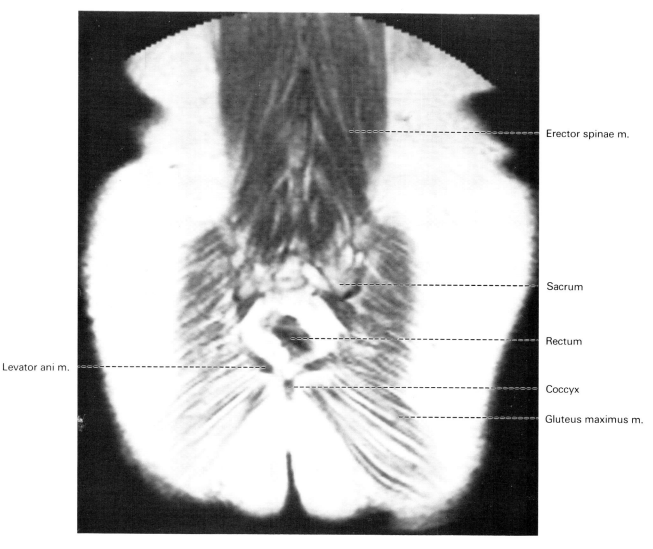

Erector spinae m.

Sacrum

Rectum

Coccyx

Gluteus maximus m.

Levator ani m.

Figure 11.2.2

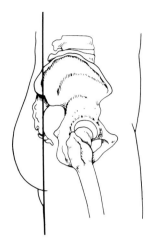

1. The anococcygeal ligament courses from the coccyx to the external anal sphincter.

2. Piriformis is exiting through the greater sciatic foramen.

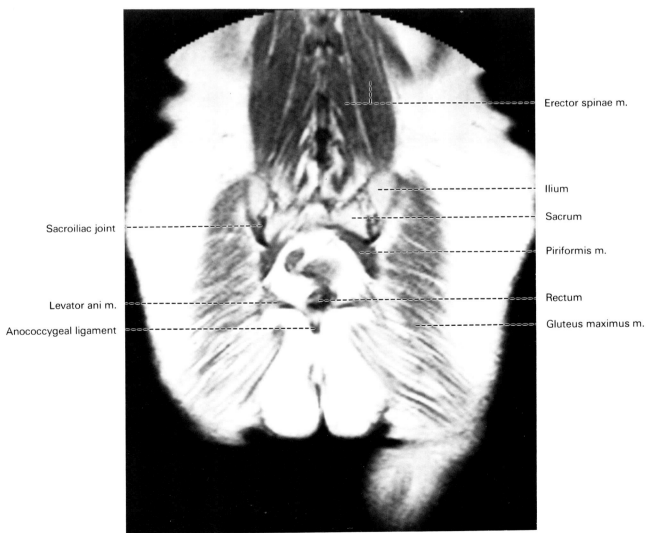

Figure 11.2.3

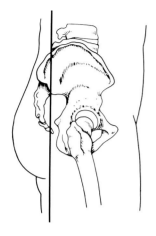

1. The uterine fundus is superior to the rectum.

2. The labia majora and the posterior wall of the vagina are seen.

3. The inferior gluteal artery exits under the piriformis muscle on the left.

4. Quadratus lumborum is lateral to the erector spinae complex.

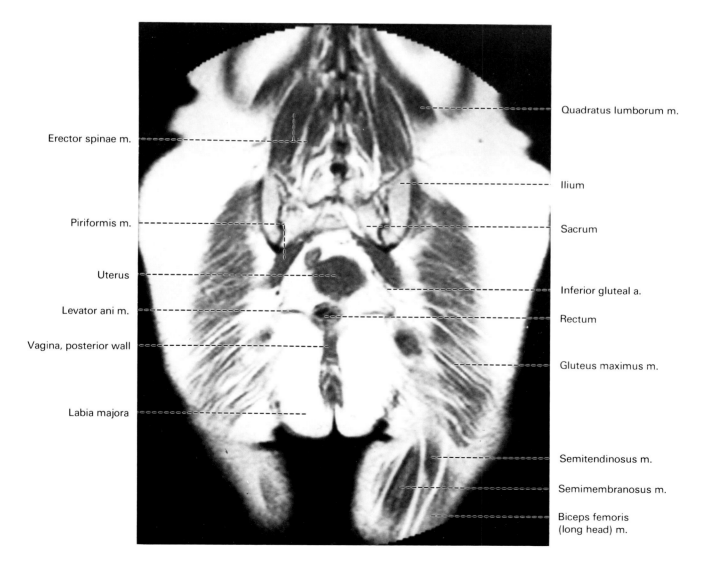

Figure 11.2.4

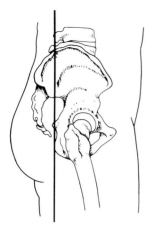

1. The vagina is again clearly identified.

2. Note levator ani arising from the tendinous arch of the obturator internus fascia.

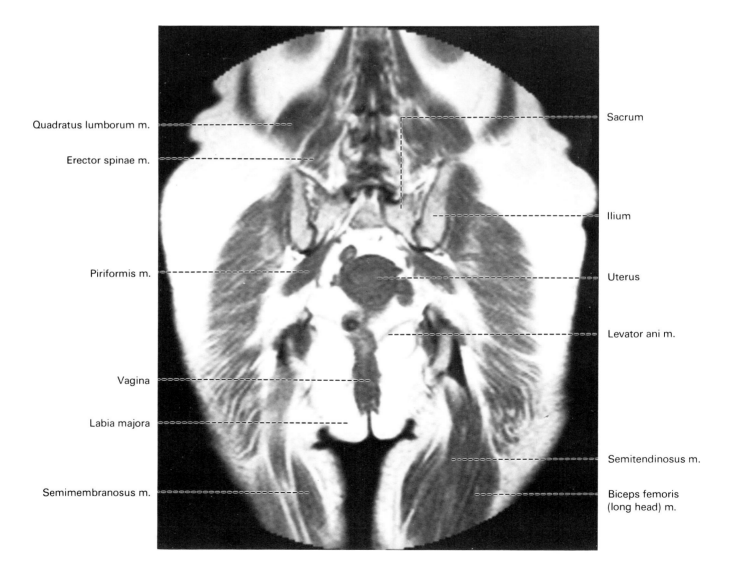

Quadratus lumborum m.

Erector spinae m.

Piriformis m.

Vagina

Labia majora

Semimembranosus m.

Sacrum

Ilium

Uterus

Levator ani m.

Semitendinosus m.

Biceps femoris (long head) m.

Figure 11.2.5

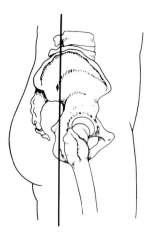

1. Note the corrugated mucosal surface of the vagina.

2. The uterovaginal vascular plexus is identified.

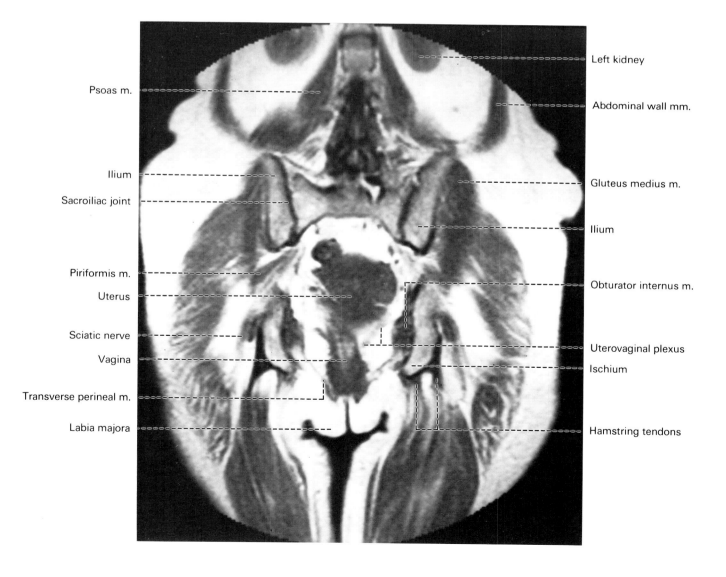

Psoas m.

Ilium

Sacroiliac joint

Piriformis m.

Uterus

Sciatic nerve

Vagina

Transverse perineal m.

Labia majora

Left kidney

Abdominal wall mm.

Gluteus medius m.

Ilium

Obturator internus m.

Uterovaginal plexus

Ischium

Hamstring tendons

Figure 11.2.6

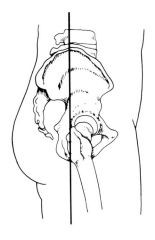

1. The superior gluteal vessels are seen exiting under the ilium through the greater sciatic notch.

2. Note the well-developed vesical plexus near the posterior wall of the urinary bladder.

3. The transverse perineal muscle lies on the inferior surface of the urogenital diaphragm.

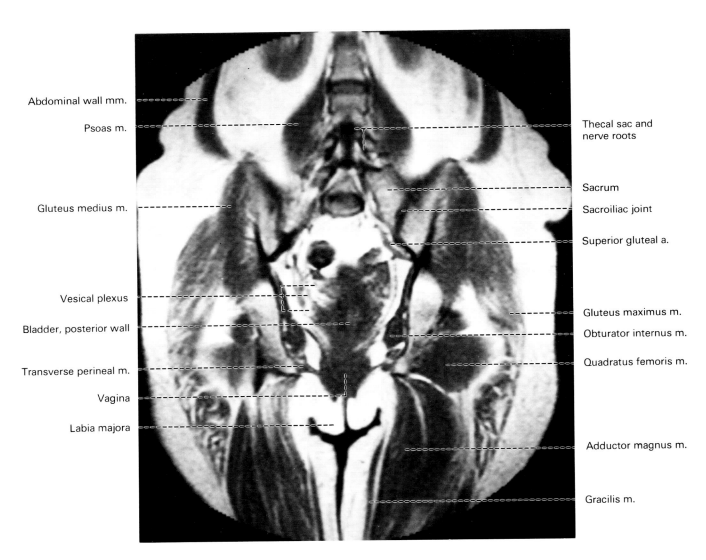

Abdominal wall mm.

Psoas m.

Gluteus medius m.

Vesical plexus

Bladder, posterior wall

Transverse perineal m.

Vagina

Labia majora

Thecal sac and nerve roots

Sacrum

Sacroiliac joint

Superior gluteal a.

Gluteus maximus m.

Obturator internus m.

Quadratus femoris m.

Adductor magnus m.

Gracilis m.

Figure 11.2.7

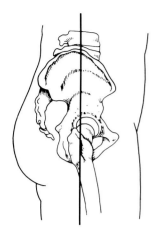

1. This section passes through the posterior portion of the urinary bladder.

2. The vesical plexus can be seen on the left.

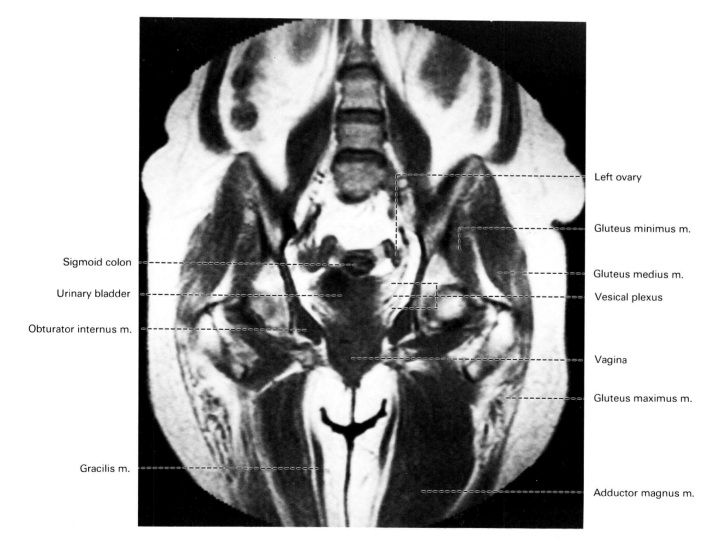

Left ovary

Gluteus minimus m.

Sigmoid colon

Gluteus medius m.

Urinary bladder

Vesical plexus

Obturator internus m.

Vagina

Gluteus maximus m.

Gracilis m.

Adductor magnus m.

Figure 11.2.8

1. The inferior portion of the vagina is seen below the bladder.

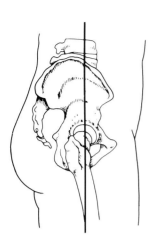

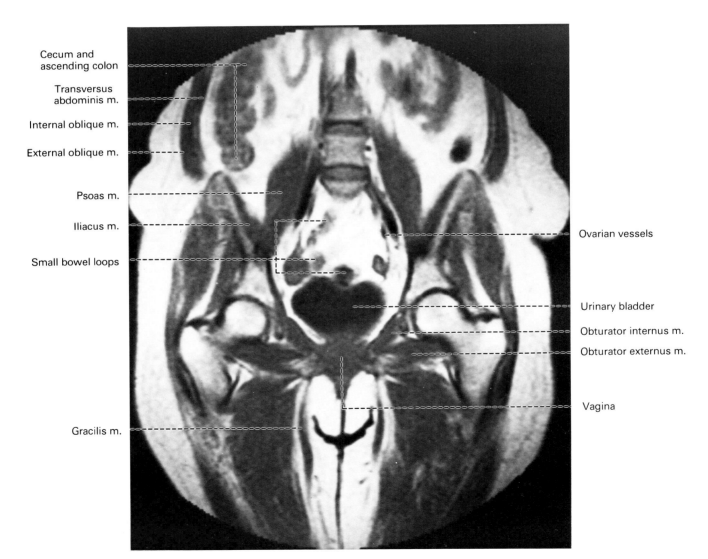

Cecum and ascending colon

Transversus abdominis m.

Internal oblique m.

External oblique m.

Psoas m.

Iliacus m.

Small bowel loops

Gracilis m.

Ovarian vessels

Urinary bladder

Obturator internus m.

Obturator externus m.

Vagina

Figure 11.3.1

1. This section passes through the obturator foramen and demonstrates the inferior and superior pubic rami.

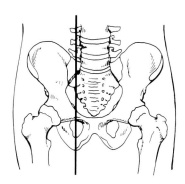

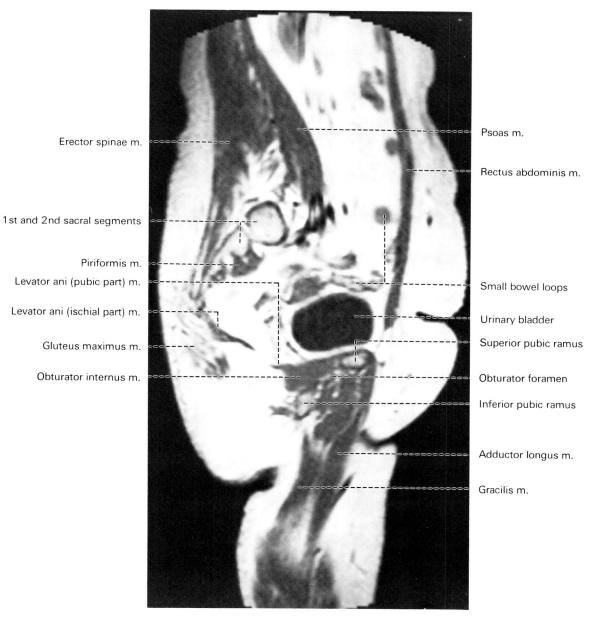

Erector spinae m.

Psoas m.

Rectus abdominis m.

1st and 2nd sacral segments

Piriformis m.

Levator ani (pubic part) m.

Small bowel loops

Levator ani (ischial part) m.

Urinary bladder

Gluteus maximus m.

Superior pubic ramus

Obturator internus m.

Obturator foramen

Inferior pubic ramus

Adductor longus m.

Gracilis m.

Figure 11.3.2

1. Note the two portions of levator ani.

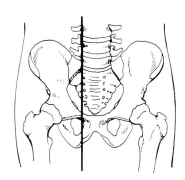

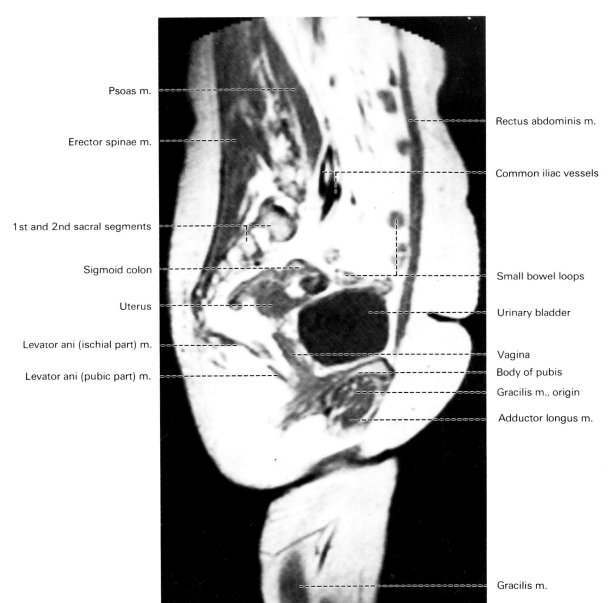

Psoas m.

Rectus abdominis m.

Erector spinae m.

Common iliac vessels

1st and 2nd sacral segments

Sigmoid colon

Small bowel loops

Uterus

Urinary bladder

Levator ani (ischial part) m.

Vagina

Levator ani (pubic part) m.

Body of pubis

Gracilis m., origin

Adductor longus m.

Gracilis m.

Figure 11.3.3

1. This section is slightly to the right of midline.

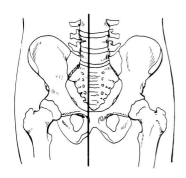

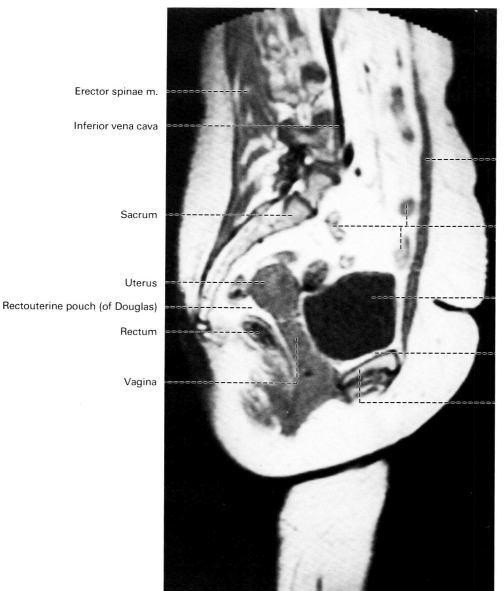

Erector spinae m.

Inferior vena cava

Rectus abdominis m.

Sacrum

Small bowel loops

Uterus

Rectouterine pouch (of Douglas)

Urinary bladder

Rectum

Retropubic (perivesical) space

Vagina

Body of pubis

Figure 11.3.4

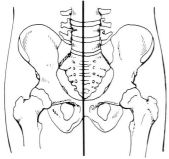

1. At this midline level the rectum and vagina are seen. Between them is the rectouterine pouch of Douglas.

2. The symphysis pubis is identified. The urethra courses posterior and inferior to the symphysis and is difficult to identify in females.

3. The external anal sphincter and anal canal are shown.

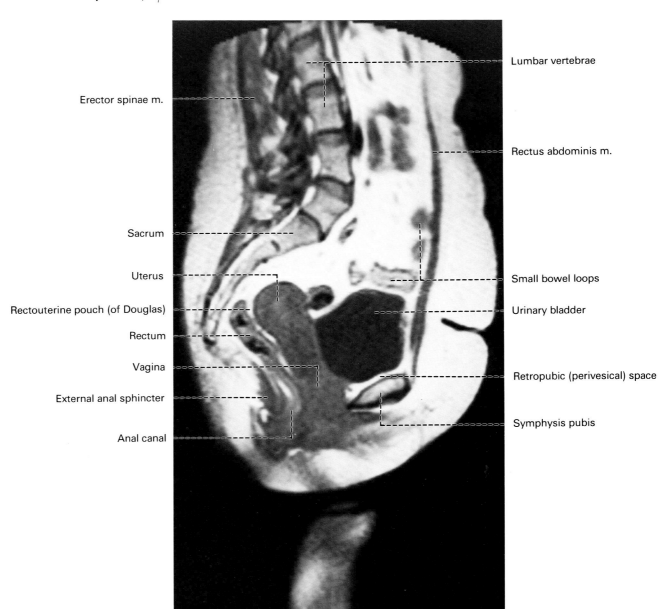

Figure 11.3.5

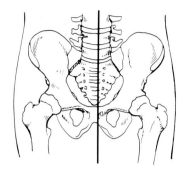

1. The vagina and uterus are clearly seen but the rectum is partially identified posterior to the uterus as this section approaches the midline.

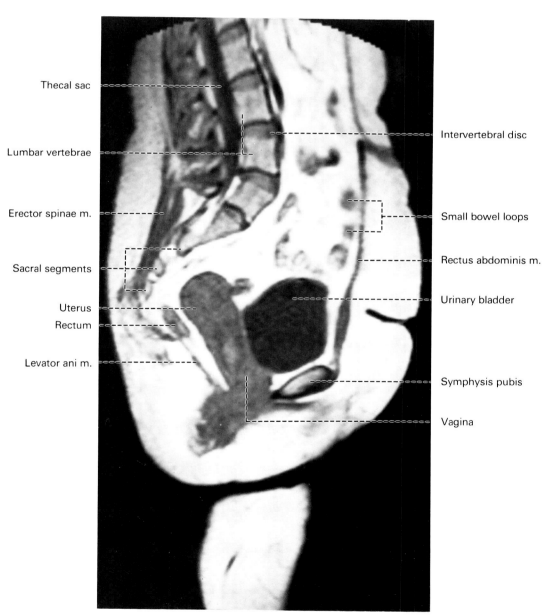

Figure 11.3.6

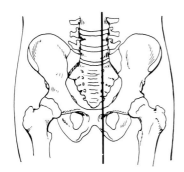

1. This image is slightly to the left of midline.

2. Note the clearly demonstrated levator ani, vagina, uterus, and bladder.

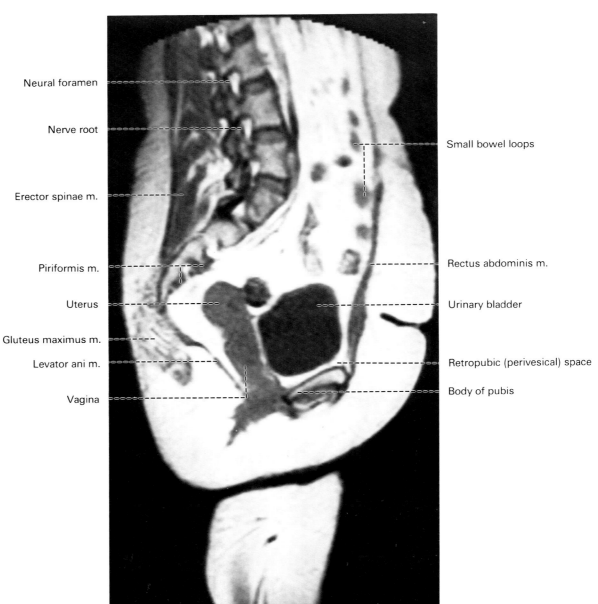

Neural foramen

Nerve root

Erector spinae m.

Piriformis m.

Uterus

Gluteus maximus m.

Levator ani m.

Vagina

Small bowel loops

Rectus abdominis m.

Urinary bladder

Retropubic (perivesical) space

Body of pubis

Figure 11.3.7

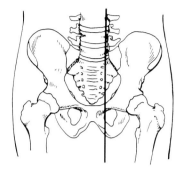

1. Both the vagina and the uterus are imaged in this section.

2. The inferior and superior pubic rami have fused to form the body of the pelvis.

3. The retropubic perivesical space is identified.

4. The nerve roots can be seen exiting the neural foramina.

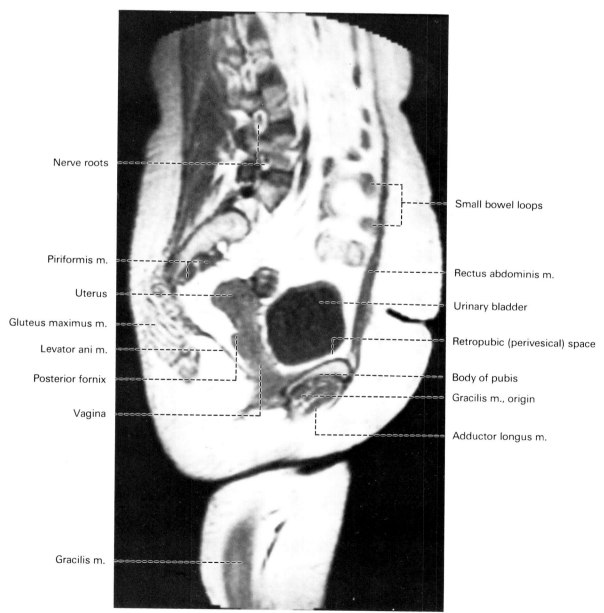

Nerve roots

Piriformis m.

Uterus

Gluteus maximus m.

Levator ani m.

Posterior fornix

Vagina

Gracilis m.

Small bowel loops

Rectus abdominis m.

Urinary bladder

Retropubic (perivesical) space

Body of pubis

Gracilis m., origin

Adductor longus m.

Figure 11.3.8

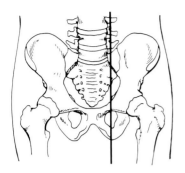

1. The urinary bladder and the uterus are partially demonstrated.

2. The iliococcygeal portion of levator ani is seen in this section with the muscle coursing toward the anus and median raphe.

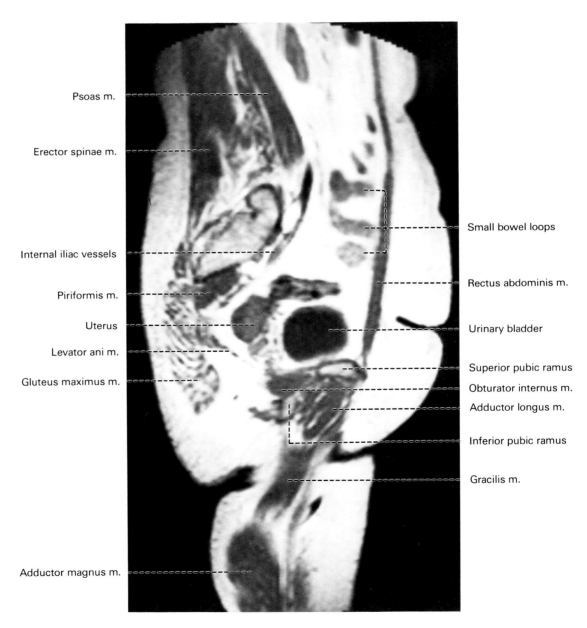

Psoas m.

Erector spinae m.

Small bowel loops

Internal iliac vessels

Rectus abdominis m.

Piriformis m.

Uterus — Urinary bladder

Levator ani m.

Gluteus maximus m. — Superior pubic ramus

Obturator internus m.

Adductor longus m.

Inferior pubic ramus

Gracilis m.

Adductor magnus m.

Figure 11.3.9

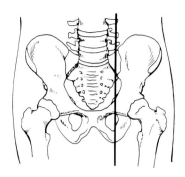

1. At this level the images are to the left of midline through the obturator foramen and obturator internus.

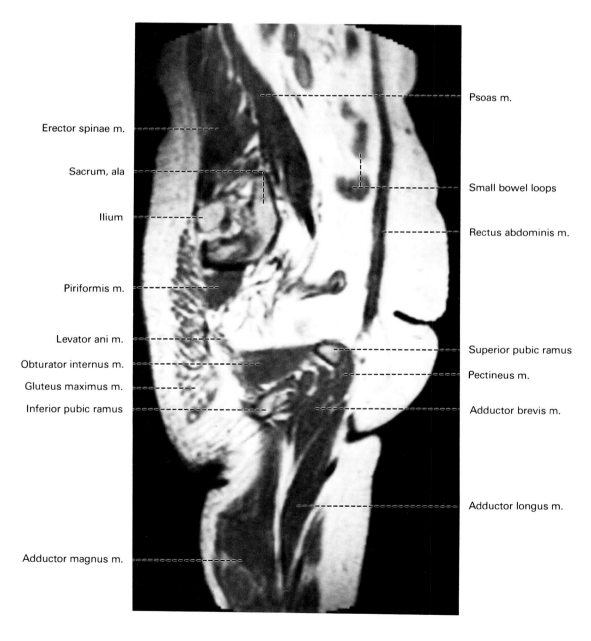

Erector spinae m.

Sacrum, ala

Ilium

Piriformis m.

Levator ani m.

Obturator internus m.

Gluteus maximus m.

Inferior pubic ramus

Adductor magnus m.

Psoas m.

Small bowel loops

Rectus abdominis m.

Superior pubic ramus

Pectineus m.

Adductor brevis m.

Adductor longus m.

V
SPINE

Chapter 12

THORACIC SPINE

Figure 12.1.1

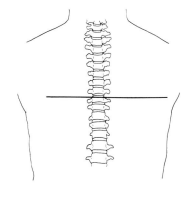

1. This section is through the upper T8 vertebral body near the superior end-plate.

2. Note the coronal orientation of T7-T8 zygapophyseal joint. This configuration is typical of these joints. The ribs, by way of the costovertebral articulations, stabilize the thoracic motion segments.

3. The azygos vein is anterior to the vertebral body but it may be to the left or right of midline.

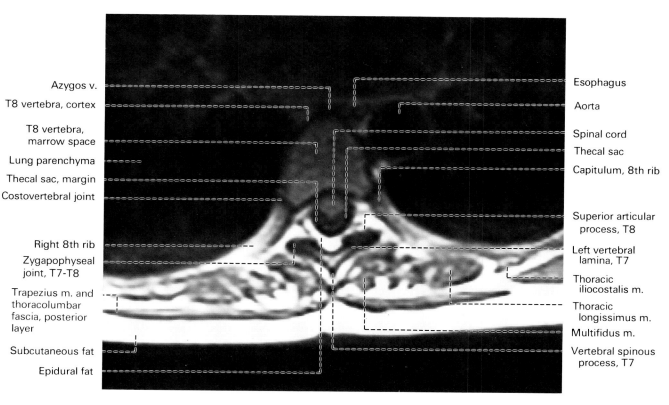

Azygos v.
T8 vertebra, cortex
T8 vertebra, marrow space
Lung parenchyma
Thecal sac, margin
Costovertebral joint
Right 8th rib
Zygapophyseal joint, T7-T8
Trapezius m. and thoracolumbar fascia, posterior layer
Subcutaneous fat
Epidural fat

Esophagus
Aorta
Spinal cord
Thecal sac
Capitulum, 8th rib
Superior articular process, T8
Left vertebral lamina, T7
Thoracic iliocostalis m.
Thoracic longissimus m.
Multifidus m.
Vertebral spinous process, T7

Figure 12.1.2

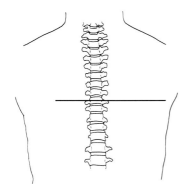

1. This section is through the upper third of the T8 body.

2. The usual thoracic kyphotic curve results in the eccentric position of the cord in the spinal canal. Note the cord is in close proximity to the T8 vertebral body. There is ample cerebrospinal fluid posterior to the cord and abundant posterior epidural fat.

3. The erector spinae muscles in the thoracic region are longissimus and iliocostalis. The longissimus is by far the bulkier of these two muscles.

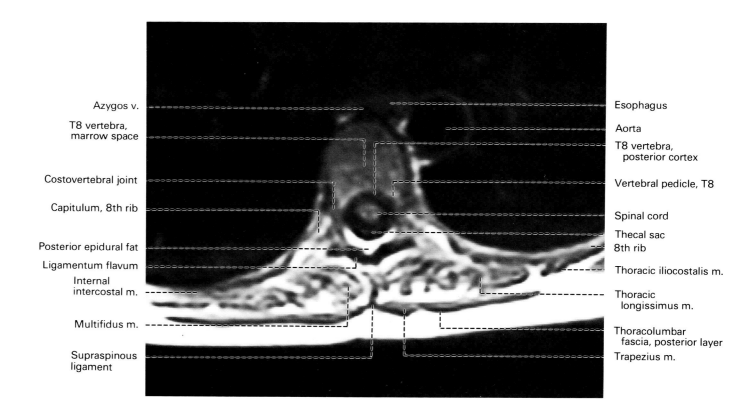

Azygos v.

T8 vertebra, marrow space

Costovertebral joint

Capitulum, 8th rib

Posterior epidural fat

Ligamentum flavum

Internal intercostal m.

Multifidus m.

Supraspinous ligament

Esophagus

Aorta

T8 vertebra, posterior cortex

Vertebral pedicle, T8

Spinal cord

Thecal sac
8th rib

Thoracic iliocostalis m.

Thoracic longissimus m.

Thoracolumbar fascia, posterior layer

Trapezius m.

Figure 12.1.3

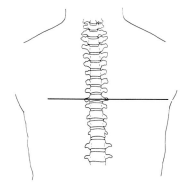

1. This section is through the middle third of the T8 body, at the level of the pedicles.

2. The hemiazygos vein joins the azygos vein, usually at the T8 level. The "hemiazygos-azygos arch" is demonstrated in this section. The variation of signal in these vessels is related to direction of flow (vertical, in the azygos and horizontal, in the hemiazygos arch).

3. A clearly defined structure adjacent to the T8 pedicle may be the sympathetic trunk.

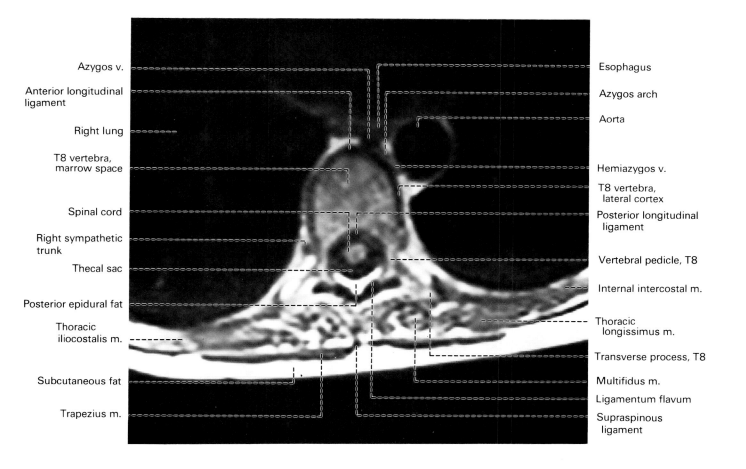

Figure 12.1.4

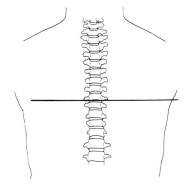

1. This section is through the lower third of the T8 body, with partial volume imaging of the inferior end-plate.

2. Fat in the vertebral marrow results in the bright signal on T1-weighted images. The end-plate (anterior) is identified by its lower signal.

3. Thoracic segmental neural elements are much smaller than the corresponding structures in the lumbar area.

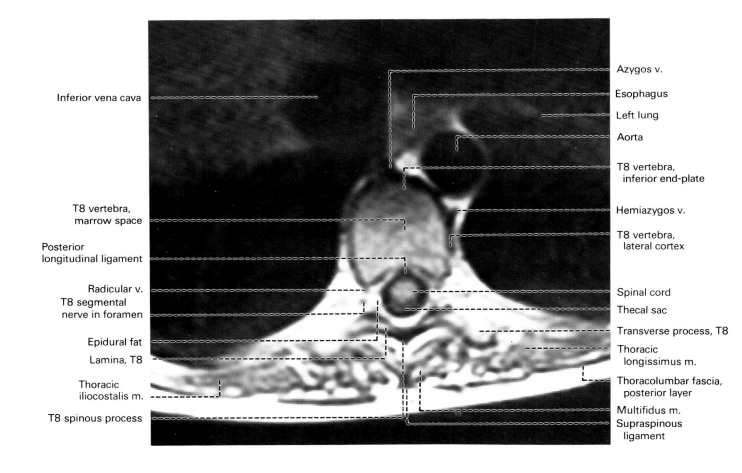

Azygos v.

Esophagus

Left lung

Aorta

T8 vertebra, inferior end-plate

Hemiazygos v.

T8 vertebra, lateral cortex

Spinal cord

Thecal sac

Transverse process, T8

Thoracic longissimus m.

Thoracolumbar fascia, posterior layer

Multifidus m.
Supraspinous ligament

Inferior vena cava

T8 vertebra, marrow space

Posterior longitudinal ligament

Radicular v.
T8 segmental nerve in foramen

Epidural fat
Lamina, T8

Thoracic iliocostalis m.

T8 spinous process

Figure 12.1.5

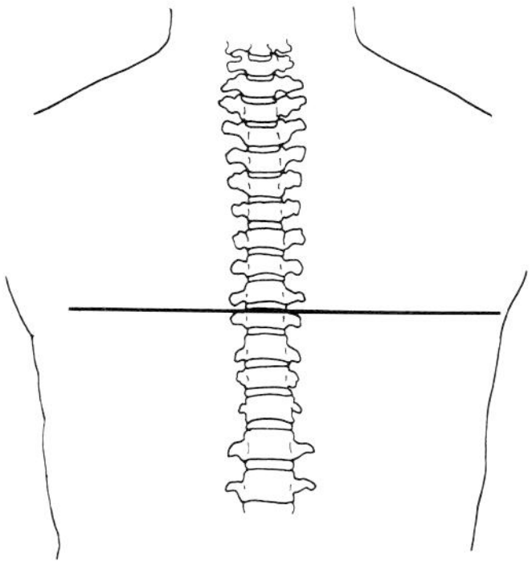

1. This section is through the T8-9 disc.

2. The thoracic longissimus muscle originates from multiple upper and midthoracic transverse processes. The thoracic iliocostalis muscle arises from the lower six or seven ribs. The distal tendons form the erector spinae aponeurosis and attach directly to the sacrum and ilium. This aponeurosis is a major component of the thoracolumbar fascia.

3. The size and configuration of the thoracic cord is uniform with the exception of the conus. At the level of the conus there is generalized enlargement of the cord.

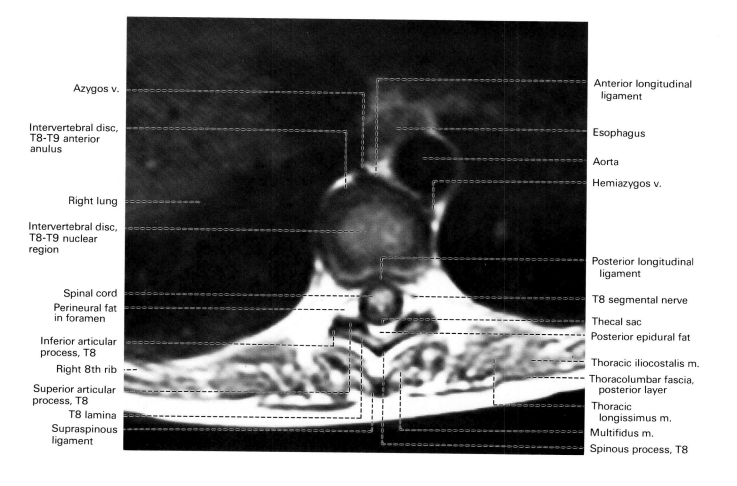

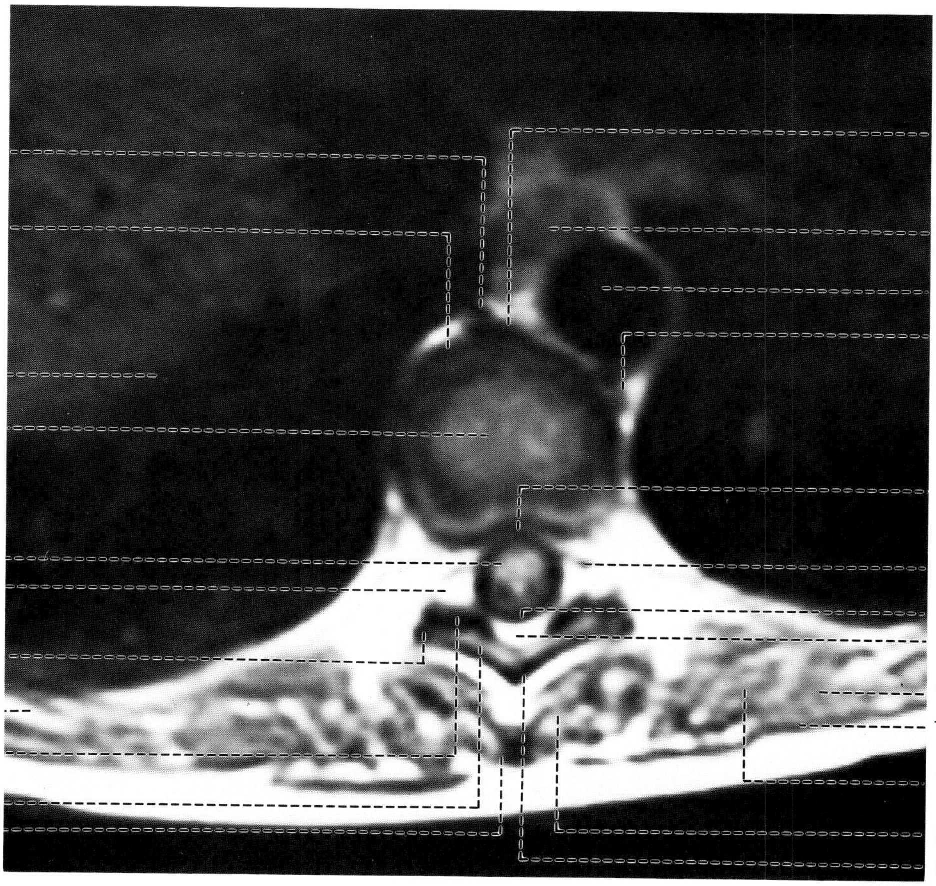
Azygos v.
Intervertebral disc, T8-T9 anterior anulus
Right lung
Intervertebral disc, T8-T9 nuclear region
Spinal cord
Perineural fat in foramen
Inferior articular process, T8
Right 8th rib
Superior articular process, T8
T8 lamina
Supraspinous ligament
Anterior longitudinal ligament
Esophagus
Aorta
Hemiazygos v.
Posterior longitudinal ligament
T8 segmental nerve
Thecal sac
Posterior epidural fat
Thoracic iliocostalis m.
Thoracolumbar fascia, posterior layer
Thoracic longissimus m.
Multifidus m.
Spinous process, T8

Figure 12.2.1

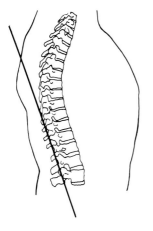

1. This section is through the spinous processes of the mid- and lower thoracic spine.

2. Fascicles of the thoracic longissimus muscle arise from the transverse processes and ribs of each segment. The distal tendon attaches to the ilium, sacrum, and spinous processes of lumbar and sacral segments.

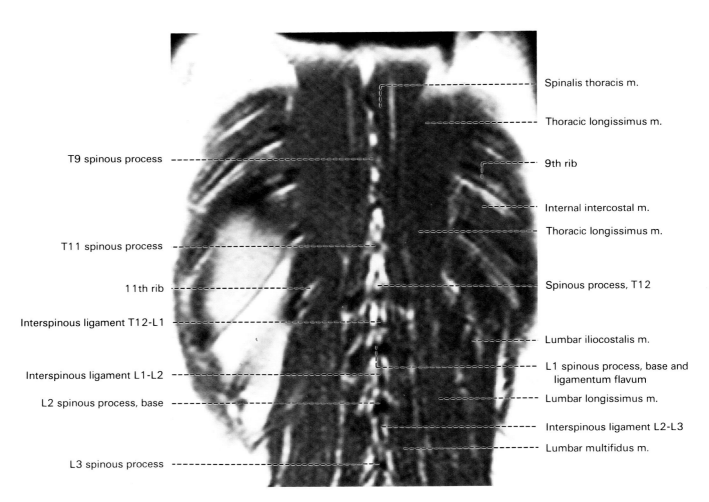

T9 spinous process

T11 spinous process

11th rib

Interspinous ligament T12-L1

Interspinous ligament L1-L2

L2 spinous process, base

L3 spinous process

Spinalis thoracis m.

Thoracic longissimus m.

9th rib

Internal intercostal m.

Thoracic longissimus m.

Spinous process, T12

Lumbar iliocostalis m.

L1 spinous process, base and ligamentum flavum

Lumbar longissimus m.

Interspinous ligament L2-L3

Lumbar multifidus m.

Figure 12.2.2

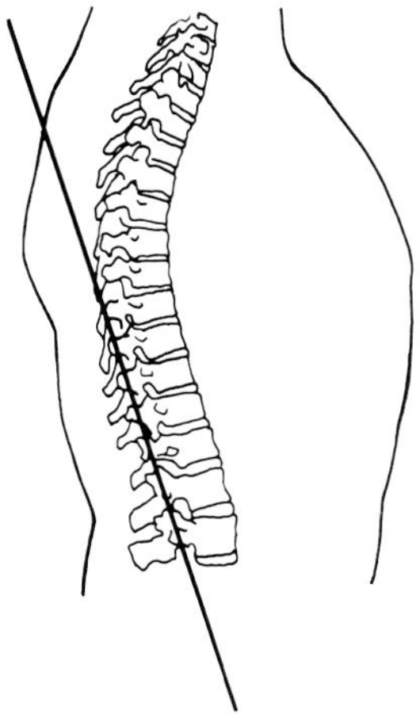

1. This section is through the posterior arches of lower thoracic segments.
2. All of the thoracic zygapophyseal joints are oriented in the coronal plane. The T12-L1 joints are usually parasagittal in orientation. The thoracic joints are not usually identifiable on coronal images.

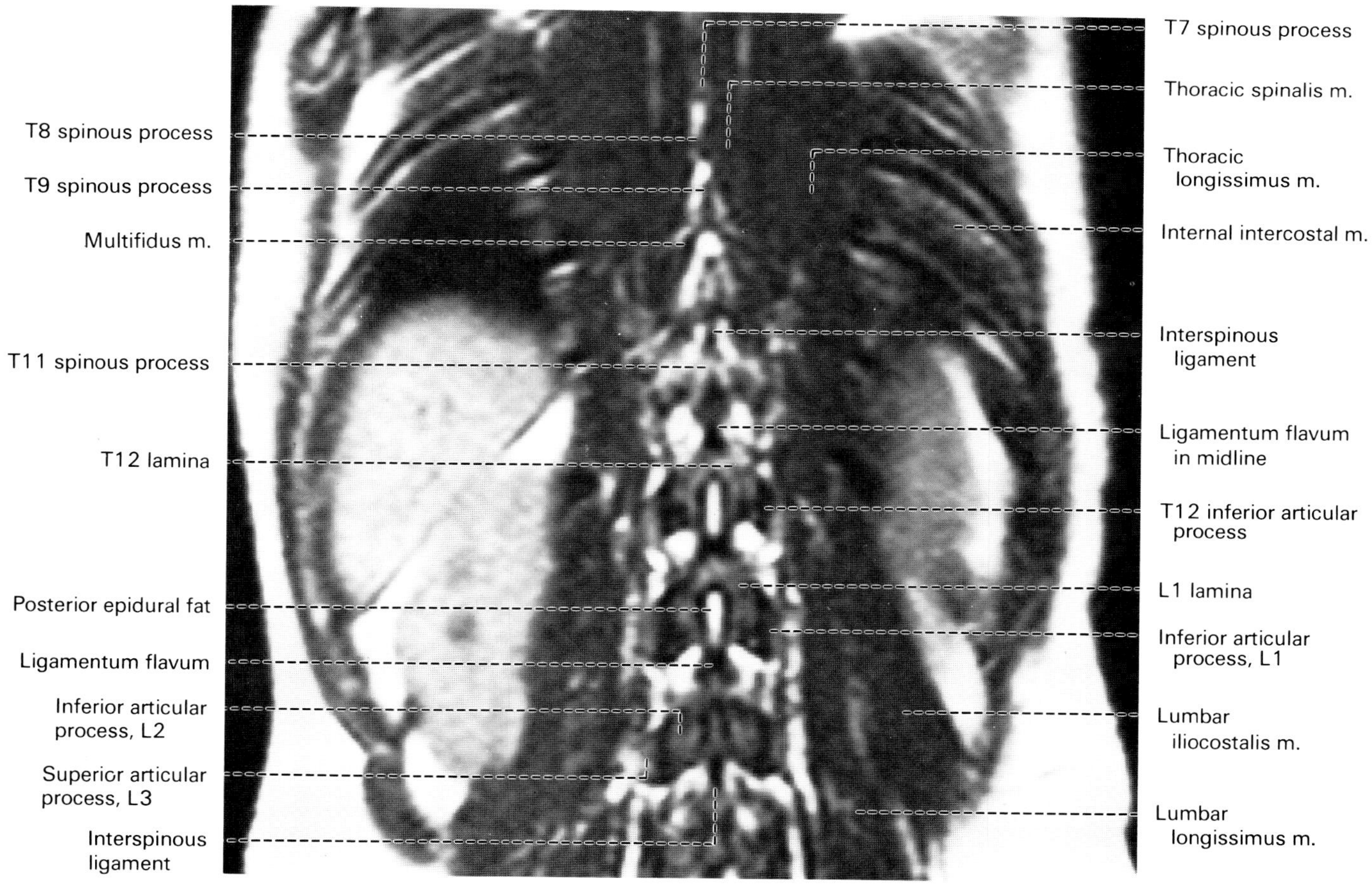
T7 spinous process
Thoracic spinalis m.
T8 spinous process
T9 spinous process
Thoracic longissimus m.
Multifidus m.
Internal intercostal m.
Interspinous ligament
T11 spinous process
Ligamentum flavum in midline
T12 lamina
T12 inferior articular process
L1 lamina
Posterior epidural fat
Inferior articular process, L1
Ligamentum flavum
Inferior articular process, L2
Lumbar iliocostalis m.
Superior articular process, L3
Lumbar longissimus m.
Interspinous ligament

Figure 12.2.3

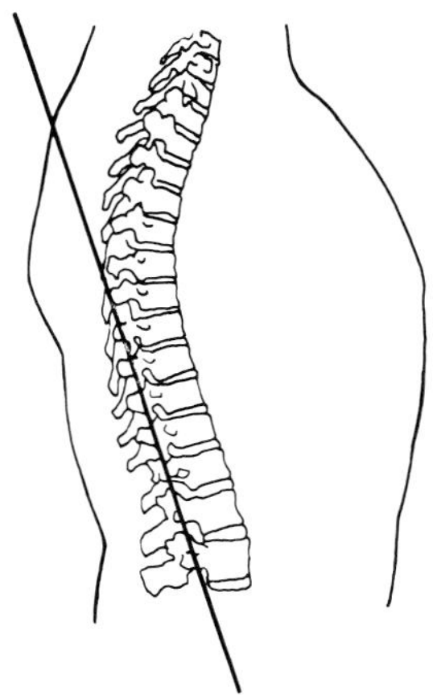

1. This section is through the transverse processes of the thoracolumbar junction.

2. The ligamentum flavum joins the laminae of adjacent vertebrae. Laterally the ligament extends in front of the articular processes to form the joint capsule of the zygapophyseal joint.

3. Paired ascending lumbar veins course just anterior to the transverse processes. They become azygos (right) and hemiazygos (left) veins in the thoracic region.

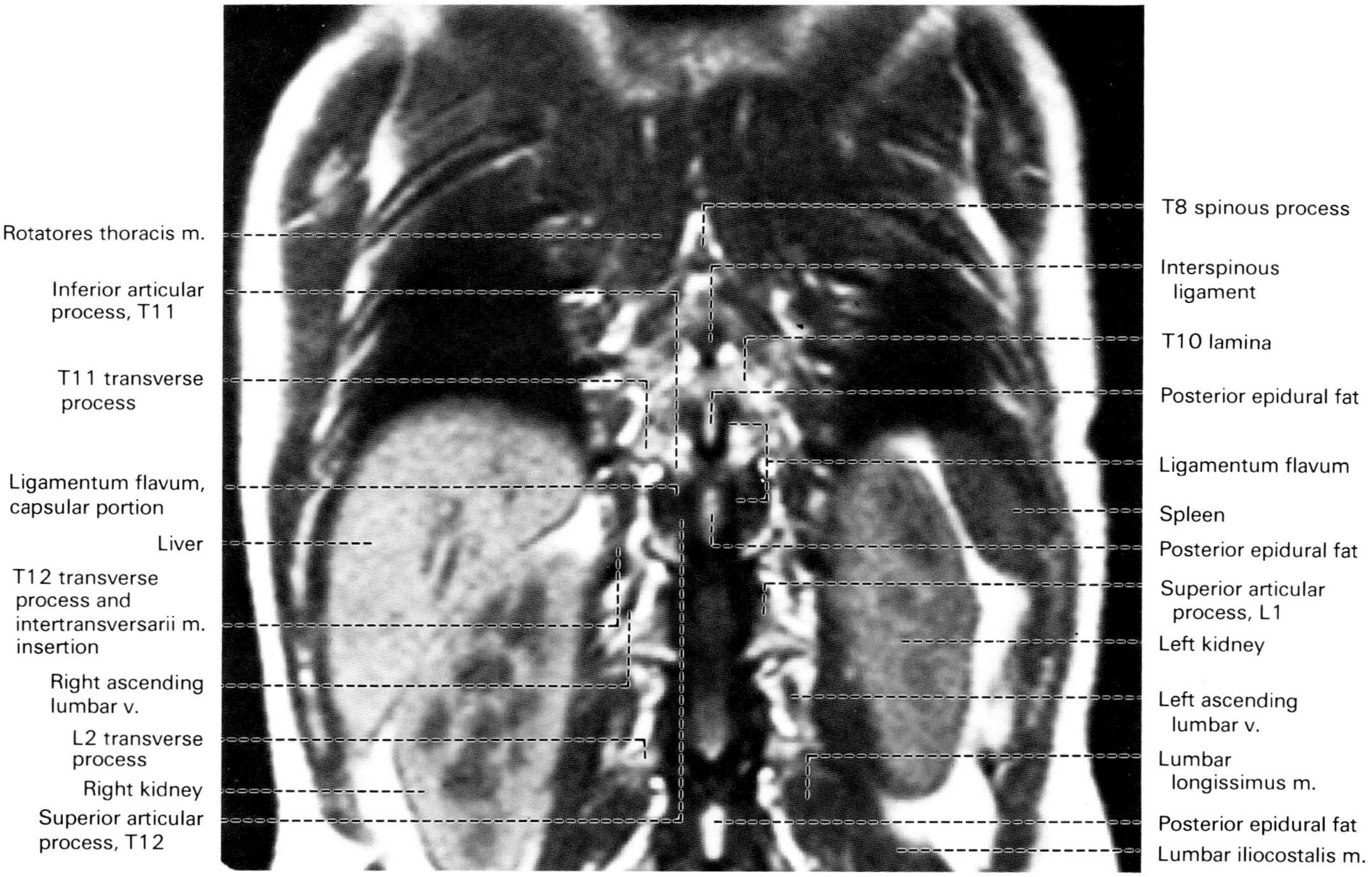

Rotatores thoracis m.
Inferior articular process, T11
T11 transverse process
Ligamentum flavum, capsular portion
Liver
T12 transverse process and intertransversarii m. insertion
Right ascending lumbar v.
L2 transverse process
Right kidney
Superior articular process, T12
T8 spinous process
Interspinous ligament
T10 lamina
Posterior epidural fat
Ligamentum flavum
Spleen
Posterior epidural fat
Superior articular process, L1
Left kidney
Left ascending lumbar v.
Lumbar longissimus m.
Posterior epidural fat
Lumbar iliocostalis m.

Figure 12.2.4

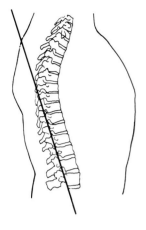

1. This section is through the mid-central canal at the level of the thoraco-lumbar junction.

2. The localized enlargement of the conus medullaris tapers to terminate between T12 and L2, in most instances.

3. Segmental neural elements are usually recognizable, and the dorsal root ganglia are frequently outlined by perineural fat.

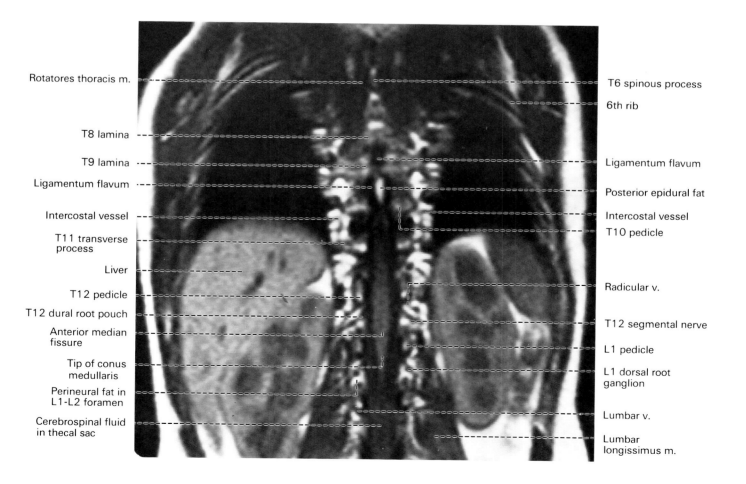

Figure 12.2.5

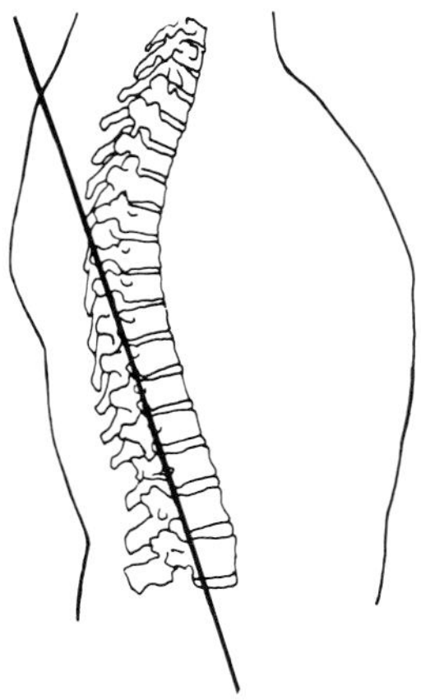

1. This section is through the anterior central canal at the thoracolumbar junction.

2. The psoas major muscle arises from transverse processes and lateral vertebral body attachments. On coronal sections the highest attachment is usually at the T12 level.

3. Paired intercostal vessels (veins and arteries) course laterally in paraspinous fat to the inferior surface of the ribs.

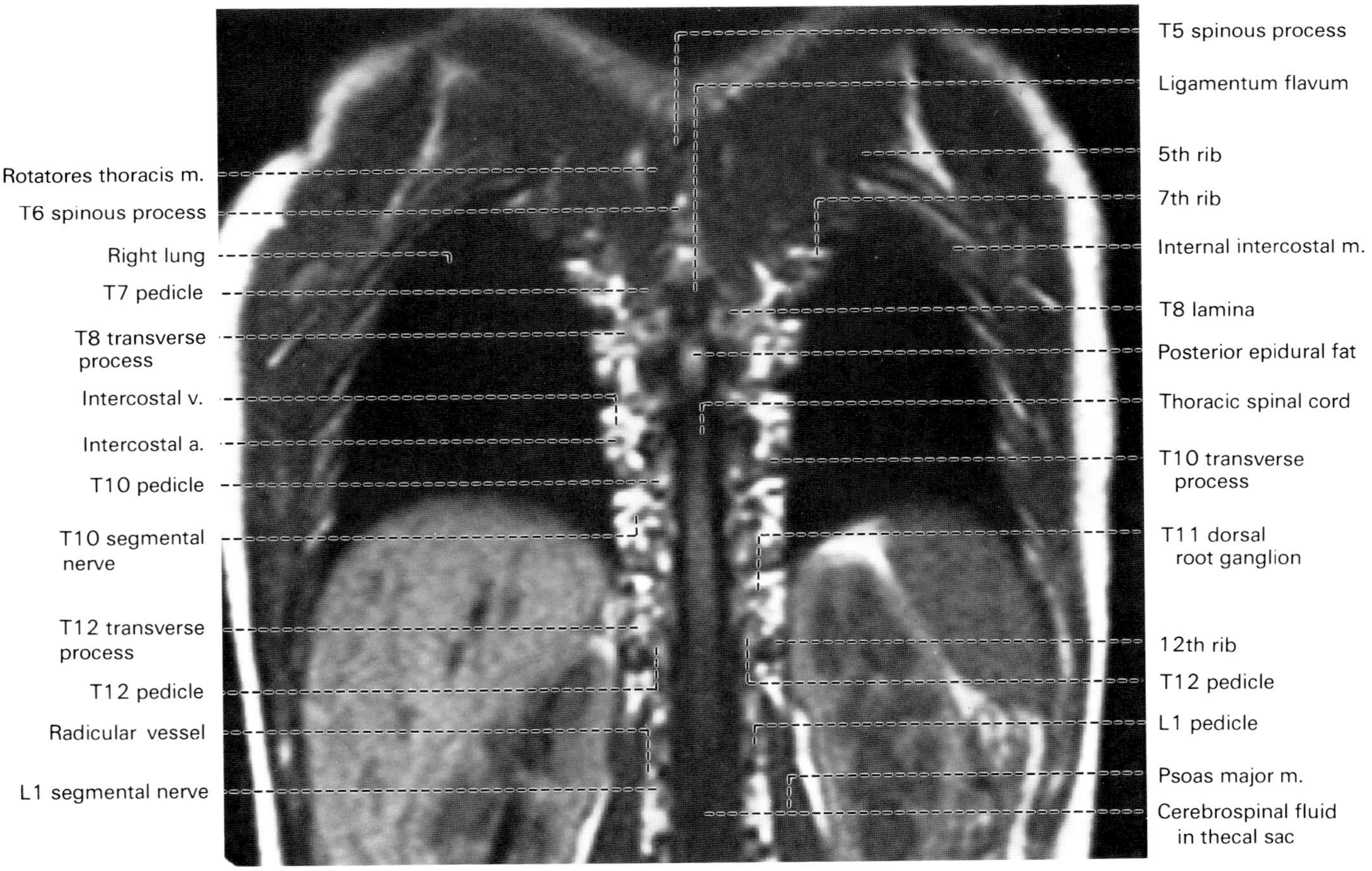
Rotatores thoracis m.
T6 spinous process
Right lung
T7 pedicle
T8 transverse process
Intercostal v.
Intercostal a.
T10 pedicle
T10 segmental nerve
T12 transverse process
T12 pedicle
Radicular vessel
L1 segmental nerve
T5 spinous process
Ligamentum flavum
5th rib
7th rib
Internal intercostal m.
T8 lamina
Posterior epidural fat
Thoracic spinal cord
T10 transverse process
T11 dorsal root ganglion
12th rib
T12 pedicle
L1 pedicle
Psoas major m.
Cerebrospinal fluid in thecal sac

Figure 12.2.6

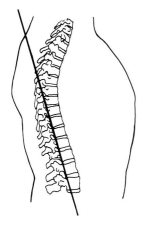

1. This section is through the posterior vertebral bodies at the thoracolumbar junction.

2. The pedicles serve to define the transverse diameter of the central canal.

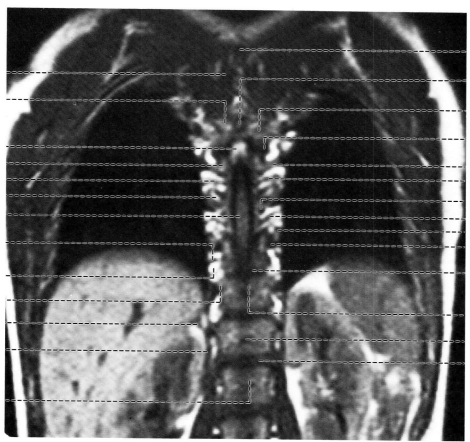

Rotatores thoracis m.

Superior articular process, T7

Posterior epidural fat

T8 pedicle

T8 segmental nerve

9th rib

Thoracic spinal cord

T10 segmental nerve

Perineural fat

T11 pedicle

Right adrenal gland

Right diaphragmatic crus

L1 vertebra, marrow space

T5 spinous process

T7 spinous process

Inferior articular process, T7

T7-T8 facet joint and capsular ligament

T8 transverse process

T8 segmental nerve

T9 pedicle

T9 segmental nerve

10th rib

Costovertebral articulation

Intervertebral disc, T10-T11 posterior anulus

T11 vertebra, marrow space

T12 vertebra

Intervertebral disc, T12-L1 posterior anulus

Figure 12.2.7

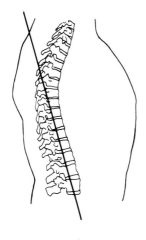

1. This section is through the posterior vertebrae of the lower thoracic spine (T9-T12).

2. The large circular collection of fat in the midvertebral bodies surrounds the basivertebral veins and is a constant feature on coronal images. These are the principal veins of the vertebral body.

3. The vertebral end-plates are usually sharply defined.

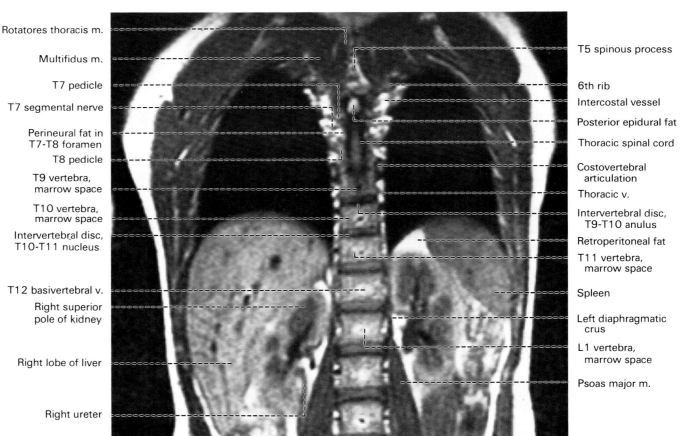

Rotatores thoracis m.

Multifidus m.

T7 pedicle

T7 segmental nerve

Perineural fat in T7-T8 foramen

T8 pedicle

T9 vertebra, marrow space

T10 vertebra, marrow space

Intervertebral disc, T10-T11 nucleus

T12 basivertebral v.

Right superior pole of kidney

Right lobe of liver

Right ureter

T5 spinous process

6th rib

Intercostal vessel

Posterior epidural fat

Thoracic spinal cord

Costovertebral articulation

Thoracic v.

Intervertebral disc, T9-T10 anulus

Retroperitoneal fat

T11 vertebra, marrow space

Spleen

Left diaphragmatic crus

L1 vertebra, marrow space

Psoas major m.

Figure 12.2.8

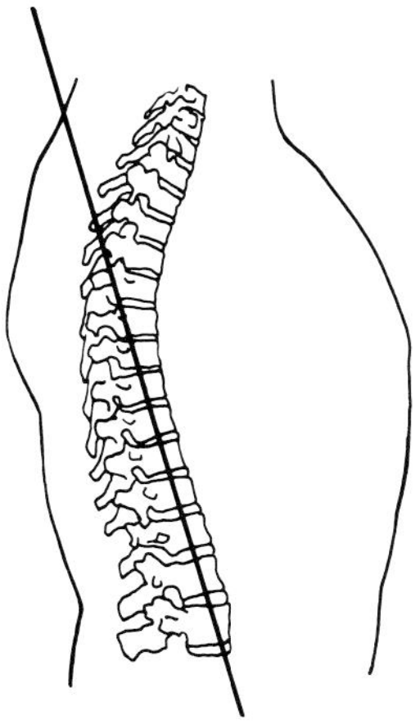

1. This section is through the mid-coronal plane of the vertebral bodies at the thoracolumbar junction.

2. Varying amounts of fat surround the basivertebral veins. The signal from the marrow space is otherwise homogeneous and of intermediate intensity.

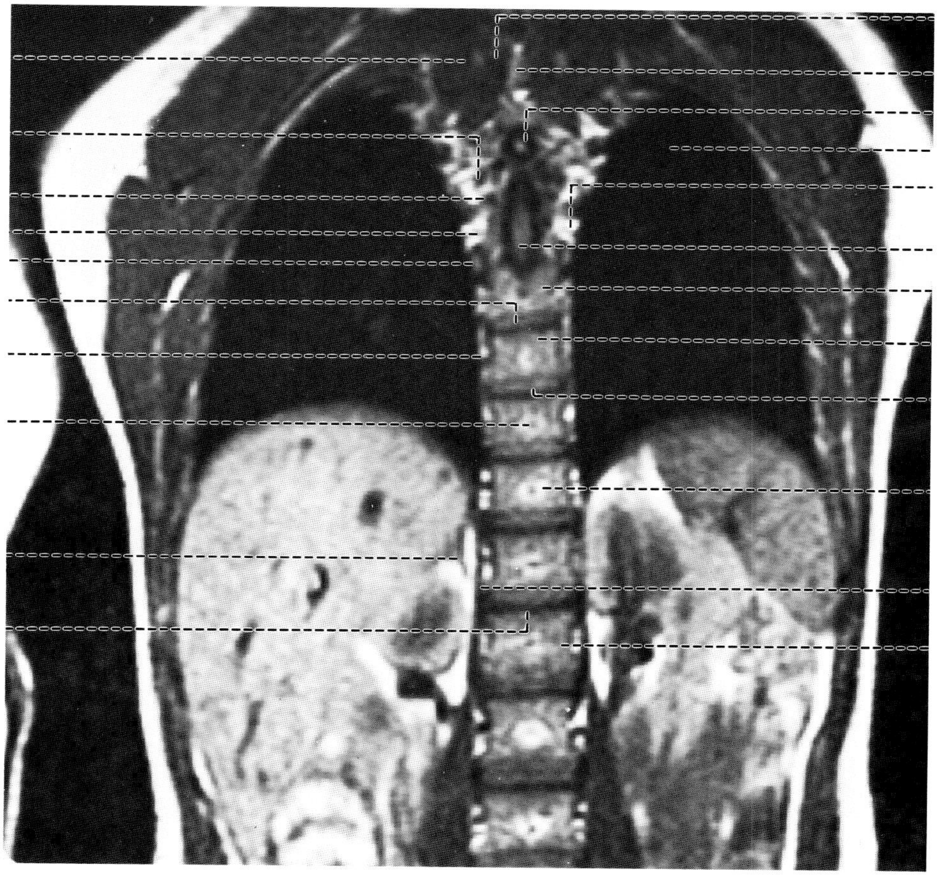

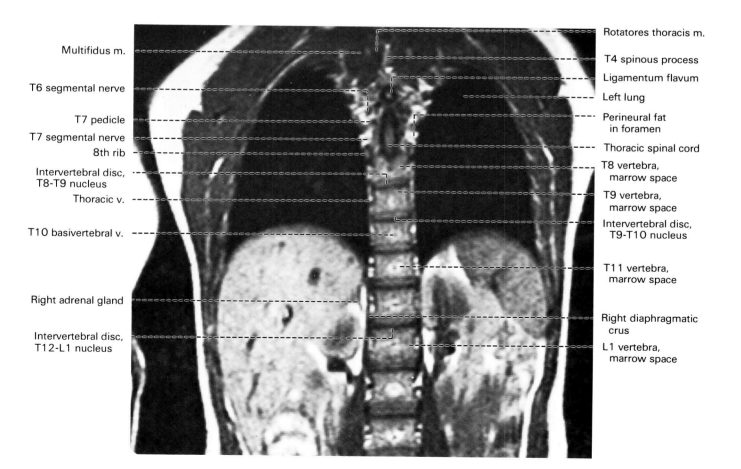

Multifidus m.
T6 segmental nerve
T7 pedicle
T7 segmental nerve
8th rib
Intervertebral disc, T8-T9 nucleus
Thoracic v.
T10 basivertebral v.
Right adrenal gland
Intervertebral disc, T12-L1 nucleus
Rotatores thoracis m.
T4 spinous process
Ligamentum flavum
Left lung
Perineural fat in foramen
Thoracic spinal cord
T8 vertebra, marrow space
T9 vertebra, marrow space
Intervertebral disc, T9-T10 nucleus
T11 vertebra, marrow space
Right diaphragmatic crus
L1 vertebra, marrow space

Figure 12.3.1

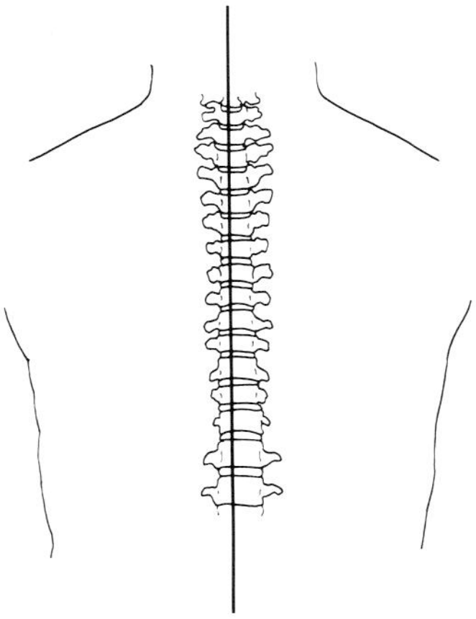

1. This right parasagittal section is through the articular processes.

2. The sagittal plane demonstrates the anatomy of the thoracic zygapophyseal joints. Note the anterior position of the superior articular processes relative to the inferior articular processes of the vertebrae above.

3. The zygapophyseal joint is enclosed by a fibrous capsule. The ligaments are redundant at the superior and inferior poles of the joint; this allows the gliding motion that is characteristic of these articulations. This ligamentous redundancy forms articular recesses. The anterior capsular ligament is formed by lateral extension of the ligamentum flavum.

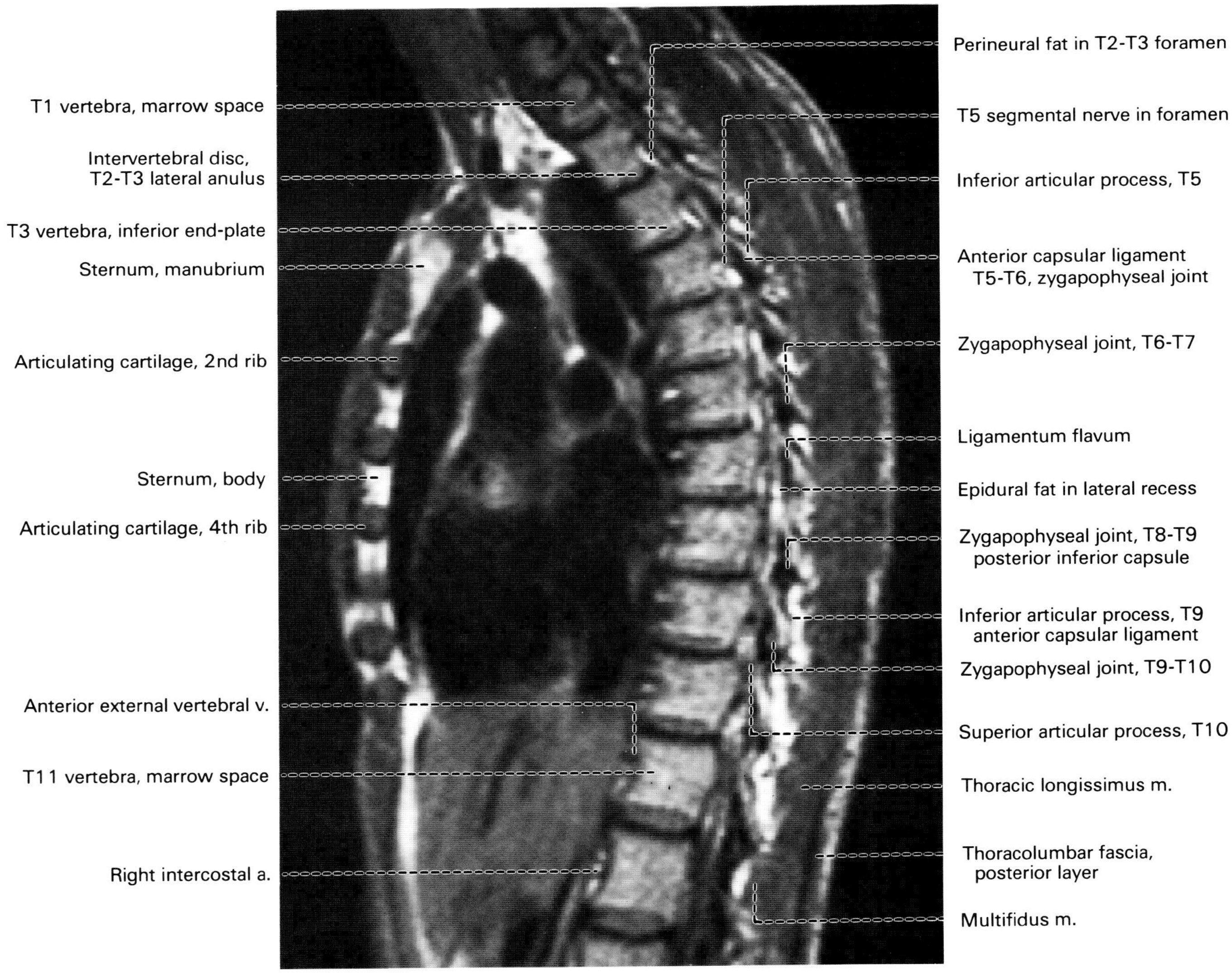
T1 vertebra, marrow space
Intervertebral disc, T2-T3 lateral anulus
T3 vertebra, inferior end-plate
Sternum, manubrium
Articulating cartilage, 2nd rib
Sternum, body
Articulating cartilage, 4th rib
Anterior external vertebral v.
T11 vertebra, marrow space
Right intercostal a.
Perineural fat in T2-T3 foramen
T5 segmental nerve in foramen
Inferior articular process, T5
Anterior capsular ligament T5-T6, zygapophyseal joint
Zygapophyseal joint, T6-T7
Ligamentum flavum
Epidural fat in lateral recess
Zygapophyseal joint, T8-T9 posterior inferior capsule
Inferior articular process, T9 anterior capsular ligament
Zygapophyseal joint, T9-T10
Superior articular process, T10
Thoracic longissimus m.
Thoracolumbar fascia, posterior layer
Multifidus m.

Figure 12.3.2

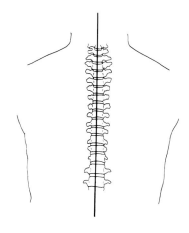

1. This right parasagittal section is through the lamina.

2. Sagittal sections best demonstrate the laminar/ligamentous relationships. The ligamentum flavum extends from the anterior surface of the upper lamina to attach on the posterior aspect of the superior surface of the lamina below.

3. "Circumferential" vessels are located at the midbody level. Both intercostal arteries and components of the anterior external vertebral venous plexus can be routinely identified. The venous structure is usually the larger of the pair.

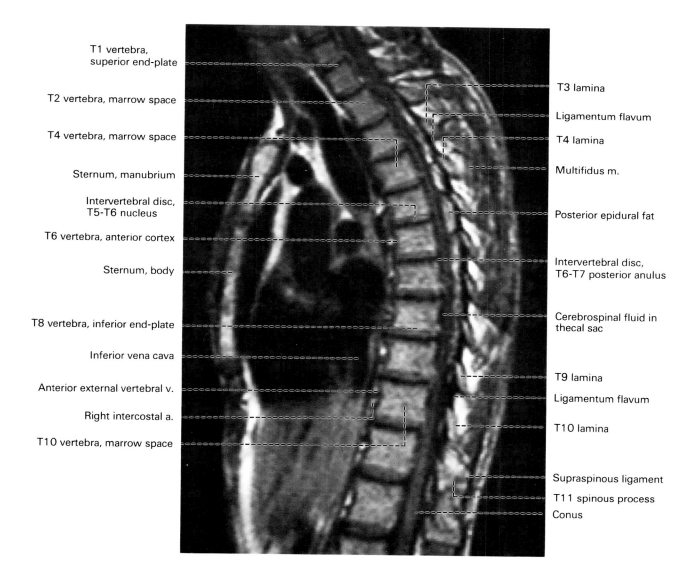

T1 vertebra, superior end-plate

T2 vertebra, marrow space

T4 vertebra, marrow space

Sternum, manubrium

Intervertebral disc, T5-T6 nucleus

T6 vertebra, anterior cortex

Sternum, body

T8 vertebra, inferior end-plate

Inferior vena cava

Anterior external vertebral v.

Right intercostal a.

T10 vertebra, marrow space

T3 lamina

Ligamentum flavum

T4 lamina

Multifidus m.

Posterior epidural fat

Intervertebral disc, T6-T7 posterior anulus

Cerebrospinal fluid in thecal sac

T9 lamina

Ligamentum flavum

T10 lamina

Supraspinous ligament

T11 spinous process

Conus

Figure 12.3.3

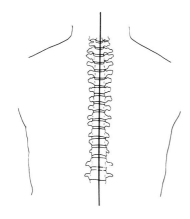

1. This section is through the midline of the dorsal spine.

2. Note the normal dorsal kyphosis. The spinal cord occupies the anterior aspect of the central canal as a result of this curve. Abundant posterior epidural fat occupies the posterior central canal.

3. Midline ligaments connect the adjacent spinous processes. The interspinous ligament is segmental, connecting the spinous processes. The supraspinous ligament is intersegmental, attaching to the tips of the spinous processes.

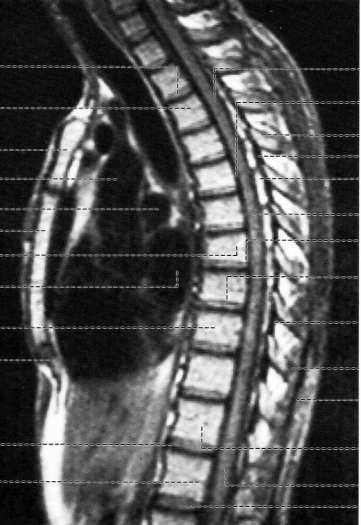

Intervertebral disc, T2-T3 nucleus

T3 vertebra, marrow space

Sternum, manubrium

Ascending aorta

Pulmonary a.

Sternum, body

T7 vertebra and basivertebral v.

Left atrium

T9 vertebra, marrow space

Tip of xiphoid process

Intervertebral disc, T11-T12 anterior nucleus

T12 vertebra and basivertebral v.

Upper thoracic spinal cord

T5 vertebra, posterior cortex

T4 spinous process

Ligamentum flavum at T4-T5

Posterior epidural fat

Thoracic cord at T6 level

Intervertebral disc, T7-T8 posterior anulus

Intervertebral disc, T8-T9 nucleus

Ligamentum flavum at T8-T9

T9 spinous process

Supraspinous ligament

T11 vertebra, marrow space at T9-T10

Conus

Intervertebral disc, T12-L1 nucleus

Figure 12.3.4

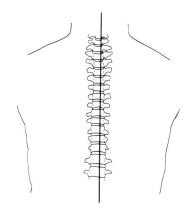

1. This left paracentral sagittal section is through the lamina.

2. The intervertebral discs are thin in the upper thoracic spine and become progressively thicker at lower levels.

3. The broad, flat thoracic laminae are angled caudally and overlap one another resulting in a "shingle"-like osseous cover for the central canal.

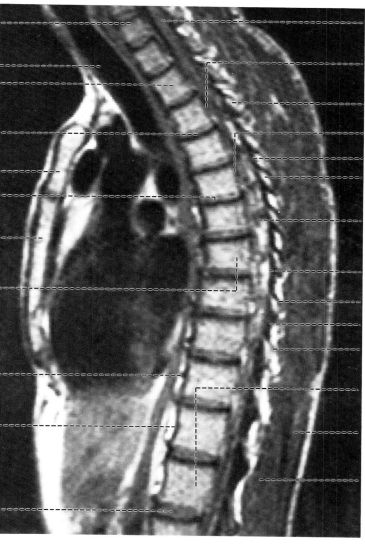

C7 vertebra, marrow space

Trachea

T2 vertebra, marrow space

T4 vertebra, superior end-plate

Sternum, manubrium

Intervertebral disc, T5-T6 nucleus

Sternum, body

T7 vertebra, marrow space

Anterior external vertebral v.

T11 vertebra, anterior cortex

Intervertebral disc, T12-L1 anterior anulus

Cervical spinal cord

T3 vertebra, posterior cortex

T3 lamina

T5 vertebra, posterior cortex

Ligamentum flavum

T5 lamina

T6 segmental nerve in foramen

Posterior epidural fat

T8 lamina

Ligamentum flavum

T9 lamina

T12 vertebra, marrow space

Thoracic longissimus m.

Lumbar longissimus m.

Figure 12.3.5

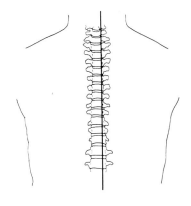

1. This left parasagittal section is through the neural foramina.

2. The thoracic segmental nerves are thin and occupy a small portion of the space available in the intervertebral foramen. Multiple radicular vessels are frequently identifiable in the abundant perineural fat in the midforamen.

3. Bone and ligamentous structures form the boundaries of the intervertebral foramen. The undersurface of the pedicle above and the superior surface of the pedicle below form the upper and lower margins of the foramen. The posterior cortex of the lower half of the vertebral body, the inferior end-plate, and the disc anulus form the anterior boundary. The anterior capsular ligament of the zygapophyseal joint and the superior articular process of the subjacent vertebra form the posterior boundary of the foramen.

Proximal esophagus	T3 pedicle
	Inferior articular process, T3
	Anterior capsular ligament, T3–T4 zygapophyseal joint
	T4 segmental nerve, dorsal root ganglion
Perineural fat in foramen	Radicular v.
	T5 pedicle
T5 vertebra, posterior cortex	T5 dorsal root ganglion
Intervertebral disc, T5–T6 posterior anulus	
	Inferior articular process, T7
Left atrium	Anterior capsular ligament, T7–T8 joint
T8 vertebra, marrow space	Superior articular process, T8
Hemiazygos v.	
	T9 pedicle, inferior cortex
	T10 vertebra, anterior cortex
Distal esophagus	T10 segmental nerve in foramen
T11 pedicle, superior cortex	T11 pedicle
	Inferior articular process, T11
Intervertebral disc, T11–T12 nucleus	T11–T12 zygapophyseal joint
T12 vertebra, marrow space	Radicular (perineural) vv.
Aorta	

Figure 12.3.6

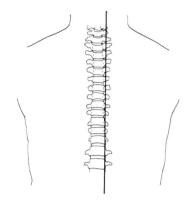

1. This left parasagittal section is lateral to the foramina.

2. The thoracic transverse processes are posterior to the costovertebral articulations. These processes serve as bony attachments for the intertransverse muscles and for fascicles of the thoracic longissimus muscle.

3. Intercostal vessels are identifiable between the ribs within the paraspinous fatty tissues. The hemiazygos vein is frequently identifiable as a large vessel posterior to the left side of the aorta forming a prominent loop or arch at the T7-T8 level.

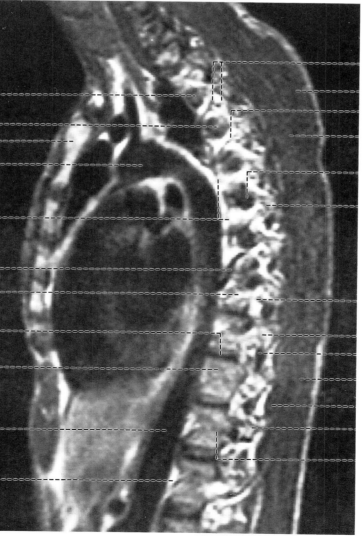

Left labels:
- Capitulum, 3rd rib
- Capitulum, 4th rib
- Sternum, manubrium
- Aortic arch
- Accessory hemiazygos v.
- Hemiazygos v.
- T8 vertebra, lateral margin
- Intervertebral disc, T9-T10 lateral anulus
- T10 vertebra, marrow space
- Abdominal aorta
- Anterior external vertebral v.

Right labels:
- Intercostal vessels
- Trapezius m.
- Intercostal vessel
- Thoracic spinalis m.
- Costovertebral joint at T6
- Transverse process, T6
- T8 segmental nerve in foramen
- Transverse process, T9
- Intertransverse ligament
- Thoracic longissimus m.
- Multifidus m.
- Transverse process, T11
- T11 vertebra, marrow space

Chapter 13

LUMBAR SPINE

AXIAL

Figure 13.1.1

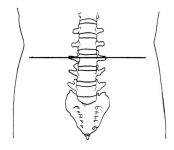

1. This section is through the middle of the L3 vertebral body.

2. Note the relation of major muscle groups — psoas and quadratus lumborum anterior — to the intrinsic back muscles (iliocostalis, longissimus, and multifidus). The back muscles lie behind the plane of the transverse processes.

3. At the midbody level, the thecal sac fills the spinal canal except for the region of the posterior epidural fat.

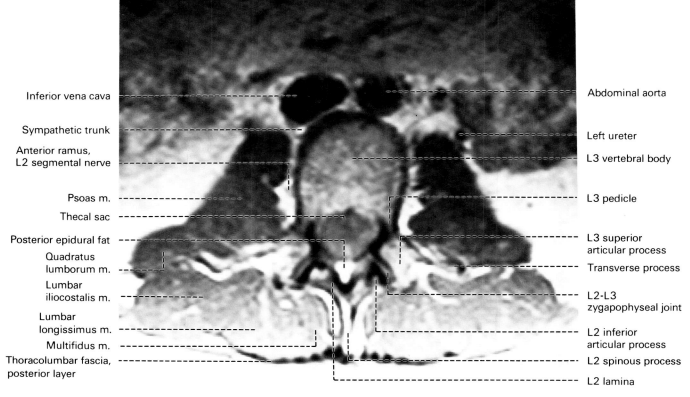

Inferior vena cava

Sympathetic trunk

Anterior ramus, L2 segmental nerve

Psoas m.

Thecal sac

Posterior epidural fat

Quadratus lumborum m.

Lumbar iliocostalis m.

Lumbar longissimus m.

Multifidus m.

Thoracolumbar fascia, posterior layer

Abdominal aorta

Left ureter

L3 vertebral body

L3 pedicle

L3 superior articular process

Transverse process

L2-L3 zygapophyseal joint

L2 inferior articular process

L2 spinous process

L2 lamina

Figure 13.1.2

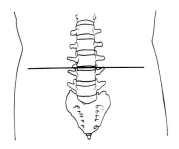

1. This section is through the inferior end-plate of L3 and the L3-L4 disc.

2. Elements of the cauda equina are seen as bright signals in the dependent part of the thecal sac.

3. The sympathetic trunk and ureters have a predictable course in relation to the other retroperitoneal structures.

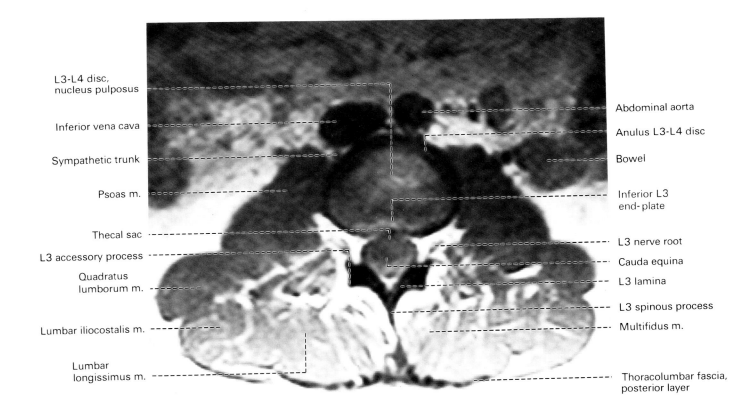

L3-L4 disc, nucleus pulposus

Inferior vena cava

Sympathetic trunk

Psoas m.

Thecal sac

L3 accessory process

Quadratus lumborum m.

Lumbar iliocostalis m.

Lumbar longissimus m.

Abdominal aorta

Anulus L3-L4 disc

Bowel

Inferior L3 end-plate

L3 nerve root

Cauda equina

L3 lamina

L3 spinous process

Multifidus m.

Thoracolumbar fascia, posterior layer

Figure 13.1.3

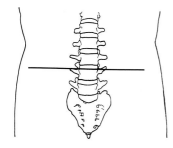

1. This section is through the lower portion of the L3-L4 disc.

2. All three layers of the thoracolumbar fascia are demonstrated.

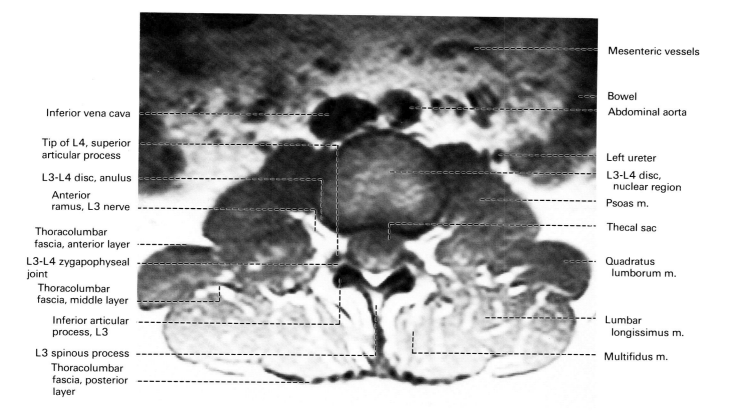

Inferior vena cava

Tip of L4, superior articular process

L3-L4 disc, anulus

Anterior ramus, L3 nerve

Thoracolumbar fascia, anterior layer

L3-L4 zygapophyseal joint

Thoracolumbar fascia, middle layer

Inferior articular process, L3

L3 spinous process

Thoracolumbar fascia, posterior layer

Mesenteric vessels

Bowel
Abdominal aorta

Left ureter

L3-L4 disc, nuclear region

Psoas m.

Thecal sac

Quadratus lumborum m.

Lumbar longissimus m.

Multifidus m.

Figure 13.1.4

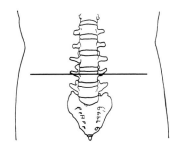

1. This section is through the upper third of the L4 vertebral body.

2. Note the neural elements within the psoas muscle. The lumbar plexus forms within the psoas muscles.

3. Ligamentum flavum extends laterally to merge with the anteromedial capsule of the zygapophyseal joints.

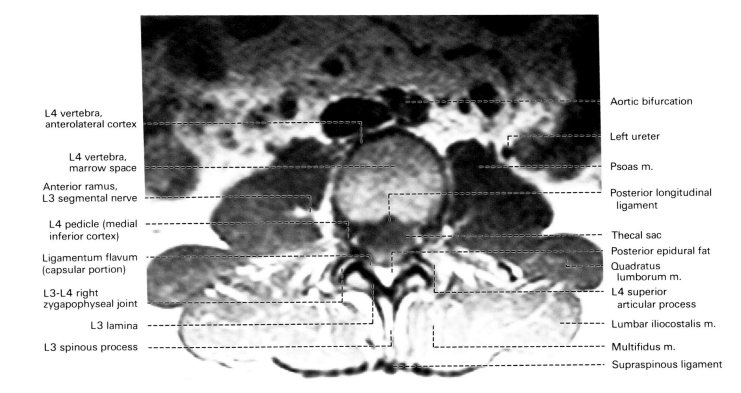

L4 vertebra, anterolateral cortex

L4 vertebra, marrow space

Anterior ramus, L3 segmental nerve

L4 pedicle (medial inferior cortex)

Ligamentum flavum (capsular portion)

L3-L4 right zygapophyseal joint

L3 lamina

L3 spinous process

Aortic bifurcation

Left ureter

Psoas m.

Posterior longitudinal ligament

Thecal sac

Posterior epidural fat

Quadratus lumborum m.

L4 superior articular process

Lumbar iliocostalis m.

Multifidus m.

Supraspinous ligament

Figure 13.1.5

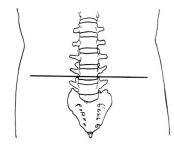

1. This section is through the lower third of the L4 vertebral body.

2. The section also passes just inferior to the pedicles and through the superior portion of the intervertebral foramen.

3. The dorsal root ganglion is seen with the superior portion of the neural foramen.

4. The middle layer of the thoracolumbar fascia extends laterally from the tips of the transverse processes to the lateral raphe. It joins the posterior layer of the thoracolumbar fascia and these two layers invest the back muscles.

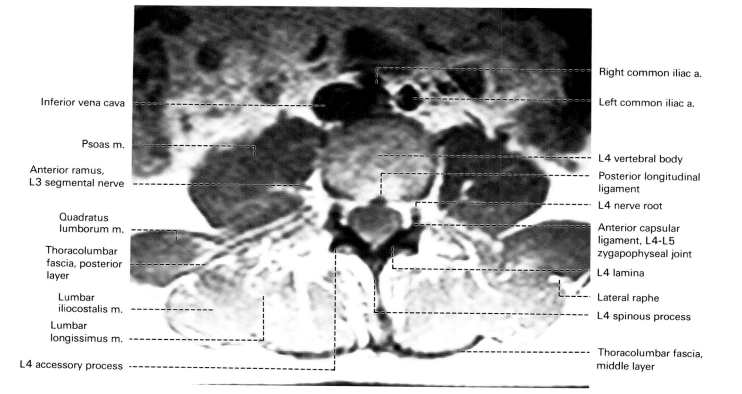

Figure 13.1.6

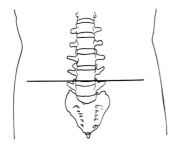

1. This section is through the inferior end-plate of L4.

2. The dorsal root ganglion is frequently identifiable as a localized swelling within the neural foramen.

3. The posterior ramus is too small to see by current imaging techniques.

4. Iliocostalis, longissimus, and spinalis are collectively referred to as the erector spinae muscle.

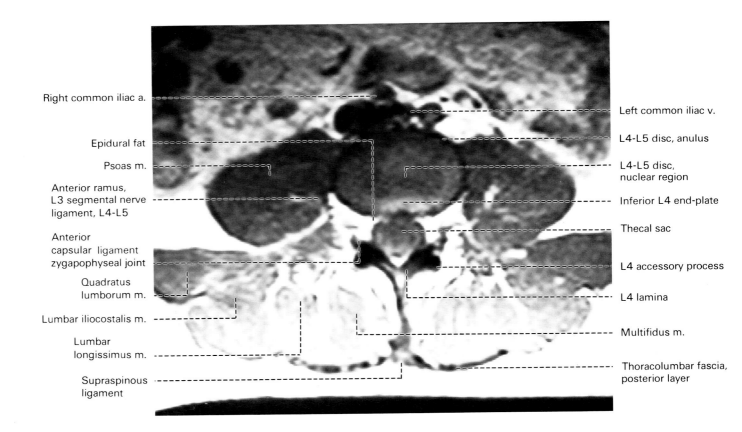

Right common iliac a.

Epidural fat

Psoas m.

Anterior ramus, L3 segmental nerve ligament, L4-L5

Anterior capsular ligament zygapophyseal joint

Quadratus lumborum m.

Lumbar iliocostalis m.

Lumbar longissimus m.

Supraspinous ligament

Left common iliac v.

L4-L5 disc, anulus

L4-L5 disc, nuclear region

Inferior L4 end-plate

Thecal sac

L4 accessory process

L4 lamina

Multifidus m.

Thoracolumbar fascia, posterior layer

Figure 13.1.7

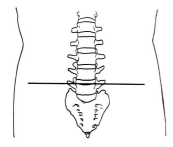

1. This section is through the L4-L5 disc.

2. Some of the nerve roots of the cauda equina can be identified within the thecal sac.

3. This section also passes through the zygapophyseal (facet) joints between L4-L5.

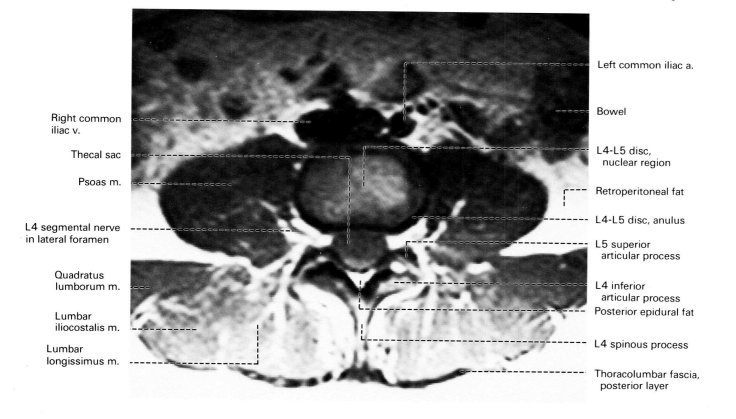

Left common iliac a.

Bowel

L4-L5 disc, nuclear region

Retroperitoneal fat

L4-L5 disc, anulus

L5 superior articular process

L4 inferior articular process

Posterior epidural fat

L4 spinous process

Thoracolumbar fascia, posterior layer

Right common iliac v.

Thecal sac

Psoas m.

L4 segmental nerve in lateral foramen

Quadratus lumborum m.

Lumbar iliocostalis m.

Lumbar longissimus m.

Figure 13.1.8

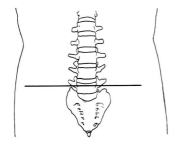

1. This section is through the upper third of the L5 vertebral body.

2. The posterior longitudinal ligament is seen as the narrow band of fibrous tissue along the back of the vertebral bodies.

3. At this level, the posterior longitudinal ligament expands laterally to cover the posterior aspect of the disc. Its fibers mesh with those of the anulus.

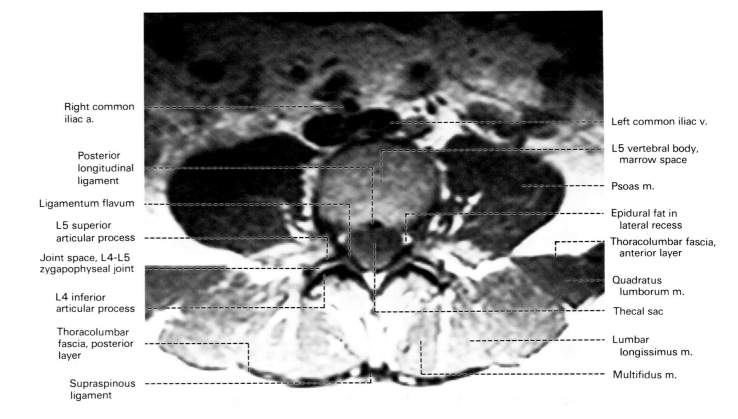

Right common iliac a.

Posterior longitudinal ligament

Ligamentum flavum

L5 superior articular process

Joint space, L4-L5 zygapophyseal joint

L4 inferior articular process

Thoracolumbar fascia, posterior layer

Supraspinous ligament

Left common iliac v.

L5 vertebral body, marrow space

Psoas m.

Epidural fat in lateral recess

Thoracolumbar fascia, anterior layer

Quadratus lumborum m.

Thecal sac

Lumbar longissimus m.

Multifidus m.

Figure 13.1.9

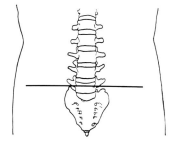

1. This section is through the middle third of the L5 vertebral body.

2. The basivertebral vein is seen at the nutrient foramen in the posterior aspect of the vertebral body.

3. The small interosseous vertebral veins (not shown in this section) drain the vertebral body and empty into the basivertebral veins, which in turn empty into the epidural anterior external venous plexus.

4. Note the triangular configuration of the spinal canal in the lower lumbar spine. Exaggeration of the triangular shape results in the commonly observed trefoil configuration.

5. The spinal canal is commonly round in the upper and midlumbar levels.

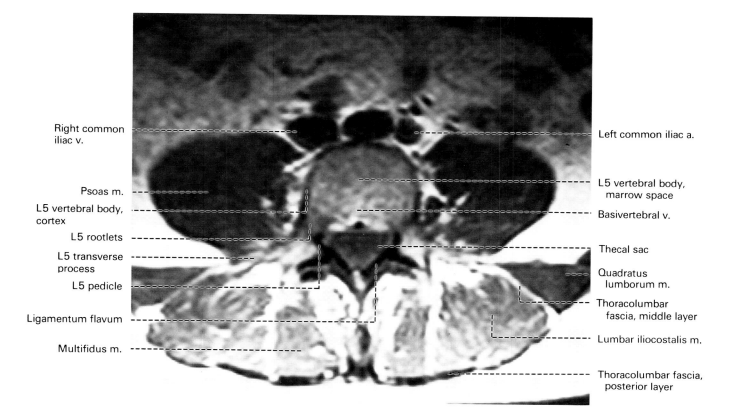

Figure 13.1.10

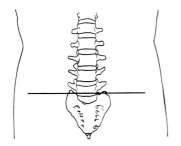

1. This section is through the lower part of the L5 vertebral body.

2. The bulge on the L5 root represents the dorsal root ganglion.

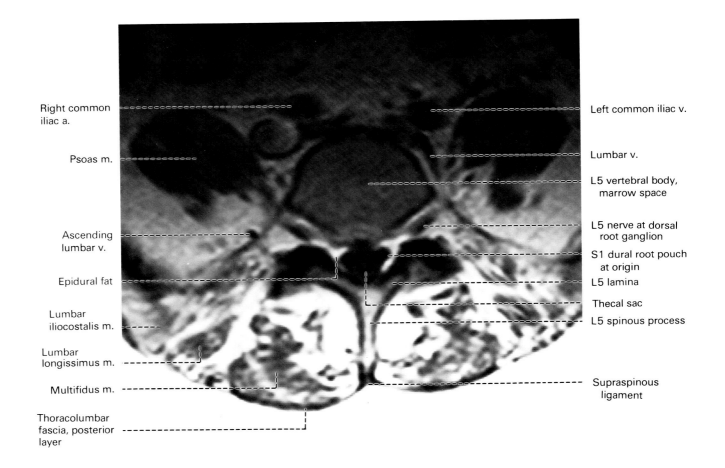

Right common iliac a.

Psoas m.

Ascending lumbar v.

Epidural fat

Lumbar iliocostalis m.

Lumbar longissimus m.

Multifidus m.

Thoracolumbar fascia, posterior layer

Left common iliac v.

Lumbar v.

L5 vertebral body, marrow space

L5 nerve at dorsal root ganglion

S1 dural root pouch at origin

L5 lamina

Thecal sac

L5 spinous process

Supraspinous ligament

Figure 13.1.11

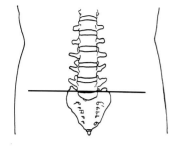

1. This section passes obliquely through the upper portion of the L5-S1, disc.

2. A plica mediana dorsalis is demonstrated in this section. It separates the epidural space into left and right compartments.

3. At this level the zygapophyseal joints are asymmetrical in orientation. This is a normal variant.

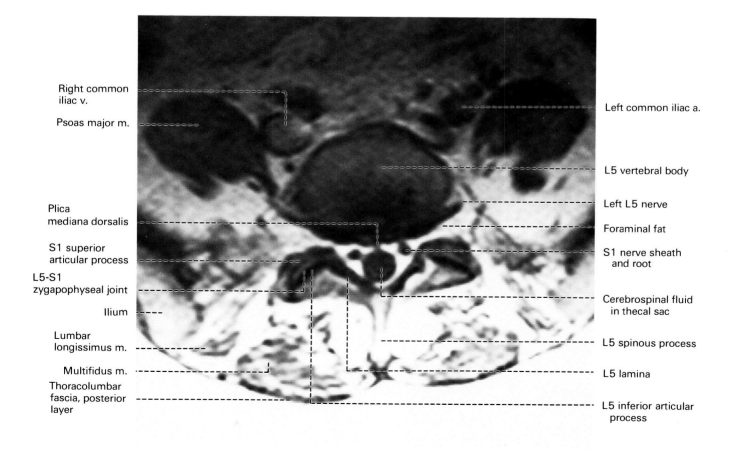

Right common iliac v.

Psoas major m.

Plica mediana dorsalis

S1 superior articular process

L5-S1 zygapophyseal joint

Ilium

Lumbar longissimus m.

Multifidus m.

Thoracolumbar fascia, posterior layer

Left common iliac a.

L5 vertebral body

Left L5 nerve

Foraminal fat

S1 nerve sheath and root

Cerebrospinal fluid in thecal sac

L5 spinous process

L5 lamina

L5 inferior articular process

Figure 13.1.12

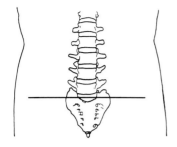

1. This section passes obliquely through the L5-S1 disc.

2. The spinal canal has a narrow sagittal diameter and a wide transverse diameter. The lateral recesses are therefore spacious.

3. Multifidus is the dominant muscle on the posterior surface of the sacrum. The posterior fascia is dense and consists of aponeurotic fibers from the erector spinae and abdominal muscles.

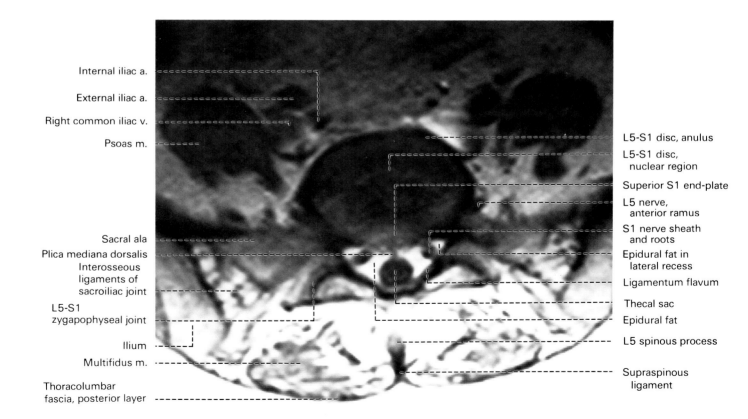

Internal iliac a.

External iliac a.

Right common iliac v.

Psoas m.

L5-S1 disc, anulus

L5-S1 disc, nuclear region

Superior S1 end-plate

L5 nerve, anterior ramus

S1 nerve sheath and roots

Sacral ala

Plica mediana dorsalis

Interosseous ligaments of sacroiliac joint

L5-S1 zygapophyseal joint

Ilium

Multifidus m.

Thoracolumbar fascia, posterior layer

Epidural fat in lateral recess

Ligamentum flavum

Thecal sac

Epidural fat

L5 spinous process

Supraspinous ligament

Figure 13.1.13

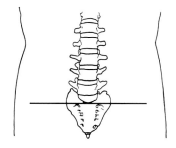

1. This section is through the upper S1 body.

2. Note that the true or synovial portion of the sacroiliac joint is anterior to the fibrous portion.

3. The S1 nerve root (bright signal) and CSF-containing (dark signal) nerve sheath around it are both clearly demonstrated.

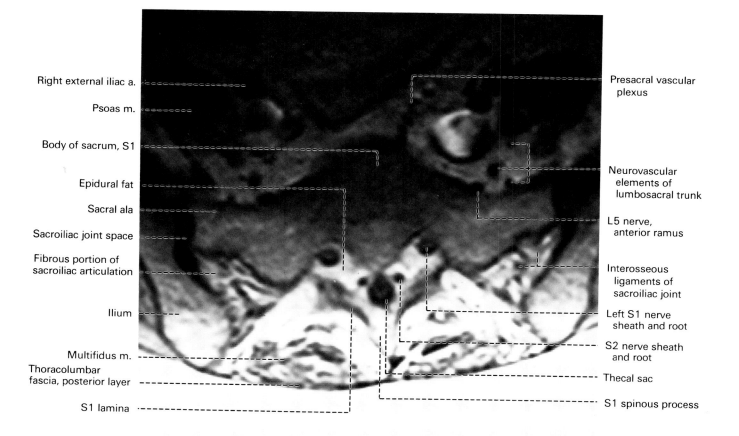

Right external iliac a.
Psoas m.
Body of sacrum, S1
Epidural fat
Sacral ala
Sacroiliac joint space
Fibrous portion of sacroiliac articulation
Ilium
Multifidus m.
Thoracolumbar fascia, posterior layer
S1 lamina

Presacral vascular plexus
Neurovascular elements of lumbosacral trunk
L5 nerve, anterior ramus
Interosseous ligaments of sacroiliac joint
Left S1 nerve sheath and root
S2 nerve sheath and root
Thecal sac
S1 spinous process

Figure 13.2.1

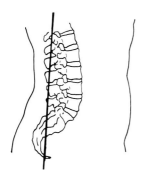

1. This section is through the posterior lumbar musculature.

2. Note the fat plane separating the erector spinae group (lumbar longissimus and iliocostalis) from the multifidi.

3. This section demonstrates the length of some of the multifidus muscles. Some fascicles extend across multiple motion segments.

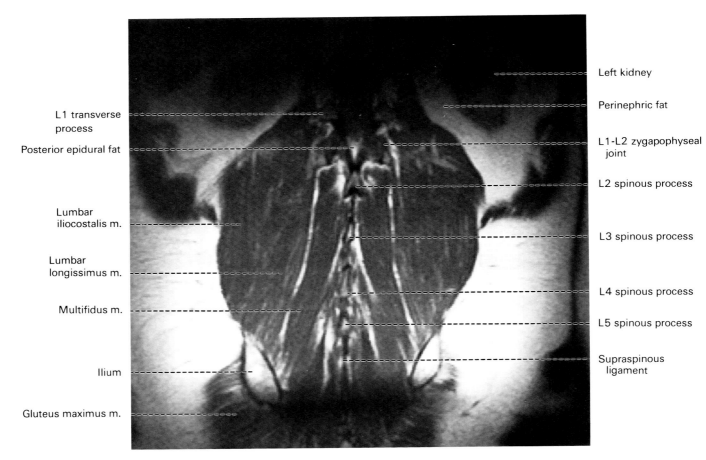

Left labels (top to bottom): L1 transverse process; Posterior epidural fat; Lumbar iliocostalis m.; Lumbar longissimus m.; Multifidus m.; Ilium; Gluteus maximus m.

Right labels (top to bottom): Left kidney; Perinephric fat; L1-L2 zygapophyseal joint; L2 spinous process; L3 spinous process; L4 spinous process; L5 spinous process; Supraspinous ligament

Figure 13.2.2

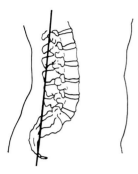

1. This section is through the lumbar spinous processes.

2. This section demonstrates muscle attachments to L2 transverse processes and several spinous processes. Shorter fascicles of lower lumbar multifidi are apparent.

3. Differentiation of components of the erector spinae group is difficult in the coronal plane; the best separation of lumbar iliocostalis and longissimus is provided on axial sections.

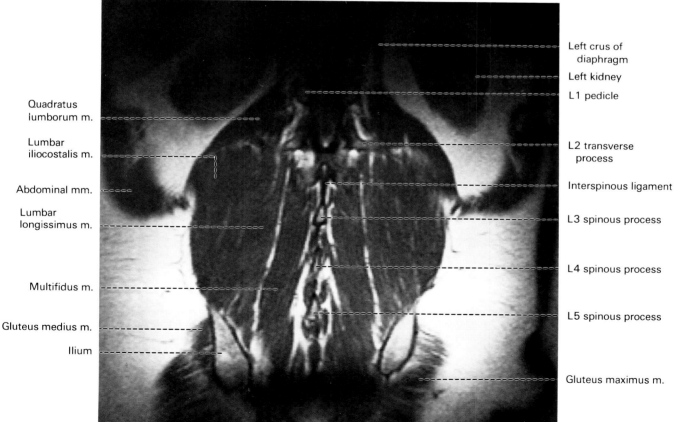

Quadratus lumborum m.

Lumbar iliocostalis m.

Abdominal mm.

Lumbar longissimus m.

Multifidus m.

Gluteus medius m.

Ilium

Left crus of diaphragm

Left kidney

L1 pedicle

L2 transverse process

Interspinous ligament

L3 spinous process

L4 spinous process

L5 spinous process

Gluteus maximus m.

Figure 13.2.3

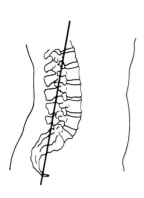

1. This section is through the base of the L3 spinous process.

2. Fat provides contrast that allows visualization of many components including segmental nerves and muscle-tendon insertions.

3. Note the posterior epidural fat. This is a constant feature of coronal images.

4. The ligamenta flava are vertically oriented low signal structures on each side of the posterior epidural fat pad.

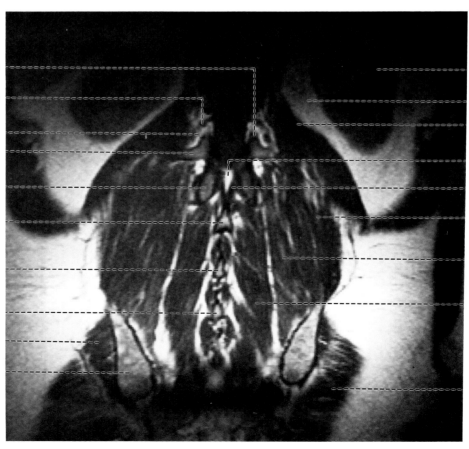

L2 superior articular process — Left kidney

L1 segmental nerve — Perinephric fat

Perineural fat — Quadratus lumborum m.

L2 transverse process — Posterior epidural fat

L2 inferior articular process — Ligamentum flavum

L3 spinous process — Lumbar iliocostalis m.

L4 spinous process — Lumbar longissimus m.

L5 spinous process — Multifidus m.

Gluteus medius m.

Ilium — Gluteus maximus m.

Figure 13.2.4

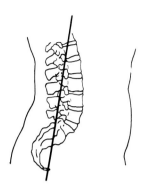

1. This section is through the base of L4 and L5 spinous processes.

2. Note the relative symmetry of the muscles.

3. The longissimus and iliocostalis muscles originate in part from the ilium.

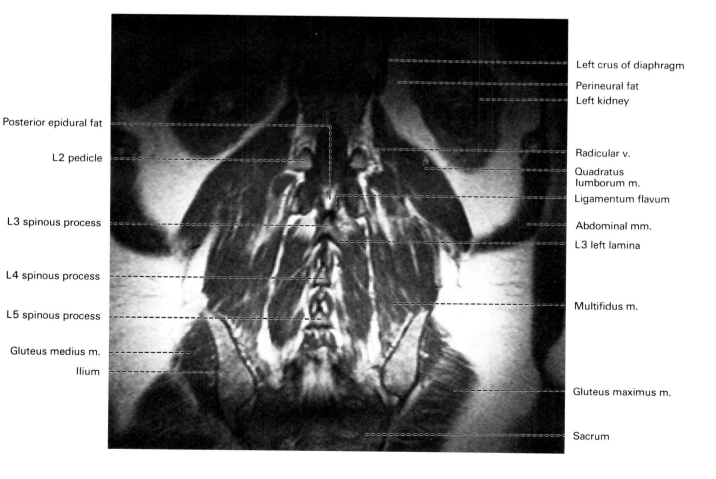

Posterior epidural fat

L2 pedicle

L3 spinous process

L4 spinous process

L5 spinous process

Gluteus medius m.

Ilium

Left crus of diaphragm

Perineural fat
Left kidney

Radicular v.

Quadratus
lumborum m.
Ligamentum flavum

Abdominal mm.
L3 left lamina

Multifidus m.

Gluteus maximus m.

Sacrum

Figure 13.2.5

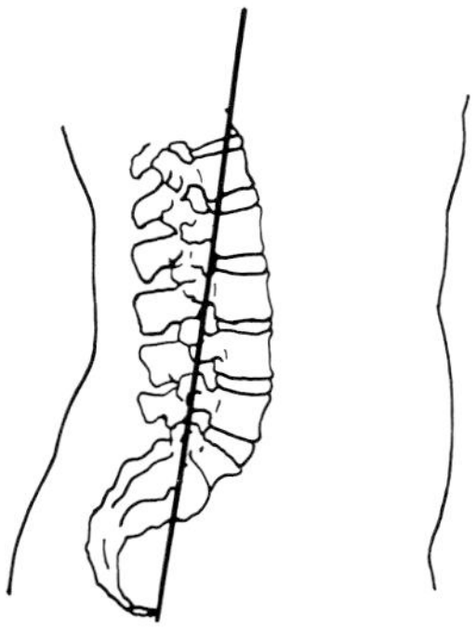

1. This section is through the L2-L3 intervertebral foramen.
2. Note the relation of the inferior and superior articular facets in the coronal plane. The inferior articular process is medial.
3. In coronal sections, the lumbar lordosis allows visualization of the dural sac at L2-L3 and L5-S1 and the posterior epidural space at L3-L4 and L4-L5.

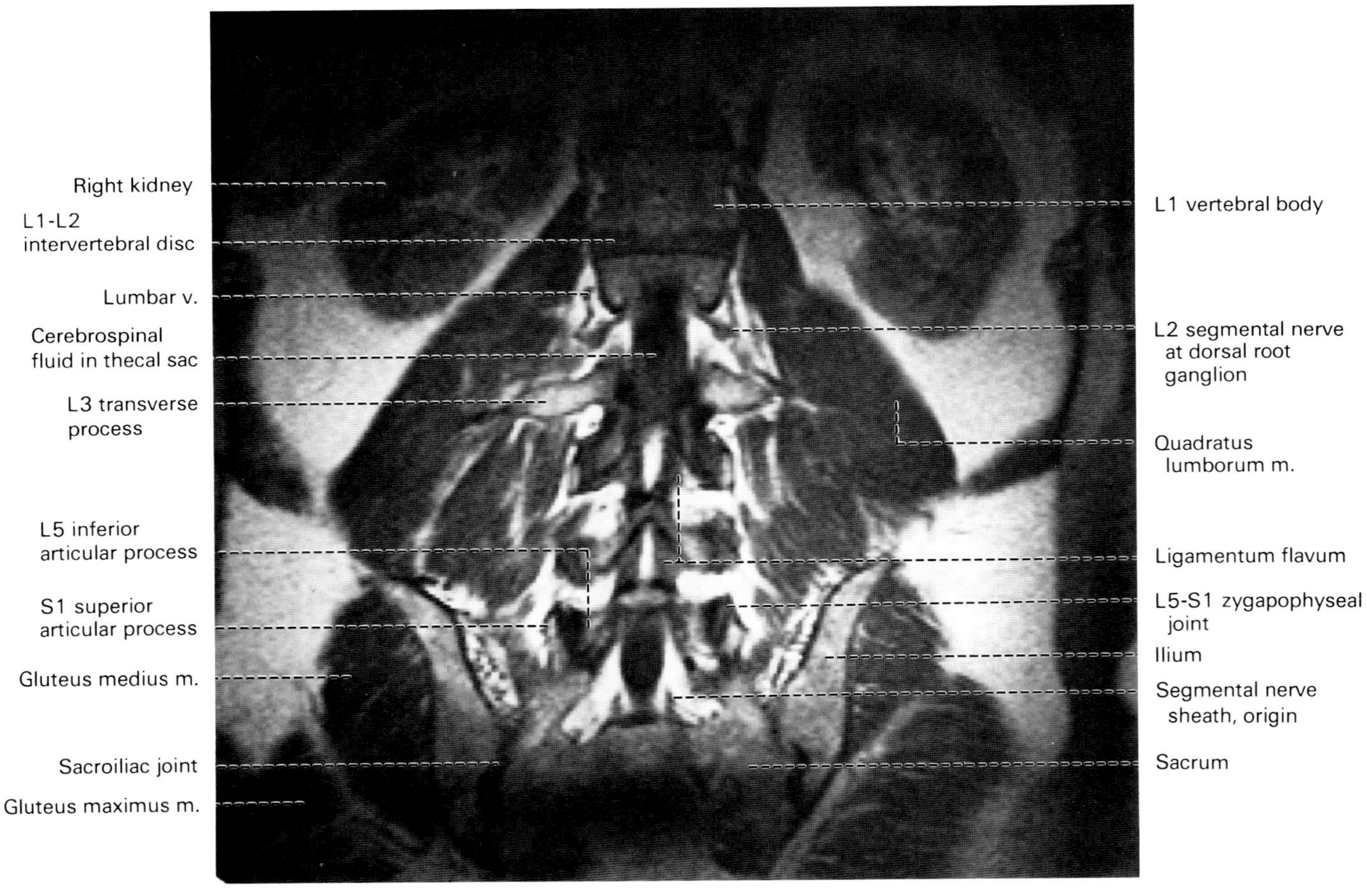
Right kidney
L1-L2 intervertebral disc
Lumbar v.
Cerebrospinal fluid in thecal sac
L3 transverse process
L5 inferior articular process
S1 superior articular process
Gluteus medius m.
Sacroiliac joint
Gluteus maximus m.
L1 vertebral body
L2 segmental nerve at dorsal root ganglion
Quadratus lumborum m.
Ligamentum flavum
L5-S1 zygapophyseal joint
Ilium
Segmental nerve sheath, origin
Sacrum

Figure 13.2.6

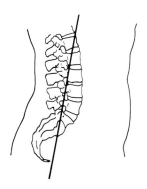

1. This section is through the L4-L5 and L5-S1 zygapophyseal joints.

2. The iliolumbar ligament is identified in this section.

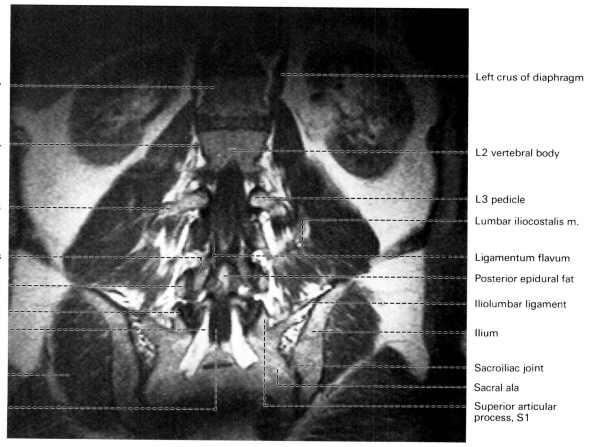

L1 vertebral body

Lumbar v.

L3 transverse process

L4 inferior
articular process

L5 superior
articular process

L5-S1
zygapophyseal joint

Perineural fat in right
S1 radicular canal

Gluteus medius m.

Thecal sac

Left crus of diaphragm

L2 vertebral body

L3 pedicle

Lumbar iliocostalis m.

Ligamentum flavum

Posterior epidural fat

Iliolumbar ligament

Ilium

Sacroiliac joint

Sacral ala

Superior articular
process, S1

Figure 13.2.7

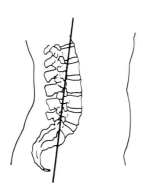

1. This section is through the midvertebral canal at the level of L4 and L5.

2. Abundant epidural/perineural fat in the lower lumbar upper sacral region is present.

3. The erector spinae muscles lie posterior to the transverse processes and are not visualized on this section. The anterior musculature (psoas major and quadratus lumborum) are the major muscles seen.

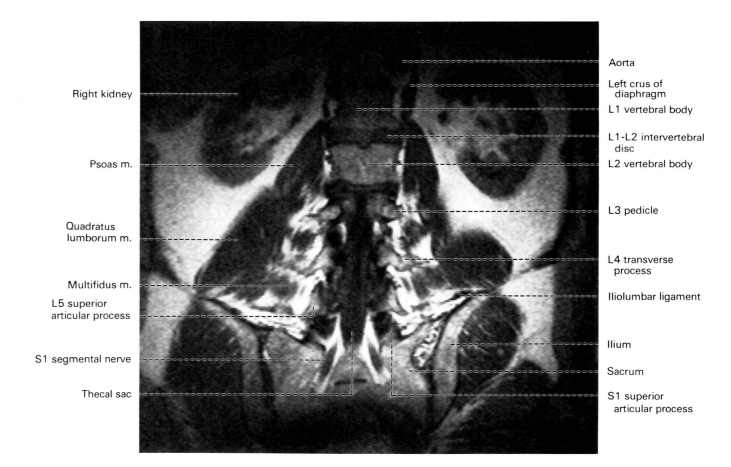

Figure 13.2.8

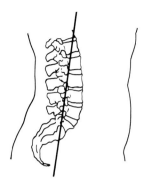

1. This section is through the anterior vertebral canal at the level of L4 and L5.

2. The lumbar veins are adjacent to the midportion of the vertebral body. These circumferential veins are valveless and allow flow between the internal epidural venous plexus and the systemic circulation via the vena cava.

3. The anterior capsules of the zygapophyseal joints are formed by lateral extensions of the ligamentum flavum.

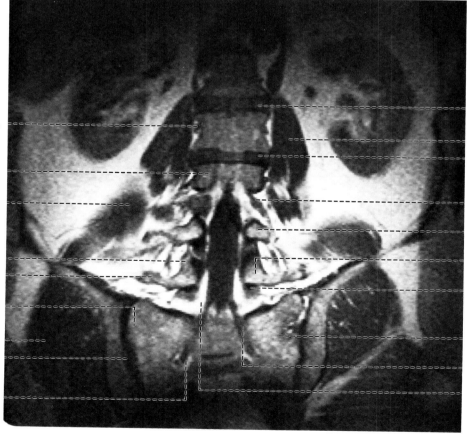

Lumbar v.

L3 pedicle base

Quadratus lumborum m.

L5 superior articular process

L5 transverse process

Sacral ala

Gluteus medius m.

Sacroiliac joint

First ventral sacral foramen

L1-L2 intervertebral disc

Psoas m.

L2-L3 intervertebral disc

L3 segmental nerve at dorsal root ganglion

L4 pedicle

L5 pedicle

Anterior capsular ligament, L5-S1 zygapophyseal joint

Sacrum

S1 segmental nerve

Epidural fat

Figure 13.2.9

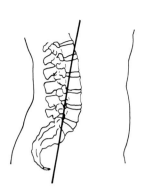

1. This section is through the L4-L5 and L5-S1 neural foramina.

2. Note the course of the neural elements from their origin through the foramina. The dural root sheath lies in close proximity medial and inferior to the pedicle. The dorsal root ganglion is in the neural foramen between the pedicles.

3. This section demonstrates the posterior longitudinal ligament at L4 and L5. This ligament is quite narrow behind the vertebral body but expands laterally at the intervertebral disc space.

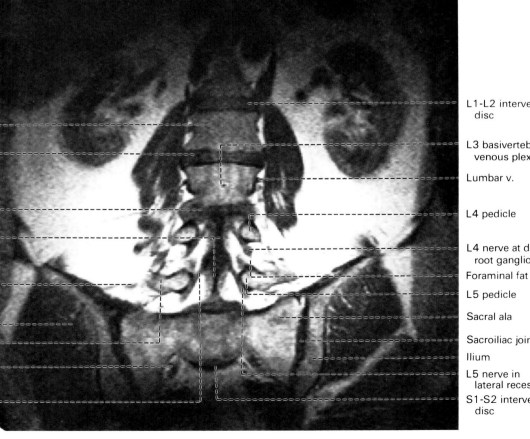

Left side labels:
- L2 vertebral body
- L2-L3 intervertebral disc
- L3-L4 intervertebral disc
- Posterior longitudinal ligament
- Iliotransverse ligament
- Gluteus medius m.
- L5 transverse process
- Anterior ramus, right S1 segmental nerve
- Right L5 nerve sheath, origin

Right side labels:
- L1-L2 intervertebral disc
- L3 basivertebral venous plexus
- Lumbar v.
- L4 pedicle
- L4 nerve at dorsal root ganglion
- Foraminal fat
- L5 pedicle
- Sacral ala
- Sacroiliac joint
- Ilium
- L5 nerve in lateral recess
- S1-S2 intervertebral disc

Figure 13.2.10

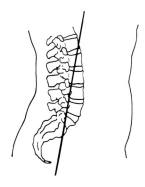

1. This section is through the posterior L4 and L5 vertebrae.

2. Note that the anulus "bulges" on each side. Mild extension of the anulus beyond the end-plate is a normal phenomenon.

3. The basivertebral plexus in the posterior aspect of the vertebral body denotes the midpoint of the body. The veins are usually surrounded by fat.

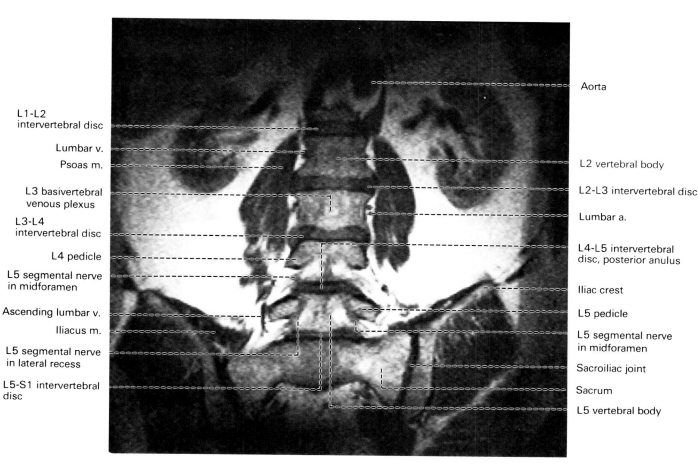

L1-L2 intervertebral disc

Lumbar v.

Psoas m.

L3 basivertebral venous plexus

L3-L4 intervertebral disc

L4 pedicle

L5 segmental nerve in midforamen

Ascending lumbar v.

Iliacus m.

L5 segmental nerve in lateral recess

L5-S1 intervertebral disc

Aorta

L2 vertebral body

L2-L3 intervertebral disc

Lumbar a.

L4-L5 intervertebral disc, posterior anulus

Iliac crest

L5 pedicle

L5 segmental nerve in midforamen

Sacroiliac joint

Sacrum

L5 vertebral body

Figure 13.2.11

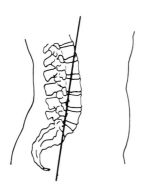

1. This section is through the posterior bodies of the lumbar vertebrae.

2. The posterior sacroiliac joint is fibrous or ligamentous. This section demonstrates the anterior portion of this articulation, which is synovial.

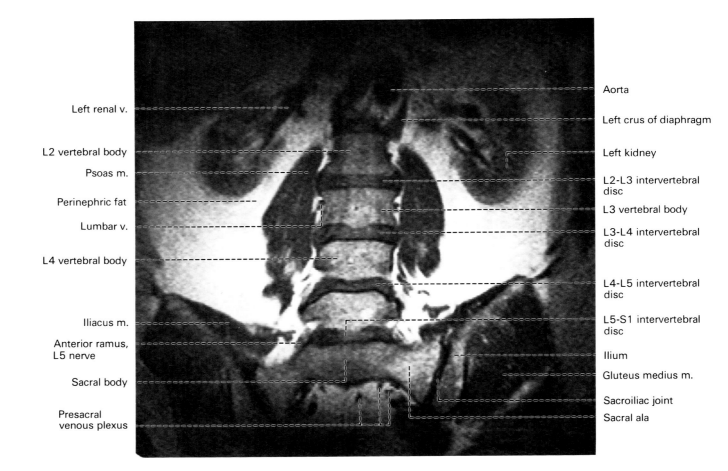

Left renal v.

L2 vertebral body

Psoas m.

Perinephric fat

Lumbar v.

L4 vertebral body

Iliacus m.

Anterior ramus, L5 nerve

Sacral body

Presacral venous plexus

Aorta

Left crus of diaphragm

Left kidney

L2-L3 intervertebral disc

L3 vertebral body

L3-L4 intervertebral disc

L4-L5 intervertebral disc

L5-S1 intervertebral disc

Ilium

Gluteus medius m.

Sacroiliac joint

Sacral ala

Figure 13.2.12

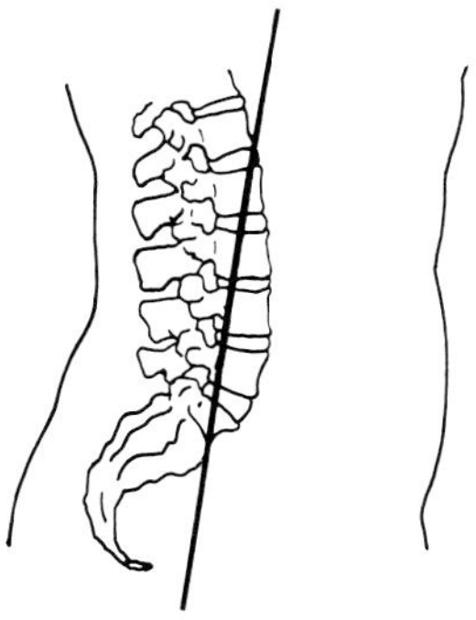

1. Note the position of the L5 nerve (anterior ramus) relative to the sacral ala. It courses across the top of the ala.

2. Note the clearly defined paraspinous space. Fat and vascular structures are interposed between the musculature and the vertebral column.

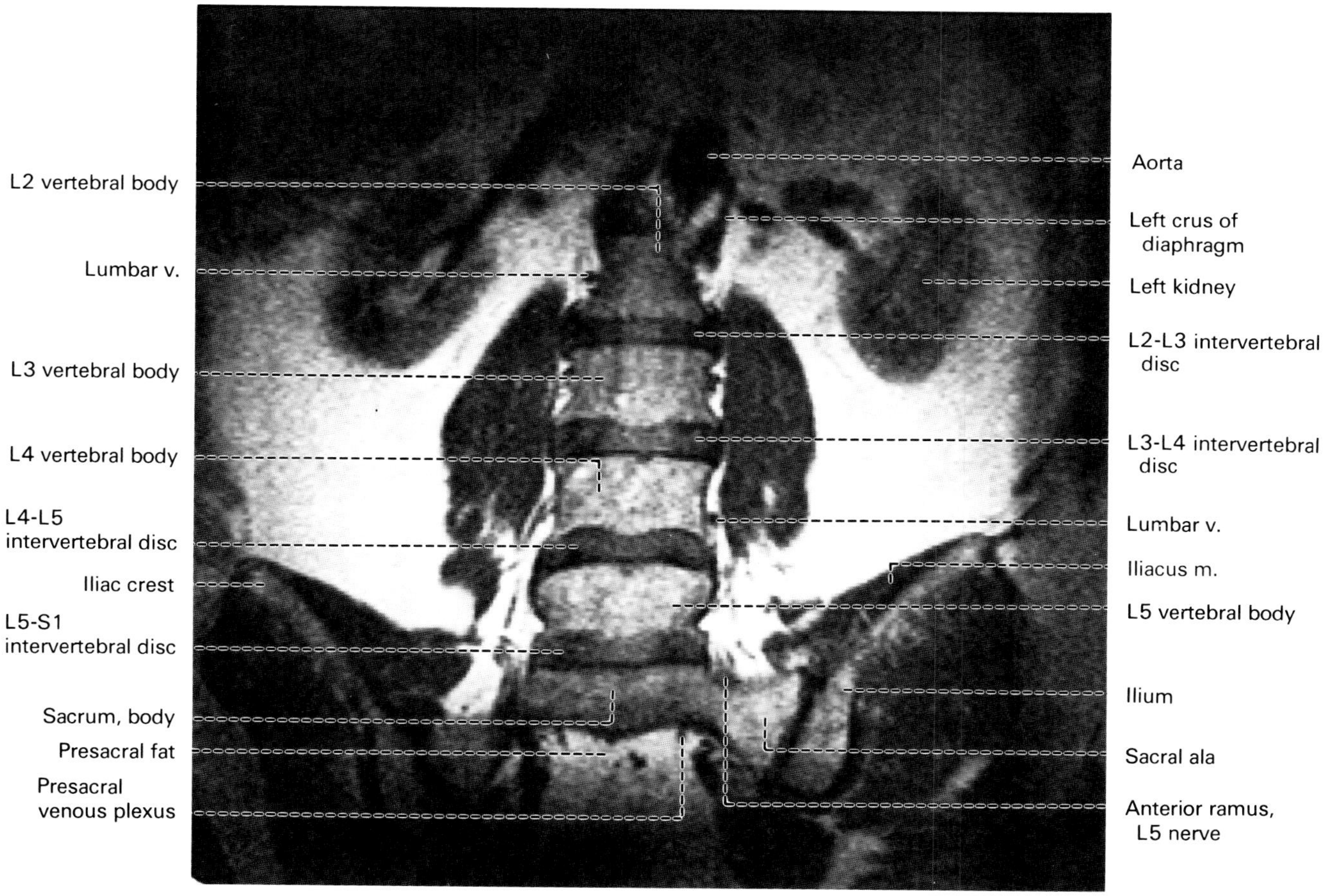
L2 vertebral body
Lumbar v.
L3 vertebral body
L4 vertebral body
L4-L5 intervertebral disc
Iliac crest
L5-S1 intervertebral disc
Sacrum, body
Presacral fat
Presacral venous plexus
Aorta
Left crus of diaphragm
Left kidney
L2-L3 intervertebral disc
L3-L4 intervertebral disc
Lumbar v.
Iliacus m.
L5 vertebral body
Ilium
Sacral ala
Anterior ramus, L5 nerve

Figure 13.3.1

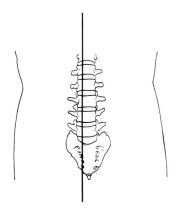

1. This right parasagittal section is through the inferior vena cava and lateral aspect of the central spinal canal.

2. This section demonstrates the lateral extension of the central canal. Multiple bundles of segmental rootlets invested by dural sheaths are identifiable in the abundant epidural fat.

3. The disc anulus has a greater diameter than the vertebral end plate.

4. Note the relation of disc anulus to dural root sheaths of segmental nerves.

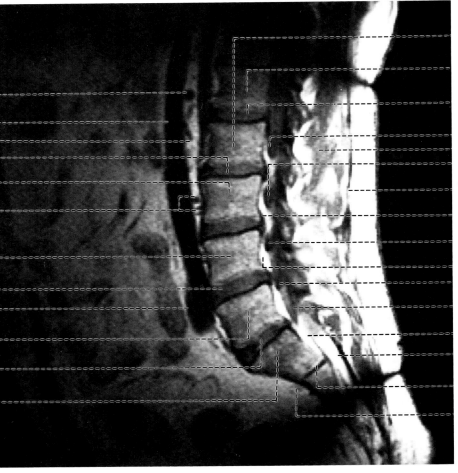

Right renal a.

Inferior vena cava

Retroperitoneal fat

L2-L3 intervertebral disc, end-plate

L3 vertebra, marrow space

Anterior external vertebral venous plexus

L4 vertebra, marrow space

L4-L5 intervertebral disc, anterior nucleus

Right common iliac a.

L5 vertebra, marrow space

L5-S1 intervertebral disc, nucleus

Sacrum, S1 segment

L2 vertebra, marrow space

L1 vertebra, marrow space

L1-L2 intervertebral disc, nucleus

L2 segmental nerve

Multifidus m.

L3 segmental nerve in lateral recess

Thoracolumbar fascia, posterior layer

L3-L4 intervertebral disc, posterior anulus

L4 segmental nerve in lateral recess

Epidural fat

L5 segmental nerve in lateral recess

S1 segmental nerve in lateral sacral canal

S2 neural elements

Sacral canal, epidural fat

S1-S2 intervertebral disc

Presacral fat

Figure 13.3.2

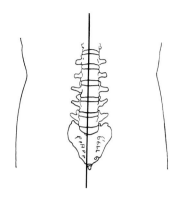

1. This paramedian sagittal section is just to the right of the midline.

2. The usually abundant epidural fat provides the contrast to define the anterior and posterior margins of the dural sac. Rootlets of the cauda equina are identifiable as linear structures of intermediate signal intensity in contrast to the low signal intensity of CSF.

3. The supraspinous and interspinous ligaments are seen between the spinous processes. These ligaments act in stabilizing the spine in flexion.

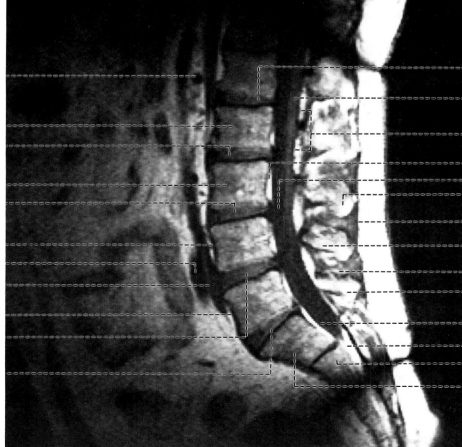

Right renal a.

L2 vertebra, marrow space

L2-L3 intervertebral disc, anterior anulus

L3 vertebra, marrow space

L3-L4 intervertebral disc

L4 vertebra, anterior cortex

Right common iliac a.

Inferior vena cava

L5 vertebra, anterior cortex

L4-L5 intervertebral disc, nucleus

L5-S1 intervertebral disc, nucleus

L1-L2 intervertebral disc

Cauda equina

Posterior epidural fat

Anterior epidural fat

Thecal sac

L3 vertebral spinous process

Supraspinous ligament

L4 vertebral spinous process

Interspinous ligament

L5 vertebral spinous process

Anterior dural margin

Sacral epidural fat

S2 vertebral body

Sacrum, S1 body

Figure 13.3.3

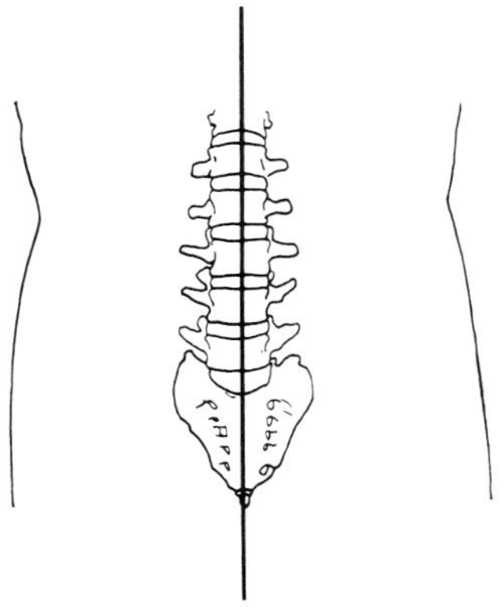

1. This is a midline sagittal section.

2. The basivertebral veins are usually identified on midline sections. The low signal of the vein is surrounded by the bright signal of the perivascular fat. This prominent venous structure denotes the center of the posterior surface of the lumbar vertebral body.

3. Posterior epidural fat is thickest in the midline. This fat provides contrast to define the posterior dura, ligamentum flavum, and the bases of the spinous processes.

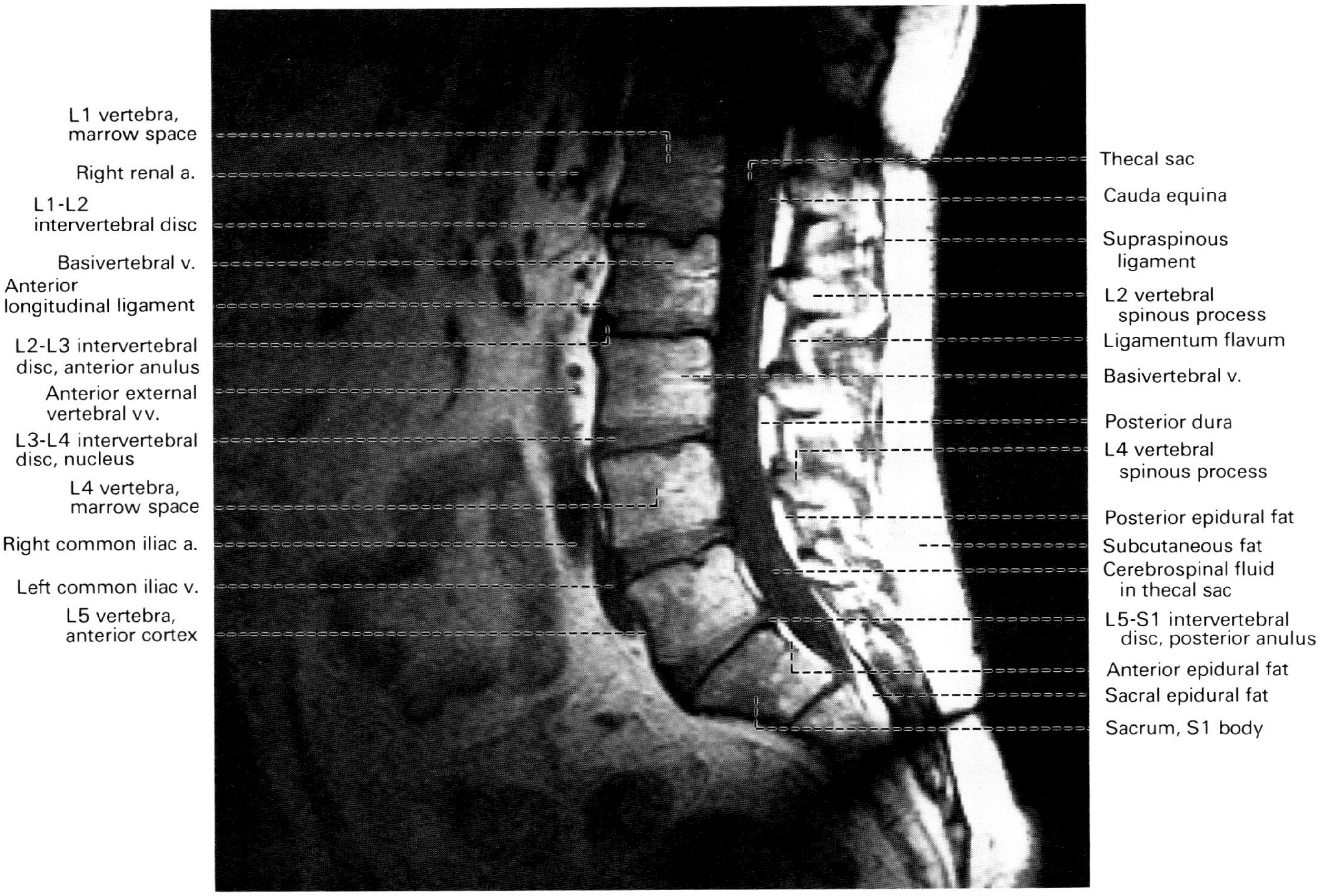

L1 vertebra, marrow space
Right renal a.
L1-L2 intervertebral disc
Basivertebral v.
Anterior longitudinal ligament
L2-L3 intervertebral disc, anterior anulus
Anterior external vertebral vv.
L3-L4 intervertebral disc, nucleus
L4 vertebra, marrow space
Right common iliac a.
Left common iliac v.
L5 vertebra, anterior cortex
Thecal sac
Cauda equina
Supraspinous ligament
L2 vertebral spinous process
Ligamentum flavum
Basivertebral v.
Posterior dura
L4 vertebral spinous process
Posterior epidural fat
Subcutaneous fat
Cerebrospinal fluid in thecal sac
L5-S1 intervertebral disc, posterior anulus
Anterior epidural fat
Sacral epidural fat
Sacrum, S1 body

Figure 13.3.4

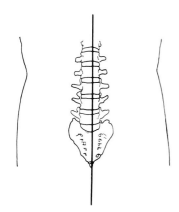

1. This parasagittal section is just to the left of the spinous processes.

2. Note the paucity of muscles on sections near the midline.

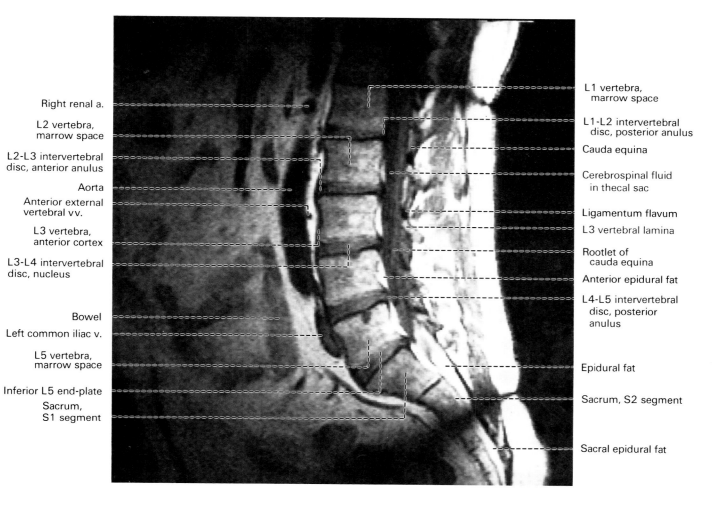

Right renal a.

L2 vertebra, marrow space

L2-L3 intervertebral disc, anterior anulus

Aorta

Anterior external vertebral vv.

L3 vertebra, anterior cortex

L3-L4 intervertebral disc, nucleus

Bowel

Left common iliac v.

L5 vertebra, marrow space

Inferior L5 end-plate

Sacrum, S1 segment

L1 vertebra, marrow space

L1-L2 intervertebral disc, posterior anulus

Cauda equina

Cerebrospinal fluid in thecal sac

Ligamentum flavum

L3 vertebral lamina

Rootlet of cauda equina

Anterior epidural fat

L4-L5 intervertebral disc, posterior anulus

Epidural fat

Sacrum, S2 segment

Sacral epidural fat

Figure 13.3.5

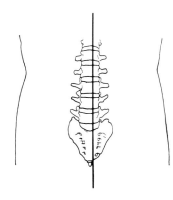

1. This parasagittal section is through the plane of the aorta and left lateral aspect of the central canal.

2. The anterior external vertebral veins are part of the anterior external vertebral plexus. They are the anterior components of the circumferential lumbar veins. These valveless veins drain into the inferior vena cava and into ascending lumbar veins.

3. This section demonstrates the left ligamentum flavum connecting the laminae of adjacent vertebrae. These elastic ligaments stretch during flexion as the laminae separate. They return to their resting thickness in neutral or extended positions and do not normally buckle into the central canal.

4. Note the proximity of the ligamentum flavum to neural elements in the lateral recesses.

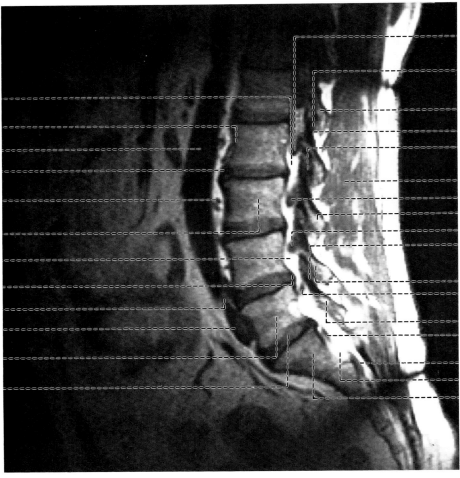

Perineural fat

L2 vertebra, anterior cortex

Aorta

L2-L3 intervertebral disc, anterior anulus

Anterior external vertebral vv.

L3 vertebra, marrow space

Epidural fat in lateral recess

L4-L5 intervertebral disc, posterior anulus

Aortic bifurcation

Left common iliac v.

L5 vertebra, marrow space

L5-S1 intervertebral disc, nucleus

L2 segmental nerve in lateral recess

Ligamentum flavum between L1-L2 lamina

L1 lamina

L2 vertebral lamina

Ligamentum flavum between L2-L3 lamina

Multifidus m.

L3 segmental nerve

L3 lamina

L4 segmental nerve

Ligamentum flavum between L4-L5 lamina

L4 lamina

L5 segmental nerve in lateral recess

L5 lamina

S1 segmental nerve in sacral canal

S2 segmental nerve

Sacral epidural fat

Sacrum, S1 segment

Figure 13.3.6

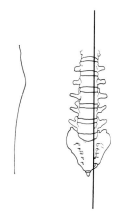

1. This left parasagittal section is through the midportion of the intervertebral foramina.

2. In the lumbar spine, neural structures occupy the upper portion of the foramina. The anulus forms the anterior wall of the foramina below the nerves.

3. Note the proximity of the superior articular processes to the neural elements.

4. The anterior capsular ligament of the zygapophyseal joints are immediately posterior to the nerves.

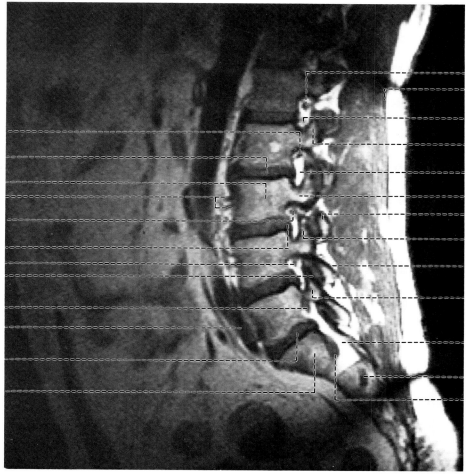

L2 segmental nerve
L2-L3 intervertebral disc
L3 vertebra, marrow space
Anterior external vertebral vv.
L3 segmental nerve
L3-L4 intervertebral disc, posterior anulus
L4 segmental nerve
L4-L5 zygapophyseal joint
L5 segmental nerve
Left common iliac v.
L5-S1 intervertebral disc, nucleus
Sacrum, S1 segment

L1 segmental nerve
Thoracolumbar fascia, posterior layer
Radicular v. in L1-L2 foramen
L2 superior articular process
Perineural fat in L2-L3 foramen
L3 vertebra, pedicle
L3 inferior articular process
L4 superior articular process
L4 inferior articular process
L5 superior articular process
Sacral epidural fat
S2 segmental nerve
S1 segmental nerve

Figure 13.3.7

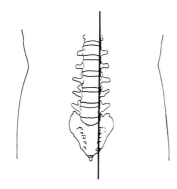

1. This parasagittal section is through the pedicles.

2. The dorsal root ganglion is the dominant neural structure visualized in the neural foramina. It is recognizable as a focal enlargement of the segmental nerve.

3. Parasagittal sections demonstrate the back muscles. Multifidius and the erector spinae group (lumbar longissimus and ileocostalis) are identifiable. The posterior layer of the thoracolumbar fascia is usually clearly defined.

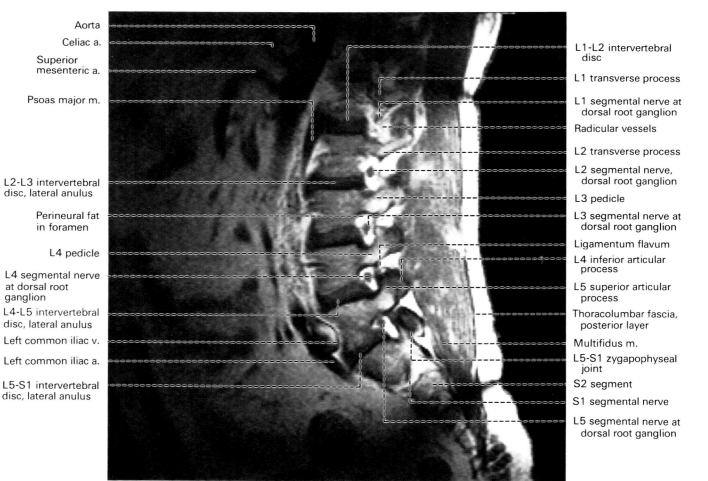

Aorta
Celiac a.
Superior mesenteric a.
Psoas major m.

L2-L3 intervertebral disc, lateral anulus
Perineural fat in foramen
L4 pedicle
L4 segmental nerve at dorsal root ganglion
L4-L5 intervertebral disc, lateral anulus
Left common iliac v.
Left common iliac a.
L5-S1 intervertebral disc, lateral anulus

L1-L2 intervertebral disc
L1 transverse process
L1 segmental nerve at dorsal root ganglion
Radicular vessels
L2 transverse process
L2 segmental nerve, dorsal root ganglion
L3 pedicle
L3 segmental nerve at dorsal root ganglion
Ligamentum flavum
L4 inferior articular process
L5 superior articular process
Thoracolumbar fascia, posterior layer
Multifidus m.
L5-S1 zygapophyseal joint
S2 segment
S1 segmental nerve
L5 segmental nerve at dorsal root ganglion

Figure 13.3.8

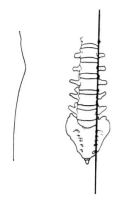

1. This left parasagittal section is through the extreme lateral aspect of the lumbar spine.

2. The true segmental spinal nerve is located in the extreme lateral aspect of the intervertebral foramina, the exit zone. In the lateral foramen the segmental nerve separates into three neural trunks. The largest trunk is the anterior ramus. The small posterior primary rami innervate the capsules of the facet joints and the "back" muscles. A tiny branch joins the gray ramus communicans of the sympathetic chain to form the sinu-vertebral nerve. This small nerve is primarily sensory in function and innervates the posterior and posterolateral anulus, the posterior longitudinal ligament, and the anterior dura.

3. There is a rich plexus of veins in the lateral foramen. The radicular perineural veins anastomose with the circumferential lumbar veins.

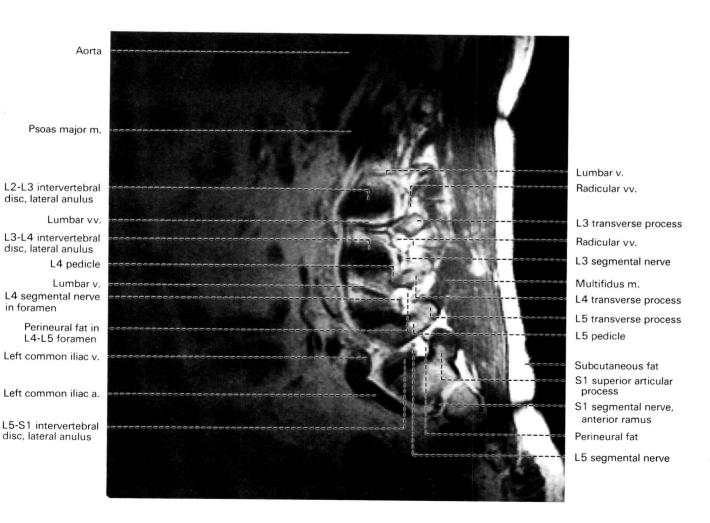

Aorta

Psoas major m.

L2-L3 intervertebral disc, lateral anulus

Lumbar vv.

L3-L4 intervertebral disc, lateral anulus

L4 pedicle

Lumbar v.

L4 segmental nerve in foramen

Perineural fat in L4-L5 foramen

Left common iliac v.

Left common iliac a.

L5-S1 intervertebral disc, lateral anulus

Lumbar v.

Radicular vv.

L3 transverse process

Radicular vv.

L3 segmental nerve

Multifidus m.

L4 transverse process

L5 transverse process

L5 pedicle

Subcutaneous fat

S1 superior articular process

S1 segmental nerve, anterior ramus

Perineural fat

L5 segmental nerve

Figure 13.3.9

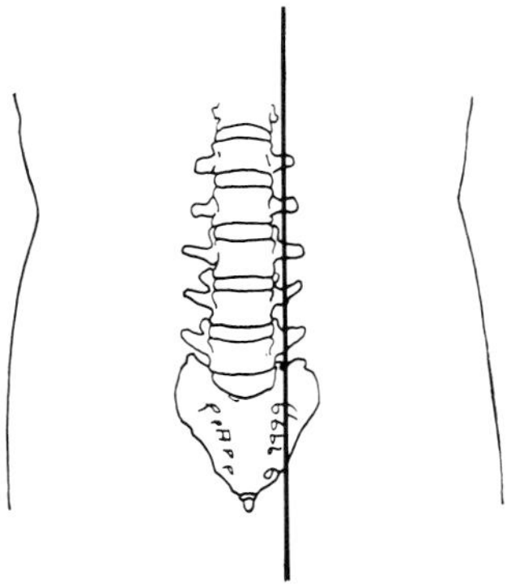

1. Parasagittal section lateral to the vertebral body through the bases of the transverse processes.

2. The back muscles (multifidi and erector spinae group) are located posterior to the transverse processes. Note the tiny lateral intertransversarii muscles. They insert on adjacent transverse processes. The psoas major muscles are anterior to the transverse processes.

3. The ascending lumbar veins course just anterior to the transverse processes. Inferiorly, these veins communicate with the common iliac veins. Superiorly, the right ascending lumbar vein becomes the azygos vein and the left becomes the hemiazygos vein.

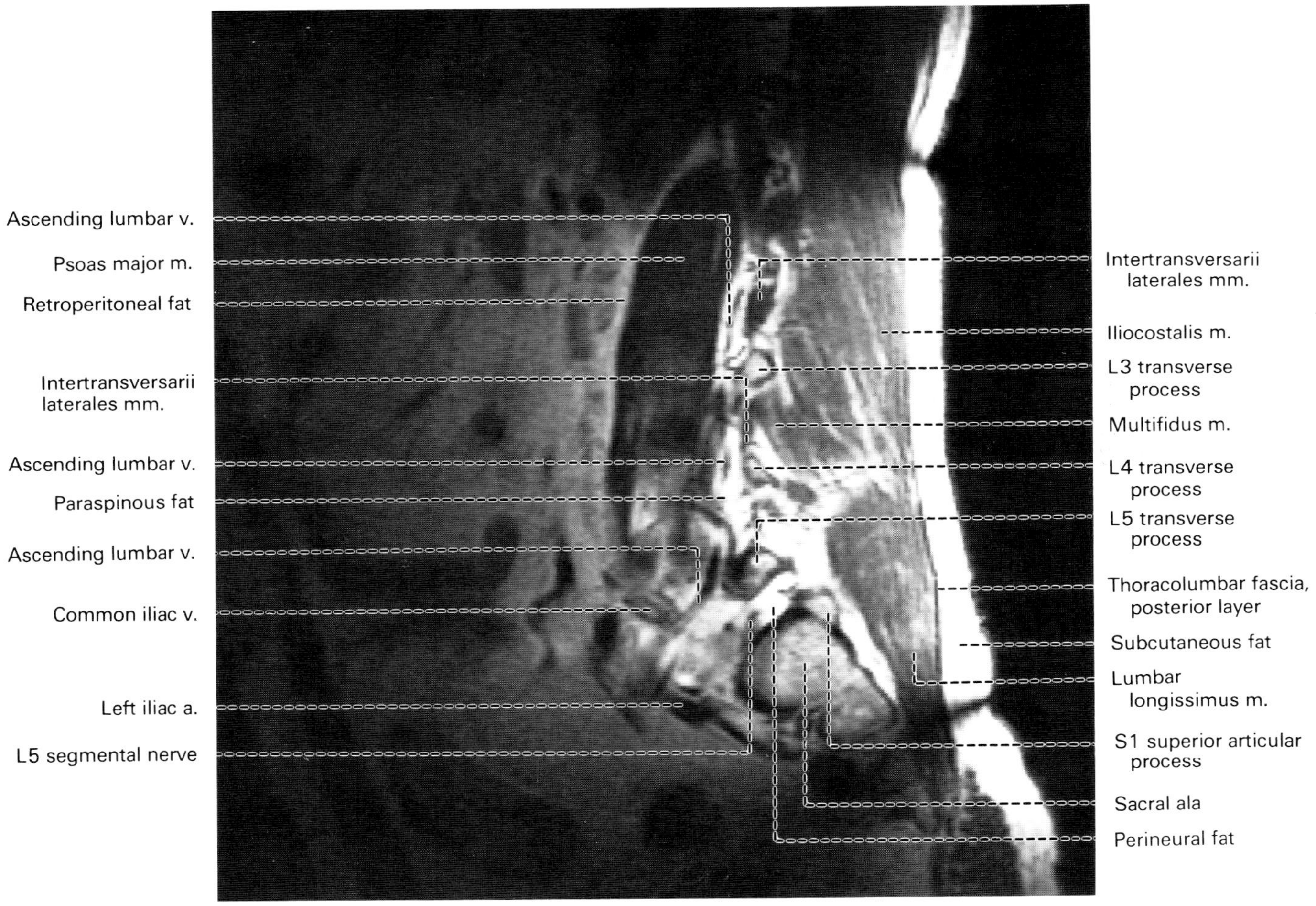
Ascending lumbar v.
Psoas major m.
Retroperitoneal fat
Intertransversarii laterales mm.
Ascending lumbar v.
Paraspinous fat
Ascending lumbar v.
Common iliac v.
Left iliac a.
L5 segmental nerve
Intertransversarii laterales mm.
Iliocostalis m.
L3 transverse process
Multifidus m.
L4 transverse process
L5 transverse process
Thoracolumbar fascia, posterior layer
Subcutaneous fat
Lumbar longissimus m.
S1 superior articular process
Sacral ala
Perineural fat

VI
LOWER LIMB

Chapter 14

THIGH

Figure 14.1.1

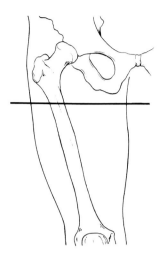

1. Note the testis on the right and the epididymis on the left.

2. Rectus femoris is distinct from the muscle mass of the vastus group, which is closely applied to the femur.

3. The hamstring group is partly tendinous and partly muscular; semitendinosus is the only fleshy portion at this level.

4. The distal fibers of gluteus maximus insert into the lateral intermuscular septum.

5. Note the medial femoral circumflex artery arising from the deep femoral artery.

6. Observe the femoral vessels close to the apex of the femoral triangle.

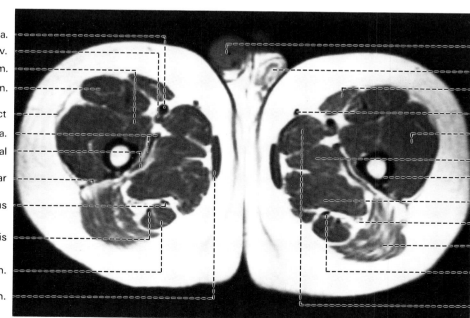

Femoral a.
Femoral v.
Vastus intermedius m.
Rectus femoris m.
Iliotibial tract
Deep femoral a.
Medial femoral circumflex a.
Lateral intermuscular septum
Semimembranosus tendon
Biceps femoris tendon
Semitendinosus m.
Gracilis m.

Testis
Epididymis
Sartorius m.
Great saphenous v.
Vastus lateralis m.
Adductor brevis m.
Femur
Adductor magnus m.
Sciatic nerve
Gluteus maximus m.
Semimembranosus tendon
Adductor longus m.

Figure 14.1.2

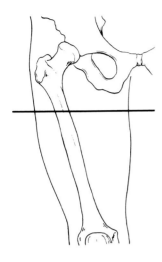

1. The femoral artery and vein course in the adductor canal of Hunter, formed by the sartorius anteriorly, the adductor longus medially, and the quadriceps group laterally.

2. This section is similar to the more proximal section.

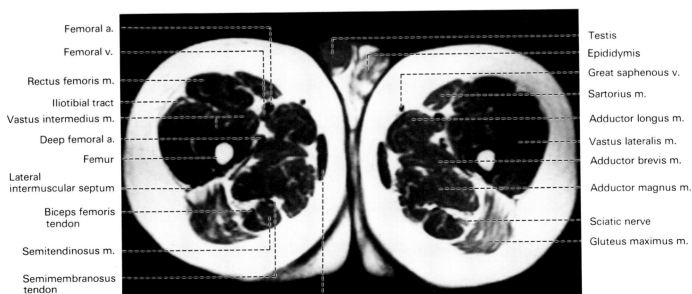

Femoral a.

Femoral v.

Rectus femoris m.

Iliotibial tract

Vastus intermedius m.

Deep femoral a.

Femur

Lateral
intermuscular septum

Biceps femoris
tendon

Semitendinosus m.

Semimembranosus
tendon

Gracilis m.

Testis

Epididymis

Great saphenous v.

Sartorius m.

Adductor longus m.

Vastus lateralis m.

Adductor brevis m.

Adductor magnus m.

Sciatic nerve

Gluteus maximus m.

Figure 14.1.3

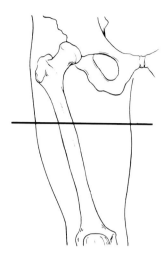

1. The muscular portion of the long head of biceps femoris is situated medial to gluteus maximus and lateral to semitendinosus.

2. Gluteus maximus diminishes in size as the sections proceed distally.

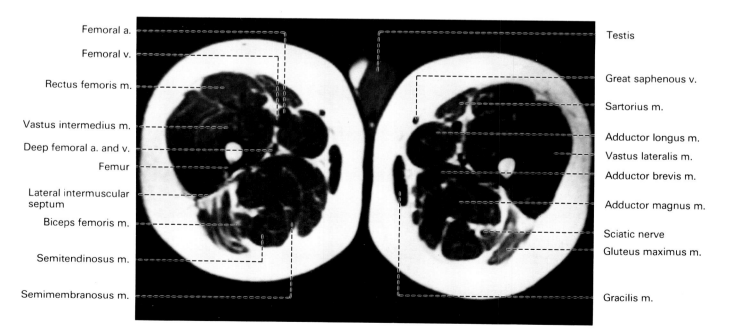

Femoral a.

Femoral v.

Rectus femoris m.

Vastus intermedius m.

Deep femoral a. and v.

Femur

Lateral intermuscular septum

Biceps femoris m.

Semitendinosus m.

Semimembranosus m.

Testis

Great saphenous v.

Sartorius m.

Adductor longus m.

Vastus lateralis m.

Adductor brevis m.

Adductor magnus m.

Sciatic nerve

Gluteus maximus m.

Gracilis m.

Figure 14.1.4

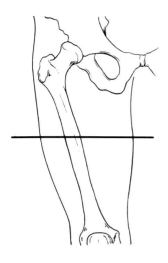

1. Note that part of semimembranosus is still tendinous at this level.

2. The sciatic nerve is interposed between adductor magnus and biceps femoris at this level.

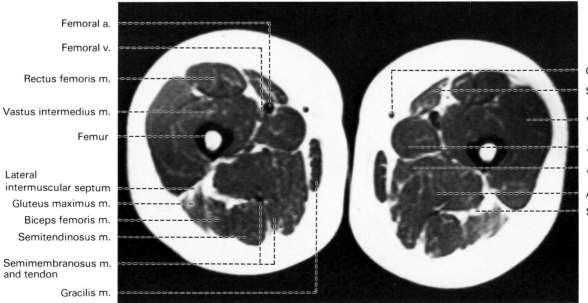

Figure 14.1.5

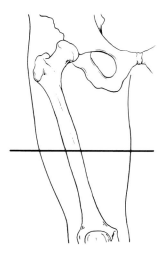

1. At this level the hamstring group is well developed; it is entirely muscular except for a small tendinous portion of semimembranosus.

2. The adductor group now consists of adductor longus and adductor magnus; adductor brevis has completed its insertion onto the upper third of the medial lip of the linea aspera.

3. The individual muscles of the vastus group are not clearly separated; they are closely applied to the femoral shaft.

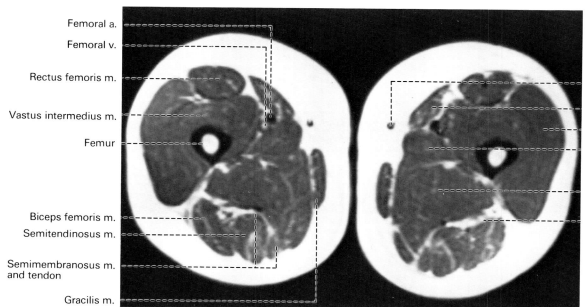

Figure 14.1.6

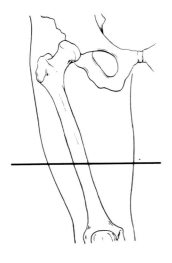

1. At this level adductor longus is decreasing in size. It forms the floor of the adductor canal of Hunter.

2. On the right the three hamstring muscles are clearly identified from medial to lateral: semimembranosus, semitendinosus, and biceps femoris.

3. The lateral intermuscular septum is sharply defined in this section.

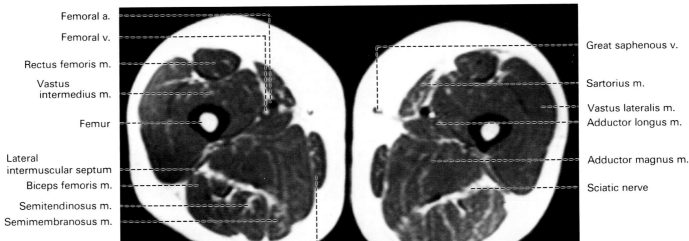

Femoral a.
Femoral v.
Rectus femoris m.
Vastus intermedius m.
Femur
Lateral intermuscular septum
Biceps femoris m.
Semitendinosus m.
Semimembranosus m.
Gracilis m.

Great saphenous v.
Sartorius m.
Vastus lateralis m.
Adductor longus m.
Adductor magnus m.
Sciatic nerve

Figure 14.1.7

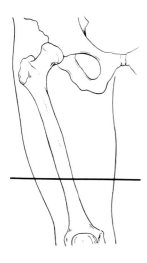

1. The femoral artery and vein lie within the fat of the medial intermuscular septum that separates the adductors from the quadriceps group. Sartorius covers these vascular structures.

2. The sciatic nerve is surrounded by biceps femoris and adductor magnus.

3. The great saphenous vein lies within the subcutaneous tissues adjacent to gracilis and sartorius.

4. Note the four components of the quadriceps group with vastus lateralis being the largest at this level.

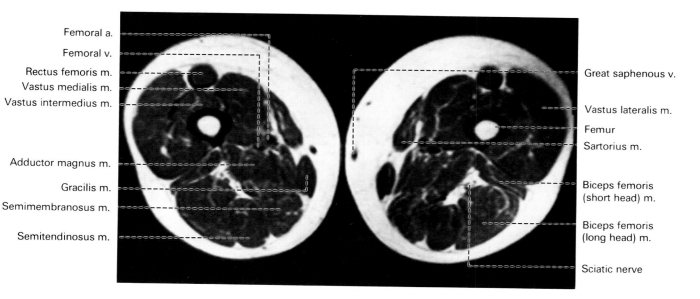

Femoral a.
Femoral v.
Rectus femoris m.
Vastus medialis m.
Vastus intermedius m.

Adductor magnus m.
Gracilis m.
Semimembranosus m.
Semitendinosus m.

Great saphenous v.

Vastus lateralis m.
Femur
Sartorius m.

Biceps femoris (short head) m.

Biceps femoris (long head) m.

Sciatic nerve

Figure 14.1.8

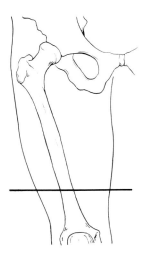

1. The vasti are incompletely separated at this level.

2. Biceps femoris is now divided into its larger long head and smaller short head.

3. In successive sections sartorius is seen coursing from its anterior lateral origin to its distal medial insertion.

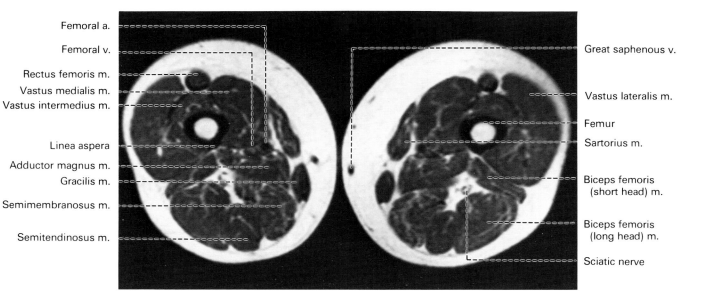

Femoral a.

Femoral v.

Rectus femoris m.
Vastus medialis m.
Vastus intermedius m.

Linea aspera
Adductor magnus m.
Gracilis m.
Semimembranosus m.

Semitendinosus m.

Great saphenous v.

Vastus lateralis m.

Femur
Sartorius m.

Biceps femoris
(short head) m.

Biceps femoris
(long head) m.

Sciatic nerve

Figure 14.1.9

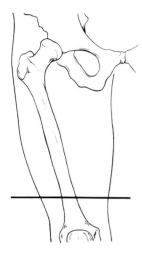

1. Note the transformation of the rectus femoris muscle into the rectus femoris tendon.

2. The posterior compartment has clearly identifiable muscular components of the hamstring group.

3. Note that the short head of biceps femoris maintains a rectangular configuration compared to the more oval appearance of the long head.

4. Note that the size of the adductor magnus decreases as the sections proceed inferiorly.

5. The linea aspera is the rough linear area on the posterior aspect of the femur providing an attachment site for vastus medialis, vastus lateralis, adductor longus, adductor magnus, adductor brevis, and the short head of biceps.

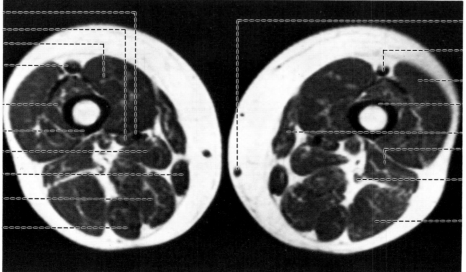

Figure 14.1.10

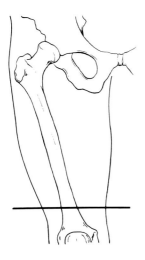

1. At this level, the femoral artery and vein are slightly superior to the adductor canal.

2. The sciatic nerve is still undivided at this level.

3. Note the relatively small size of semitendinosus compared to the much larger semimembranosus in this section.

4. Gracilis is decreasing in size.

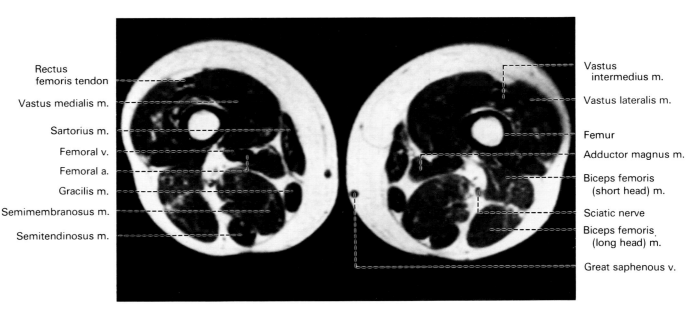

Rectus femoris tendon
Vastus medialis m.
Sartorius m.
Femoral v.
Femoral a.
Gracilis m.
Semimembranosus m.
Semitendinosus m.

Vastus intermedius m.
Vastus lateralis m.
Femur
Adductor magnus m.
Biceps femoris (short head) m.
Sciatic nerve
Biceps femoris (long head) m.
Great saphenous v.

Figure 14.1.11

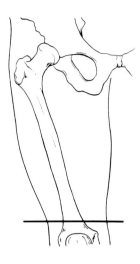

1. This image is at the level of the adductor hiatus. A small portion of adductor magnus remains and the femoral artery and vein are adjacent to it. Inferior to this, the femoral vein and artery become the popliteal vein and artery.

2. At this level the sciatic divides into the tibial and common peroneal nerves.

3. Vastus intermedius is becoming tendinous.

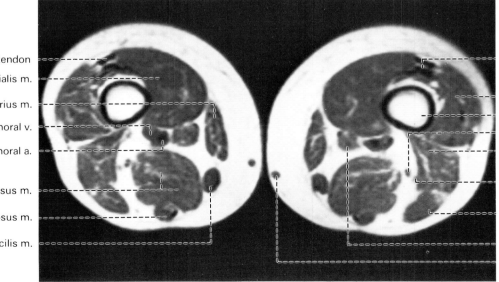

Rectus femoris tendon
Vastus medialis m.
Sartorius m.
Femoral v.
Femoral a.
Semimembranosus m.
Semitendinosus m.
Gracilis m.

Vastus intermedius tendon
Vastus lateralis m.
Femur
Tibial nerve
Biceps femoris (short head) m.
Common peroneal nerve
Biceps femoris (long head) m.
Adductor magnus m.
Great saphenous v.

Figure 14.1.12

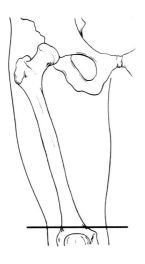

1. This section is at the level of the superior aspect of the popliteal space.

2. Note that the popliteal artery is medial to the popliteal vein.

3. From this level down to the knee the vastus medialis remains the most prominent member of the quadriceps group.

4. At this level, biceps femoris is predominantly composed of the short head.

5. Gracilis and semitendinosus are tendinous from this level to their insertion.

6. The tendons of vastus intermedius and rectus femoris are starting to fuse forming the proximal portion of the quadriceps tendon.

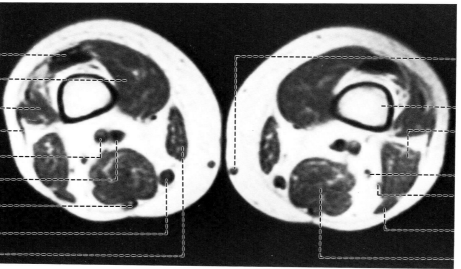

Quadriceps femoris tendon
Vastus medialis m.
Vastus lateralis m.
Iliotibial tract
Popliteal v.
Popliteal a.
Semitendinosus tendon
Gracilis m.
Sartorius m.

Great saphenous v.
Femur
Biceps femoris (short head) m.
Tibial nerve
Common peroneal nerve
Biceps femoris (long head) m.
Semimembranosus m.

Figure 14.1.13

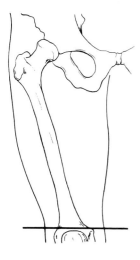

1. This level is superior to the patella, and the low signal of the quadriceps tendon is identifiable.

2. The great saphenous vein is clearly identified as a large vascular structure, superficially located adjacent to sartorius.

3. Vastus lateralis inserts into the lateral patellar retinaculum.

4. Note the significant thickness of the iliotibial tract, which lies adjacent to vastus lateralis.

5. The common peroneal nerve is adjacent to the medial surface of the short head of biceps femoris.

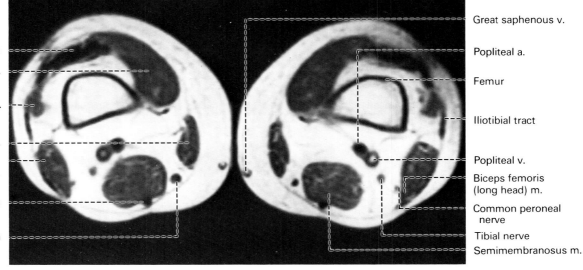

Quadriceps tendon
Vastus medialis m.
Vastus lateralis m.
Sartorius m.
Biceps femoris (short head) m.
Semitendinosus tendon
Gracilis tendon

Great saphenous v.
Popliteal a.
Femur
Iliotibial tract
Popliteal v.
Biceps femoris (long head) m.
Common peroneal nerve
Tibial nerve
Semimembranosus m.

Figure 14.1.14

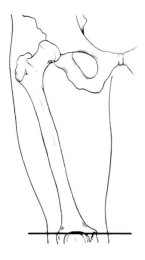

1. The synovial space is demonstrated at this level.

2. The only muscle of the quadriceps group identified at this level is vastus medialis.

3. Note the thick linear structure of the iliotibial tract.

4. The neurovascular bundle is seen posterior to the distal femur. At this level of the popliteal space, the artery is the most anterior, followed by the vein, and the tibial nerve as the most posterior. The more lateral common peroneal nerve is deep to biceps femoris posterolaterally.

5. Note the origin of the medial head of gastrocnemius arising from the posterior aspect of the medial femoral condyle.

6. Of the three muscles that constitute the pes anserinus (sartorius, gracilis, and semitendinosus), only sartorius remains fleshy at this level.

7. Note the origin of the plantaris muscle from the posterior aspect of the lateral femoral condyle.

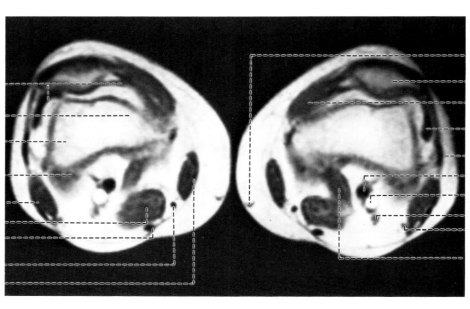

CORONAL

Figure 14.2.1

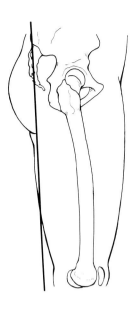

1. This section passes through the most posterior aspect of the buttocks.

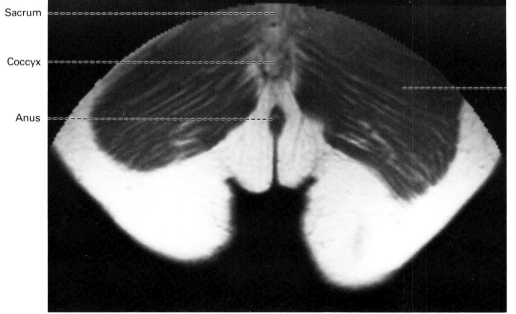

Sacrum

Coccyx

Anus

Gluteus maximus m.

Figure 14.2.2

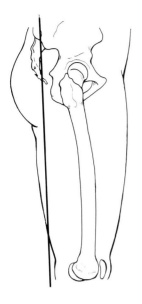

1. The hamstring muscles are partially seen in this section.

2. Gluteus maximus covers the origin of the hamstring group.

3. Adductor magnus is partially imaged medial to the hamstring group.

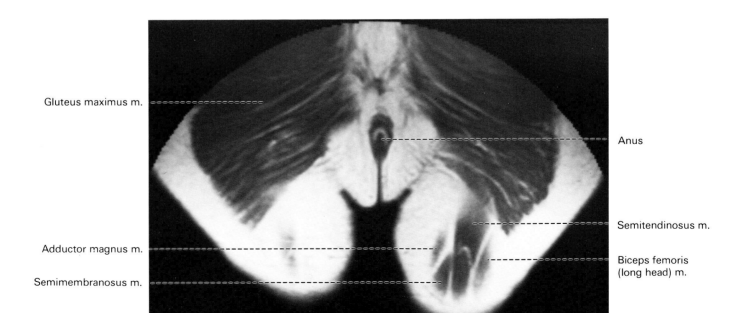

Gluteus maximus m.

Adductor magnus m.

Semimembranosus m.

Anus

Semitendinosus m.

Biceps femoris (long head) m.

Figure 14.2.3

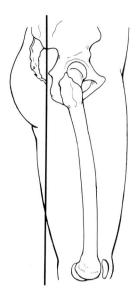

1. The external anal sphincter is noted around the anus.

2. The ischiorectal fossa is filled with fat.

3. The levator ani courses toward the anus and its two halves insert (in part) onto the anococcygeal ligament.

4. Note the posterior portion of adductor magnus that functions as a hamstring muscle and is innervated by the sciatic nerve.

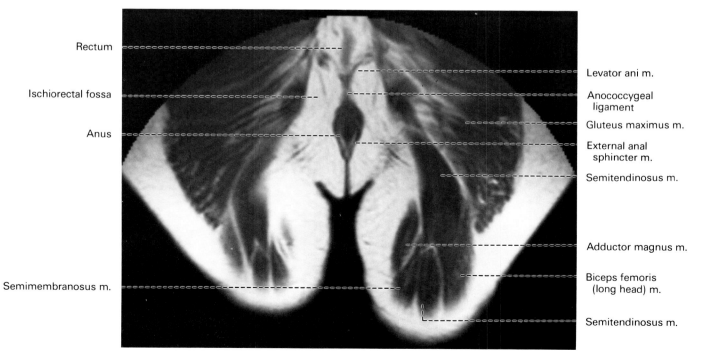

Figure 14.2.4

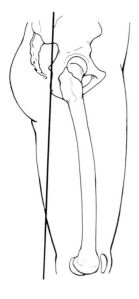

1. The conjoint tendon of the hamstring group arises from the ischium.

2. The ischial tuberosity gives rise to the more vertically oriented posterior portion of adductor magnus.

3. The rectum and superior rectal vessels are demonstrated.

4. The fat of the ischiorectal fossa is in continuity with the medial subcutaneous fat of the proximal thigh.

5. Obturator internus is seen medial to the ischium.

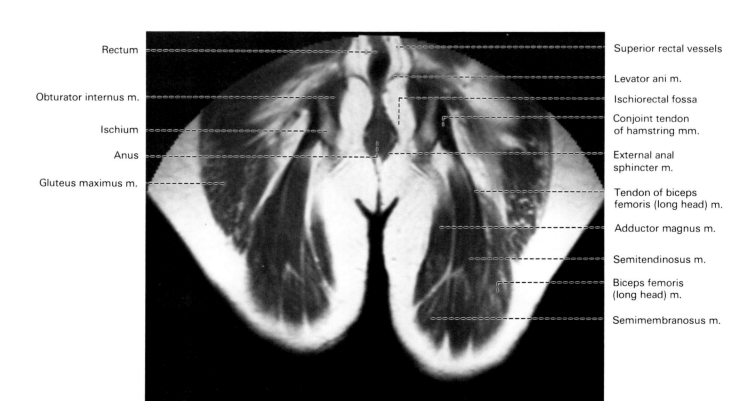

Rectum

Obturator internus m.

Ischium

Anus

Gluteus maximus m.

Superior rectal vessels

Levator ani m.

Ischiorectal fossa

Conjoint tendon of hamstring mm.

External anal sphincter m.

Tendon of biceps femoris (long head) m.

Adductor magnus m.

Semitendinosus m.

Biceps femoris (long head) m.

Semimembranosus m.

Figure 14.2.5

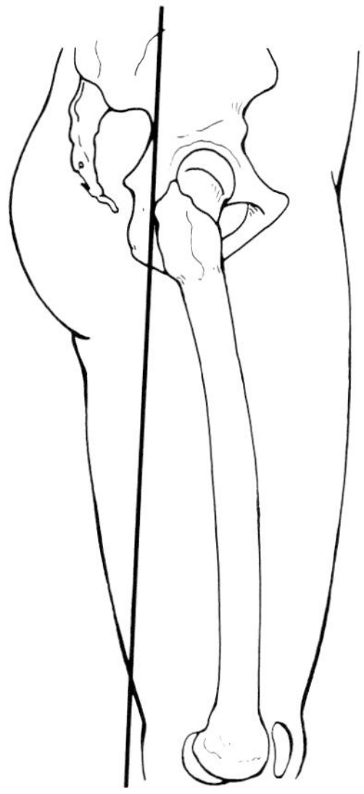

1. The sciatic nerve is seen exiting the greater sciatic foramen.
2. Note the fibers of gluteus maximus inserting into the iliotibial tract.
3. The short external rotators (piriformis, gemelli, obturator internus tendon, and quadratus femoris) are demonstrated just lateral to the ischium on the left. Obturator internus lines the medial surface of the ischium.

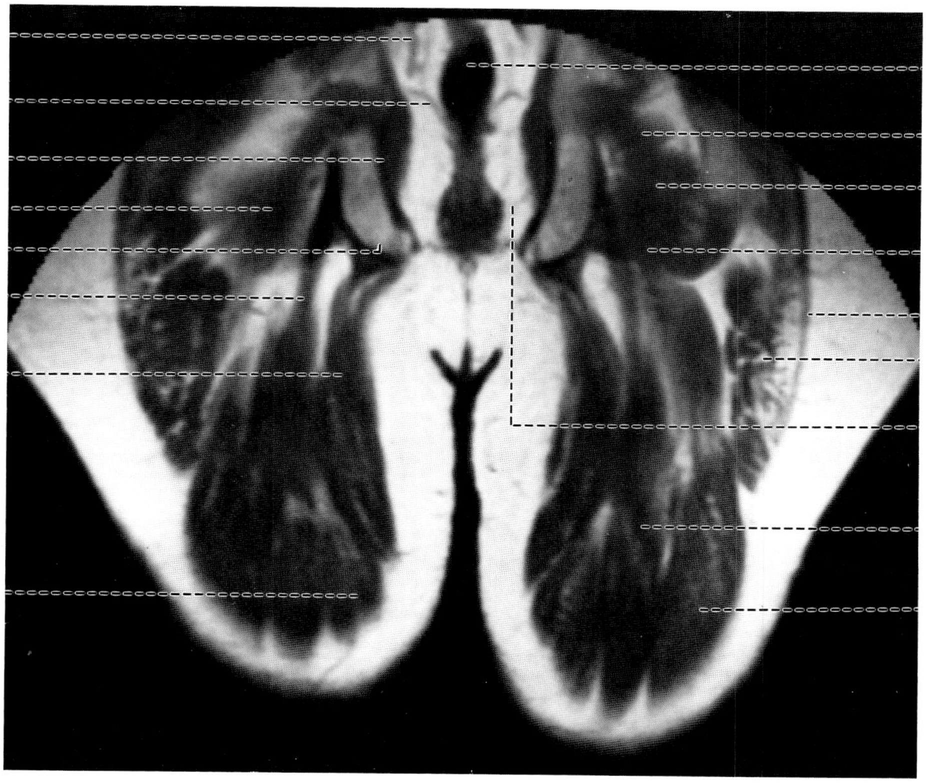
Superior rectal vessels
Levator ani m.
Obturator internus m.
Sciatic nerve
Ischium
Semitendinosus tendon
Adductor magnus m.
Semimembranosus m.
Rectum
Piriformis m.
Obturator internus and gemelli mm.
Quadratus femoris m.
Iliotibial tract
Gluteus maximus m.
Ischiorectal fossa
Semitendinosus m.
Biceps femoris m.

Figure 14.2.6

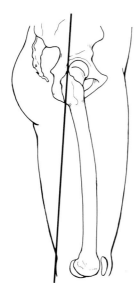

1. Adductor brevis courses obliquely toward its insertion on the medial lip of the linea aspera.

2. The posterior position of the greater trochanter can be identified at this level. The short external rotators converge toward it to insert.

3. The posterior portion of the prostate can be seen.

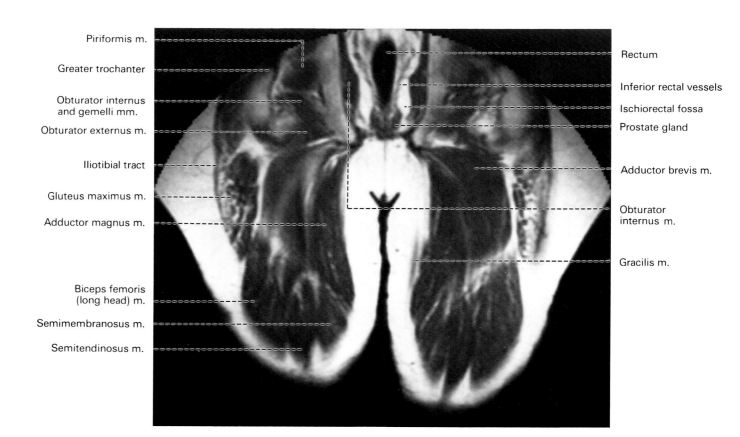

Piriformis m.

Greater trochanter

Obturator internus and gemelli mm.

Obturator externus m.

Iliotibial tract

Gluteus maximus m.

Adductor magnus m.

Biceps femoris (long head) m.

Semimembranosus m.

Semitendinosus m.

Rectum

Inferior rectal vessels

Ischiorectal fossa

Prostate gland

Adductor brevis m.

Obturator internus m.

Gracilis m.

Figure 14.2.7

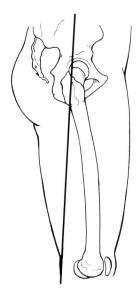

1. The greater trochanter, intertrochanteric crest, and lesser trochanter are posterior structures.

2. The seminal vesicles are identified on either side of the prostate gland.

3. The ureter is identified on the right coming into the posterior aspect of the bladder.

4. On the left, the origin of the vastus lateralis from the lateral lip of the linea aspera is seen as far superiorly as the greater trochanter.

5. Obturator externus is seen coursing toward its insertion in the trochanteric fossa.

6. Semitendinosus becomes tendinous in the inferior aspect of the thigh.

Greater trochanter
Intertrochanteric crest
Lesser trochanter
Adductor brevis m.
Gluteus maximus m.
Biceps femoris m.
Semimembranosus m.
Semitendinosus m.

Inferior vesical vessels
Obturator internus m.
Obturator externus m.
Pectineus m.
Prostate gland
Seminal vesicle
Vastus lateralis m.
Adductor magnus m.
Gracilis m.
Semitendinosus tendon

Figure 14.2.8

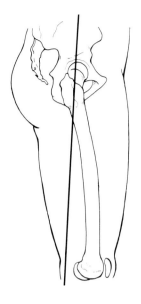

1. The semitendinosus tendon courses posterior to semimembranosus.

2. Obturator internus and obturator externus originate on opposite sides of the obturator foramen.

3. Gracilis originates from the inferior pubic ramus near the symphysis.

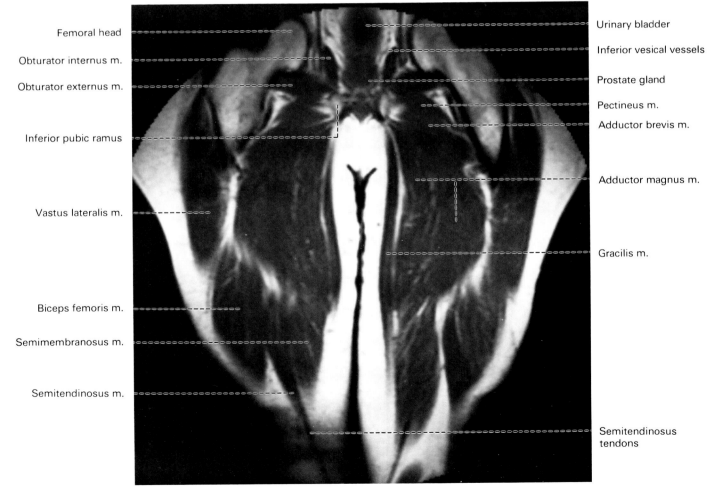

Femoral head

Obturator internus m.

Obturator externus m.

Inferior pubic ramus

Vastus lateralis m.

Biceps femoris m.

Semimembranosus m.

Semitendinosus m.

Urinary bladder

Inferior vesical vessels

Prostate gland

Pectineus m.

Adductor brevis m.

Adductor magnus m.

Gracilis m.

Semitendinosus tendons

Figure 14.2.9

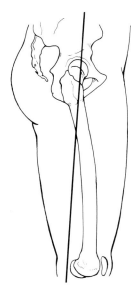

1. Semimembranosus, semitendinosus, gracilis, and sartorius become tendinous in the distal thigh.

2. The ejaculatory ducts can be seen coursing toward the prostate.

3. Gracilis is demonstrated in its entire length.

4. The obturator vessels emerge from the obturator canal and course inferiorly beneath pectineus.

5. Sartorius is partially seen in the distal thigh on the left.

6. Iliopsoas courses toward its insertion on the lesser trochanter.

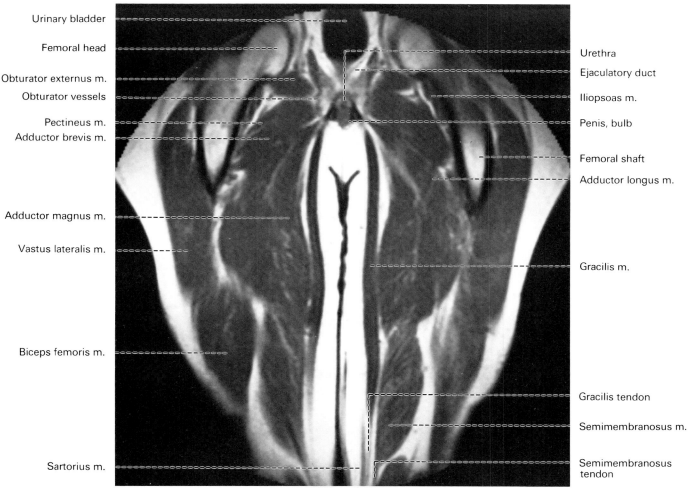

Urinary bladder
Femoral head
Obturator externus m.
Obturator vessels
Pectineus m.
Adductor brevis m.
Adductor magnus m.
Vastus lateralis m.
Biceps femoris m.
Sartorius m.

Urethra
Ejaculatory duct
Iliopsoas m.
Penis, bulb
Femoral shaft
Adductor longus m.
Gracilis m.
Gracilis tendon
Semimembranosus m.
Semimembranosus tendon

Figure 14.2.10

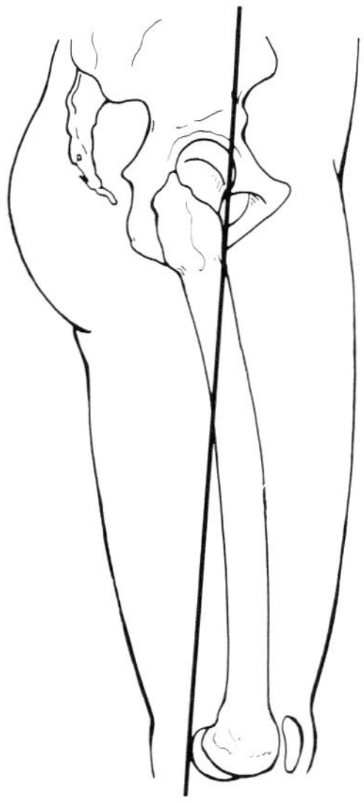

1. The perivesical space is clearly seen.
2. The superior pubic ramus gives origin to pectineus and part of obturator externus.
3. Note the convergence of the long and short heads of biceps femoris. The short head of the biceps originates from the lower half of the lateral lip of the linea aspera.
4. The femoral head and neck are covered anteriorly by iliopsoas. The iliopsoas does not have a significant tendinous component.
5. Note the origins of the medial and lateral heads of gastrocnemius from the posterior aspects of the femoral condyles.

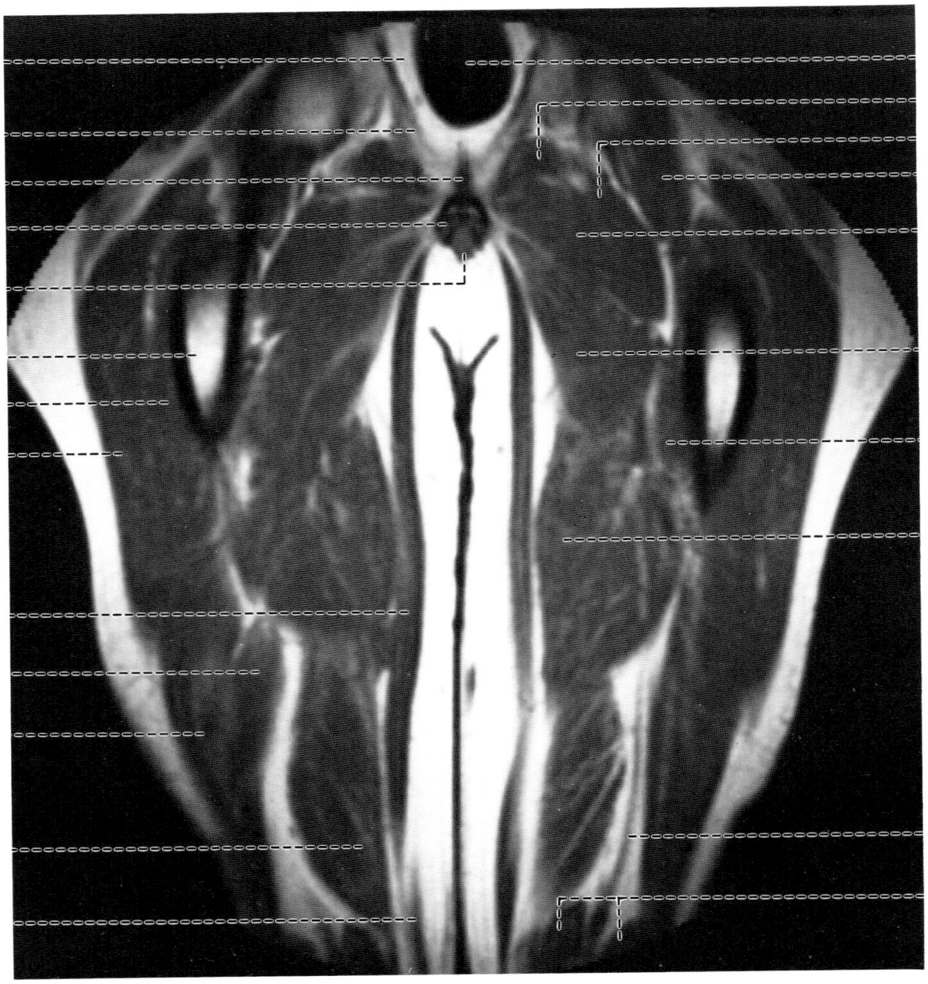
Perivesical space
Superior pubic ramus
Symphysis pubis
Corpus cavernosum
Corpus spongiosum
Femoral shaft
Vastus intermedius m.
Vastus lateralis m.
Gracilis m.
Biceps femoris (short head) m.
Biceps femoris (long head) m.
Semimembranosus m.
Sartorius m.
Urinary bladder
Obturator externus m.
Pectineus m.
Iliopsoas m.
Adductor brevis m.
Adductor longus m.
Vastus intermedius m.
Adductor magnus m.
Popliteal a.
Gastrocnemius m., medial and lateral heads

Figure 14.2.11

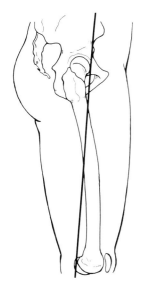

1. Note the femoral vessels coursing medial to iliopsoas and anterior to pectineus.

2. Sartorius muscles are only partially seen because of their oblique course in the thigh.

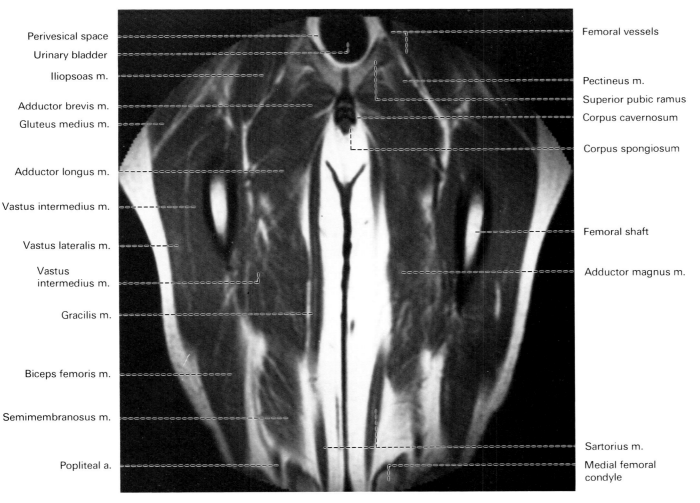

Perivesical space
Urinary bladder
Iliopsoas m.
Adductor brevis m.
Gluteus medius m.
Adductor longus m.
Vastus intermedius m.
Vastus lateralis m.
Vastus intermedius m.
Gracilis m.
Biceps femoris m.
Semimembranosus m.
Popliteal a.

Femoral vessels
Pectineus m.
Superior pubic ramus
Corpus cavernosum
Corpus spongiosum
Femoral shaft
Adductor magnus m.
Sartorius m.
Medial femoral condyle

Figure 14.2.12

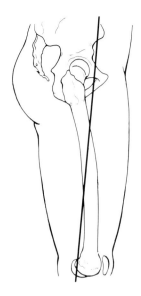

1. The femoral artery and vein can be seen in the distal thigh; the artery is medial to the vein. After exiting the adductor hiatus they are renamed the popliteal artery and vein.

2. The femoral vessels can be seen superiorly at the level of the groin; the artery is lateral to the vein.

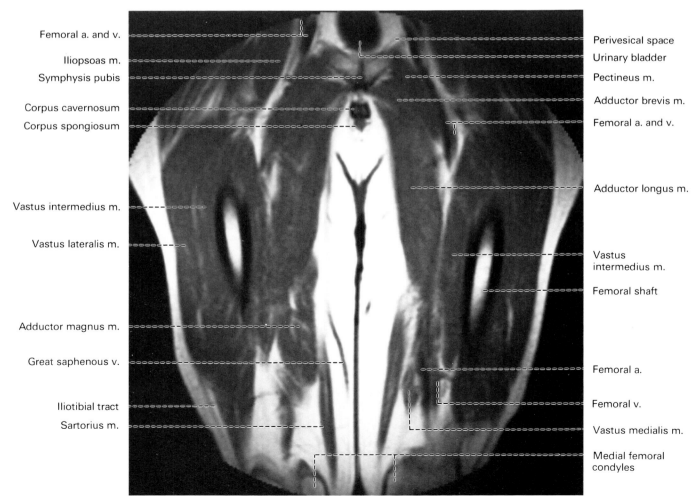

Femoral a. and v.
Iliopsoas m.
Symphysis pubis
Corpus cavernosum
Corpus spongiosum
Vastus intermedius m.
Vastus lateralis m.
Adductor magnus m.
Great saphenous v.
Iliotibial tract
Sartorius m.

Perivesical space
Urinary bladder
Pectineus m.
Adductor brevis m.
Femoral a. and v.
Adductor longus m.
Vastus intermedius m.
Femoral shaft
Femoral a.
Femoral v.
Vastus medialis m.
Medial femoral condyles

Figure 14.2.13

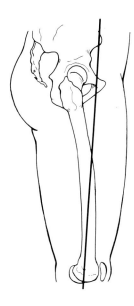

1. The femoral artery and vein are seen in the groin.

2. At this level tensor fasciae latae is demonstrated.

3. Vastus medialis is seen lateral to sartorius.

4. Note the perforating veins between the great saphenous and femoral veins. In healthy subjects they carry blood from the superficial to the deep system.

5. The iliotibial tract is seen in the distal thigh.

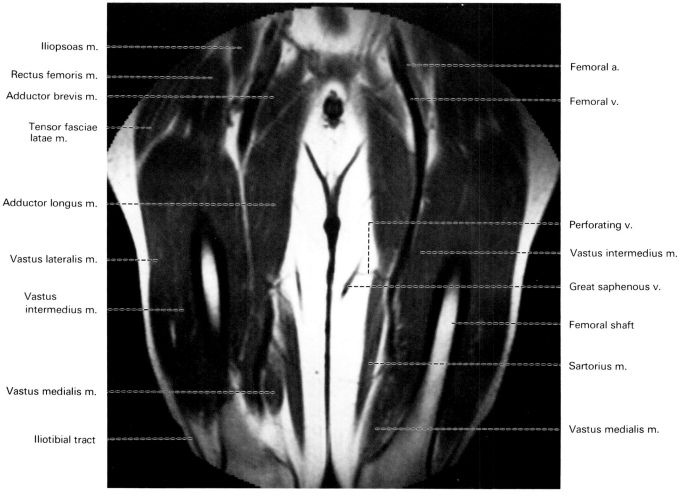

Figure 14.2.14

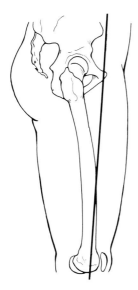

1. In the superior part of the image note sartorius coursing inferiorly from its origin at the anterior superior iliac spine.

2. Rectus femoris is coursing inferiorly from its origin at the anterior inferior iliac spine and acetabular margin.

3. The great saphenous vein ascends to drain into the femoral vein just distal to the inguinal ligament.

4. This section passes through the anterior abdominal wall and demonstrates rectus abdominis. The linea alba is the anterior midline aponeurosis between the two rectus abdominis muscles.

5. Note the spermatic cords coursing superolaterally toward the inguinal canal.

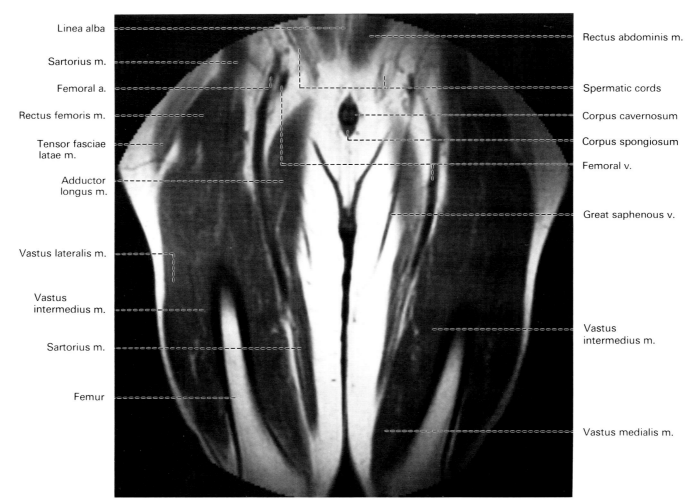

Linea alba
Sartorius m.
Femoral a.
Rectus femoris m.
Tensor fasciae latae m.
Adductor longus m.
Vastus lateralis m.
Vastus intermedius m.
Sartorius m.
Femur

Rectus abdominis m.
Spermatic cords
Corpus cavernosum
Corpus spongiosum
Femoral v.
Great saphenous v.
Vastus intermedius m.
Vastus medialis m.

Figure 14.2.15

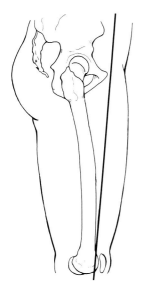

1. Vastus medialis becomes prominent medially in the distal thigh.

2. Note the inguinal lymph nodes, which are demonstrated bilaterally.

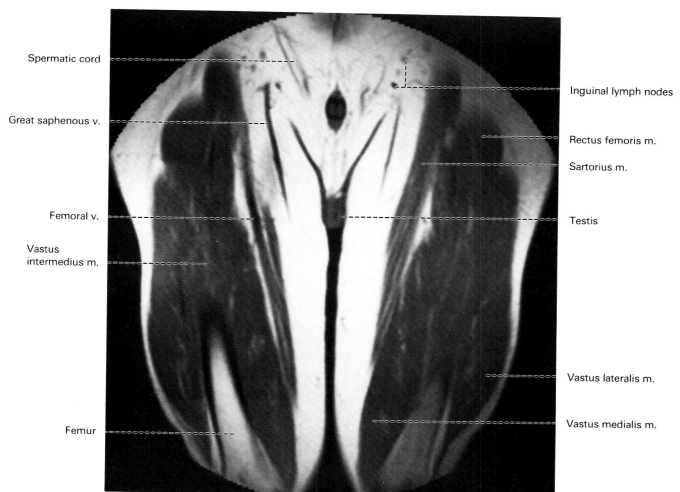

Spermatic cord

Great saphenous v.

Femoral v.

Vastus
intermedius m.

Femur

Inguinal lymph nodes

Rectus femoris m.

Sartorius m.

Testis

Vastus lateralis m.

Vastus medialis m.

Figure 14.2.16

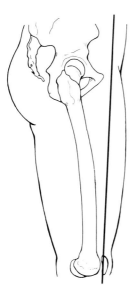

1. The quadriceps muscles and sartorius are well demonstrated in this section.

2. The spermatic cord is seen coursing from the testes toward the inguinal canal.

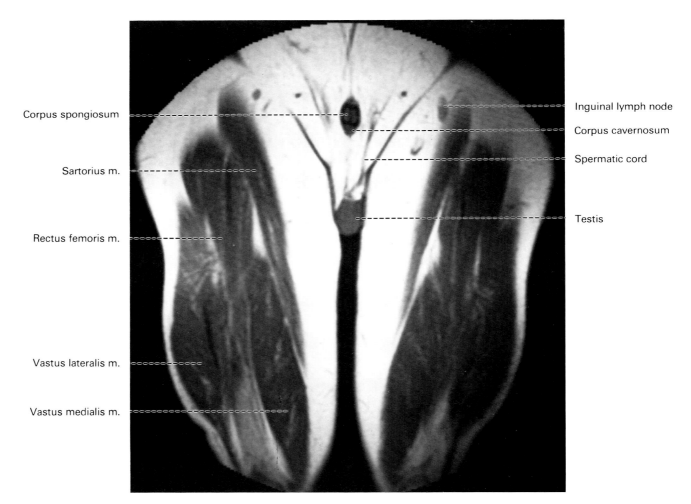

Figure 14.2.17

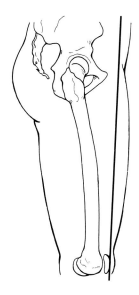

1. Inguinal lymph nodes are demonstrated in the subcutaneous fat of the inguinal region.

2. The spermatic cord and head of epididymis are seen.

3. Note the conversion and insertion of the quadriceps muscles into the quadriceps tendon.

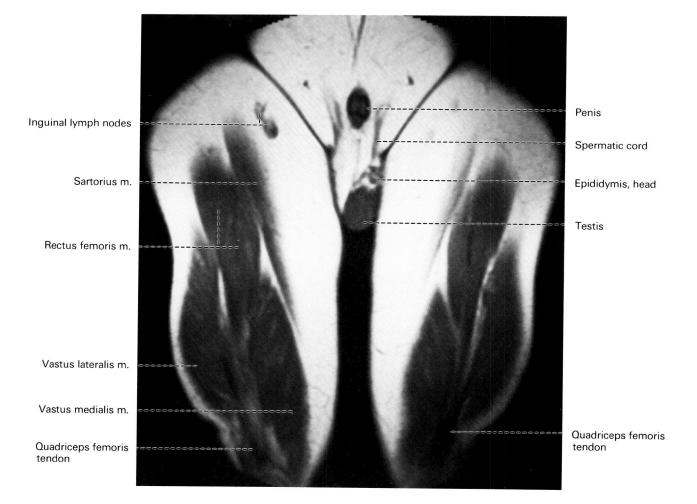

Inguinal lymph nodes

Sartorius m.

Rectus femoris m.

Vastus lateralis m.

Vastus medialis m.

Quadriceps femoris tendon

Penis

Spermatic cord

Epididymis, head

Testis

Quadriceps femoris tendon

Figure 14.2.18

1. The quadriceps femoris tendon is seen inferiorly in the right thigh.

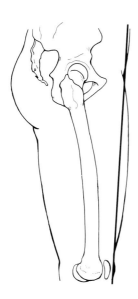

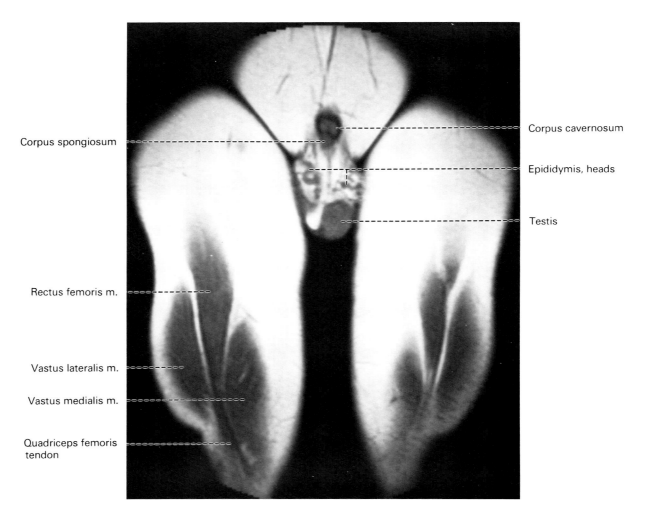

Corpus spongiosum

Corpus cavernosum

Epididymis, heads

Testis

Rectus femoris m.

Vastus lateralis m.

Vastus medialis m.

Quadriceps femoris tendon

SAGITTAL

Figure 14.3.1

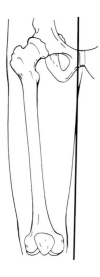

1. This section passes sagittally through the most medial aspect of the thigh.

2. Gracilis is partially demonstrated.

3. Gluteus maximus arises in part from the coccyx.

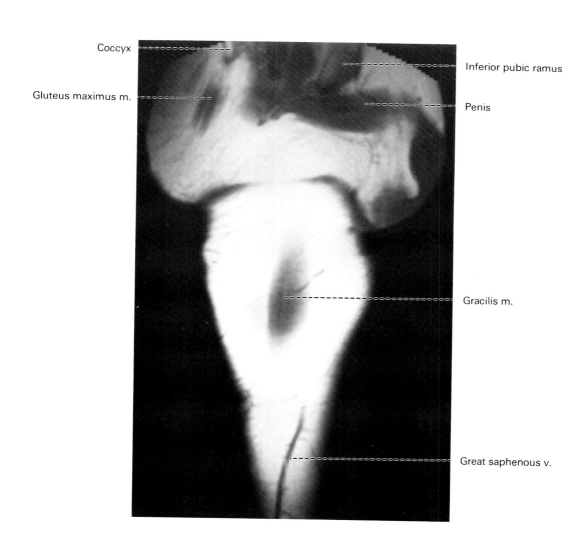

Coccyx

Inferior pubic ramus

Gluteus maximus m.

Penis

Gracilis m.

Great saphenous v.

Figure 14.3.2

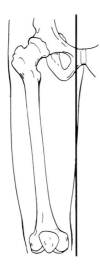

1. Gracilis arises from the inferior pubic ramus inferior to the symphysis pubis.

2. Adductor magnus is partially seen posterior to gracilis.

3. The great saphenous vein ascends in the subcutaneous tissues on the anteromedial aspect of the thigh.

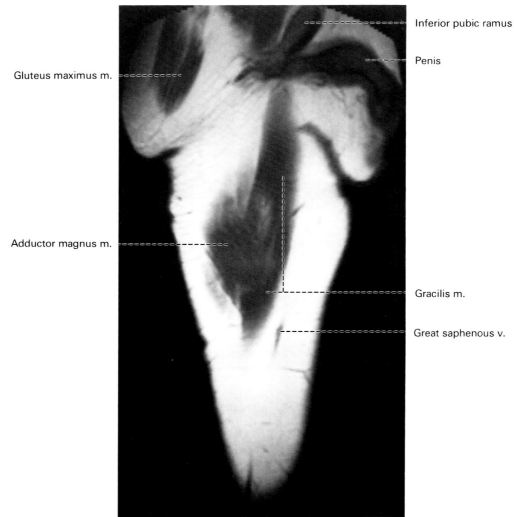

Figure 14.3.3

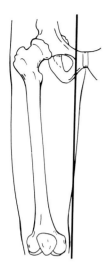

1. Gracilis, adductor longus, and adductor brevis arise from the inferior pubic ramus.

2. Adductor magnus arises from the inferior pubic ramus and ischium. Its most posterior portion functions as a hamstring muscle and is innervated by the sciatic nerve.

3. Note the relation of sartorius and gracilis in the distal thigh. Along with semitendinosus they form the so-called pes anserinus tendon.

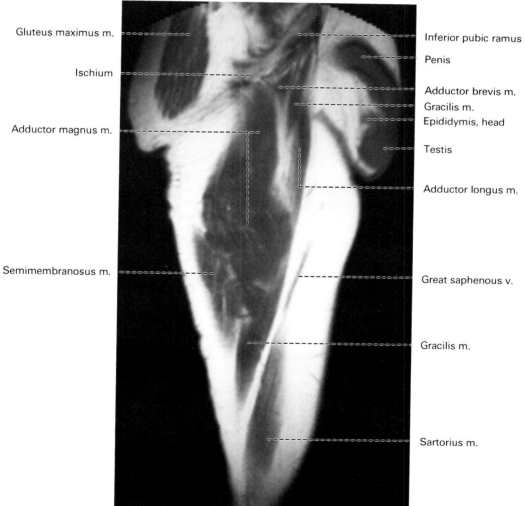

Figure 14.3.4

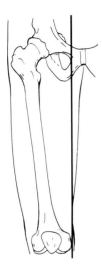

1. Obturator internus and externus are partially demonstrated on opposite sides of the inferior pubic ramus.

2. At the level of the knee the components of the pes anserinus become tendinous. The tendon of gracilis is well demonstrated in this section.

3. Semimembranosus is partially seen posterior to adductor magnus.

4. Note the part of adductor magnus that originates from the ischial tuberosity.

5. The great saphenous vein continues to ascend on the anteromedial aspect of the thigh.

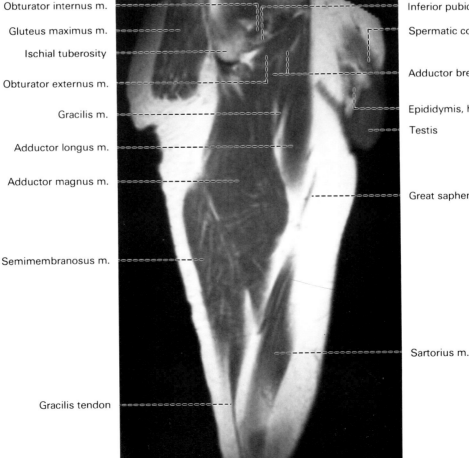

Obturator internus m.
Gluteus maximus m.
Ischial tuberosity
Obturator externus m.
Gracilis m.
Adductor longus m.
Adductor magnus m.
Semimembranosus m.
Gracilis tendon

Inferior pubic ramus
Spermatic cord
Adductor brevis and pectineus mm.
Epididymis, head
Testis
Great saphenous v.
Sartorius m.

Figure 14.3.5

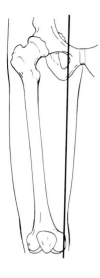

1. Pectineus arises from the pectin on the superior pubic ramus and courses posterolaterally to insert on the pectineal line of the femur. It forms the medial floor of the femoral triangle.

2. Vastus medialis is partially demonstrated above the medial femoral condyle.

3. Adductor magnus becomes tendinous at the adductor hiatus. The tendon continues distally to insert at the medial supracondylar line of the femur.

4. The semitendinosus tendon courses distally posterior to the semimembranosus muscle. It forms the posterior component of the pes anserinus complex, which inserts on the anteromedial aspect of the proximal tibia.

5. Note the origin of semitendinosus from the ischial tuberosity.

6. The spermatic cord courses toward the inguinal canal.

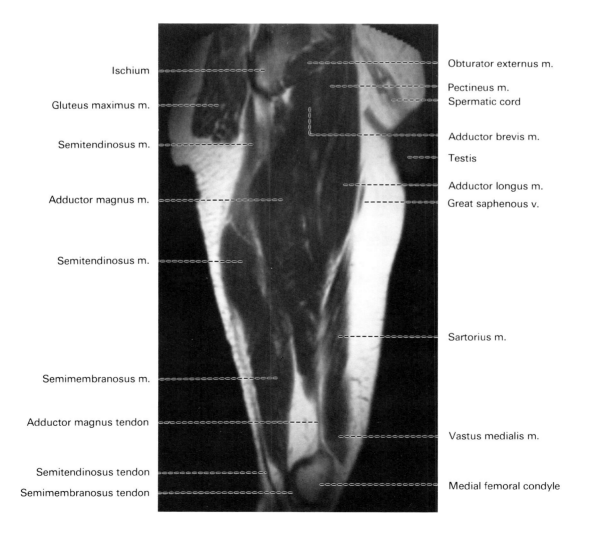

Figure 14.3.6

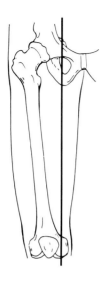

1. The origin of pectineus from the superior pubic ramus is demonstrated.

2. Obturator externus covers the anterior surface of the obturator foramen.

3. The femoral vessels course distally in the adductor canal.

4. The semimembranosus tendon is seen at its origin from the ischial tuberosity. The conjoint tendon of semitendinosus and biceps femoris is posterior to the origin of the semimembranosus tendon.

5. Gluteus maximus covers the origin of the hamstring muscles.

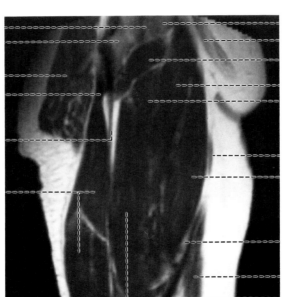

Obturator foramen
Ischium

Gluteus maximus m.

Semitendinosus and biceps femoris conjoint tendon

Semimembranosus tendon

Semitendinosus m.

Adductor magnus m.

Semimembranosus m.

Gastrocnemius (medial head) m.

Superior pubic ramus
Spermatic cord
Obturator externus m.

Pectineus m.
Adductor brevis m.

Great saphenous v.
Adductor longus m.

Adductor canal

Sartorius m.
Superficial femoral vessels

Vastus medialis m.

Medial femoral condyle

Figure 14.3.7

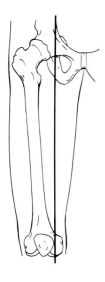

1. Sartorius, in its distal half, forms the roof of the adductor canal.

2. In the thigh the superficial femoral artery is anterior in position to the superficial femoral vein.

3. Observe the superficial femoral vessels crossing the adductor hiatus to enter the popliteal fossa. They become the popliteal artery and vein.

4. Note that the muscular portion of adductor magnus ends distally at the adductor hiatus; from there on it becomes tendinous.

5. The inferior gluteal artery exits from the pelvis inferior to the piriformis.

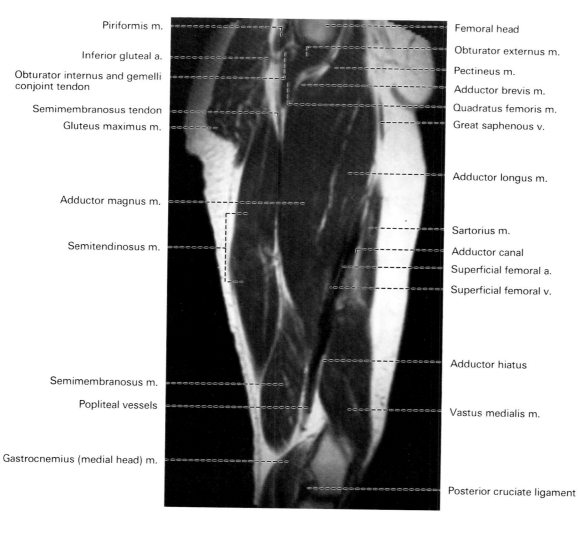

Figure 14.3.8

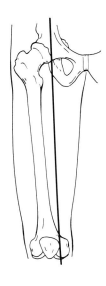

1. In this section the great saphenous vein is shown draining into the femoral vein.

2. Iliopsoas passes anterior to the femoral head.

3. The medial femoral circumflex artery passes toward the femoral neck.

4. Note the course of the superficial femoral vessels within the adductor canal.

5. The sciatic nerve courses distally on the posterior surface of the adductor magnus.

Obturator internus and gemelli conjoint tendon
Obturator externus m.
Quadratus femoris m.
Adductor brevis m.

Sciatic nerve
Gluteus maximus m.

Adductor magnus m.

Semitendinosus m.

Semimembranosus m.

Popliteal v.
Popliteal a.
Posterior cruciate ligament

Femoral head
Iliopsoas m.
Great saphenous v.
Femoral v.

Pectineus m.
Medial femoral circumflex a.
Adductor longus m.

Adductor canal

Superficial femoral a.

Sartorius m.

Superficial femoral v.

Vastus medialis m.

Quadriceps tendon

Intercondylar notch

Figure 14.3.9

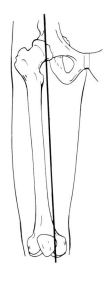

1. Observe iliopsoas inserting on the lesser trochanter.

2. The common femoral artery divides into the deep and superficial branches.

3. In the proximal thigh the sciatic nerve is covered posteriorly by gluteus maximus.

4. The long head of biceps femoris is seen in this section.

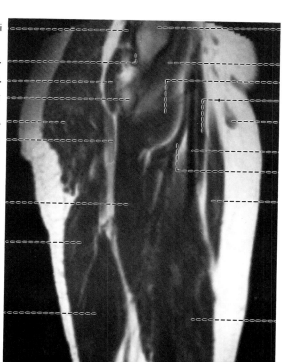

Obturator internus and gemelli conjoint tendon

Obturator externus m.

Quadratus femoris m.

Lesser trochanter

Gluteus maximus m.

Sciatic nerve

Adductor magnus m.

Semitendinosus m.

Biceps femoris (long head) m.

Femoral head

Iliopsoas m.

Pectineus m.

Superficial femoral a.

Inguinal lymph node

Superficial femoral v.

Deep femoral vessels

Sartorius m.

Vastus medialis m.

Femoral shaft

Patella

Patellar ligament

Figure 14.3.10

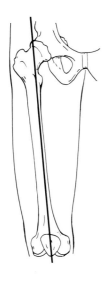

1. The lateral femoral circumflex artery and its descending branch are depicted in this section. The medial and lateral femoral circumflex arteries together supply the femoral head.

2. Vastus intermedius is anterior to the femoral shaft.

3. All four components of the quadriceps muscle converge on the quadriceps tendon.

4. The sciatic nerve divides at a variable distance above the knee into the tibial and common peroneal nerves.

5. Quadratus femoris inserts on the quadrate line inferior to the intertrochanteric crest.

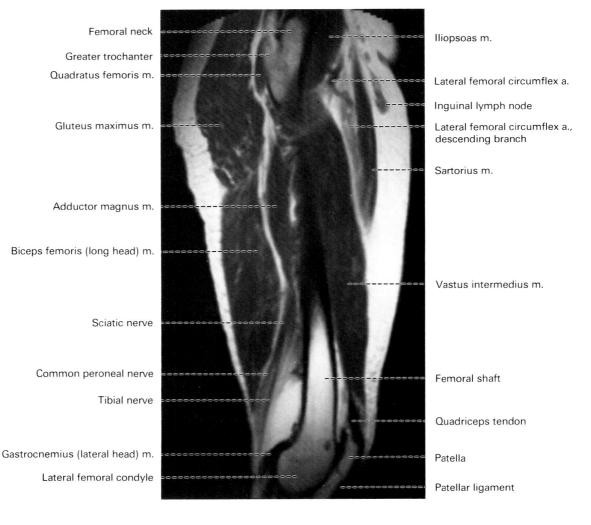

Figure 14.3.11

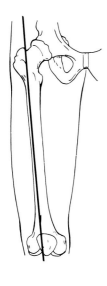

1. Rectus femoris is partially demonstrated in this section. In the proximal thigh it lies posterior to sartorius.

2. Rectus femoris lies above vastus intermedius.

3. Note the origin of the short head of biceps femoris from the posterior aspect of the femur.

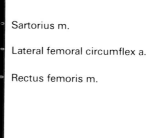

Greater trochanter

Quadratus femoris m.

Gluteus maximus m.

Biceps femoris (long head) m.

Biceps femoris (short head) m.

Sartorius m.

Lateral femoral circumflex a.

Rectus femoris m.

Vastus intermedius m.

Femoral shaft

Quadriceps tendon

Patella

Figure 14.3.12

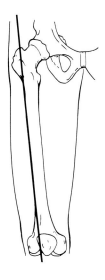

1. Vastus lateralis is partially demonstrated as the sections move more laterally.

2. The long and short heads of the biceps femoris merge in the distal thigh.

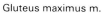

Sartorius m.

Rectus femoris m.

Gluteus maximus m.

Vastus intermedius m.

Femoral shaft

Biceps femoris (long head) m.

Vastus lateralis m.

Biceps femoris (short head) m.

Quadriceps tendon

Figure 14.3.13

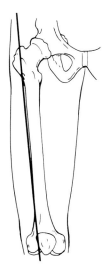

1. Gluteus medius and minimus are identified close to their insertion on the greater trochanter.

2. The superficial fibers of gluteus maximus insert into the iliotibial tract.

3. The short head of biceps femoris is seen posterior to the vastus lateralis.

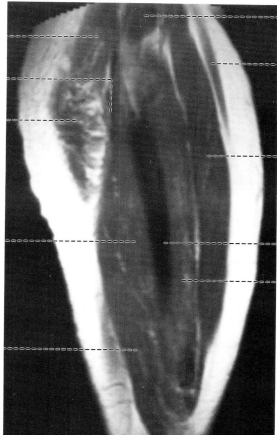

Gluteus medius m.

Iliotibial tract

Gluteus maximus m.

Vastus lateralis m.

Biceps femoris (short head) m.

Gluteus minimus m.

Sartorius m.

Rectus femoris m.

Femoral shaft, lateral cortex

Vastus intermedius m.

Figure 14.3.14

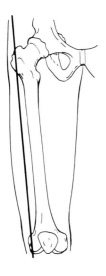

1. Tensor fasciae latae is partially demonstrated in this lateral section of the thigh.

2. Vastus lateralis makes up the majority of the lateral musculature of the thigh.

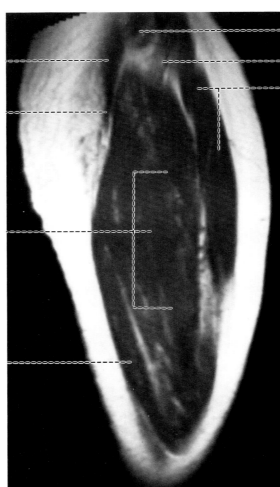

Gluteus medius m.

Iliotibial tract

Vastus lateralis m.

Biceps femoris (short head) m.

Gluteus minimus m.

Tensor fasciae latae m.

Rectus femoris m.

Figure 14.3.15

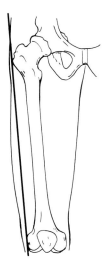

1. A longitudinal section of the iliotibial tract is observed.

2. The marbled fascicles of tensor fasciae latae are demonstrated.

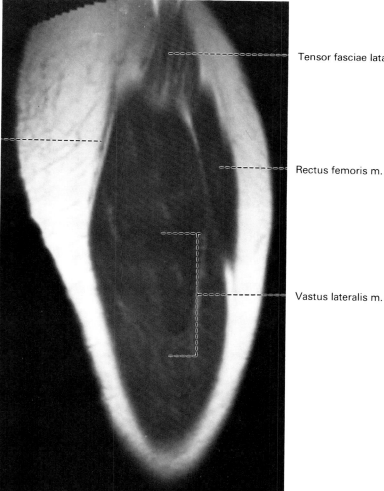

Tensor fasciae latae m.

Iliotibial tract

Rectus femoris m.

Vastus lateralis m.

Figure 14.3.16

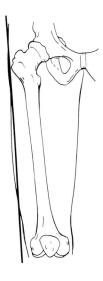

1. Rectus femoris originates deep to tensor fasciae latae from the anterior superior iliac spine (straight head) and supra-acetabular area (reflected head).

2. This section cuts through the most lateral aspect of the thigh passing through vastus lateralis.

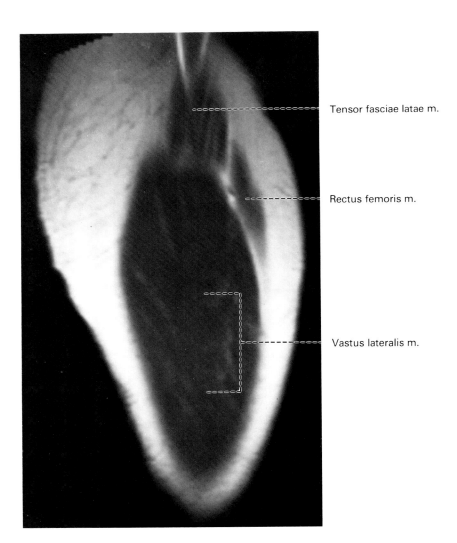

Tensor fasciae latae m.

Rectus femoris m.

Vastus lateralis m.

KNEE AND CALF

Figure 15.1.1

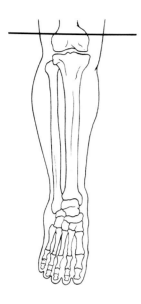

1. This section passes through the intercondylar groove and notch. The patella is seated within the groove.

2. The synovial space in the left knee is mildly distended with fluid. In the right knee the synovial space is collapsed.

3. Immediately posterior to biceps femoris, the common peroneal nerve is demonstrated.

4. The medial and lateral heads of gastrocnemius are seen at their origins from the posterior aspect of the femoral condyles.

5. Plantaris originates medial to the lateral head of gastrocnemius.

6. Medial to the patella the most distal portion of vastus medialis is identified; on the opposite side of the patella, the lateral patellar retinaculum is demonstrated.

7. Of the three muscles forming the pes anserinus tendon, semitendinosus and gracilis are already tendinous in this section whereas sartorius is still muscular.

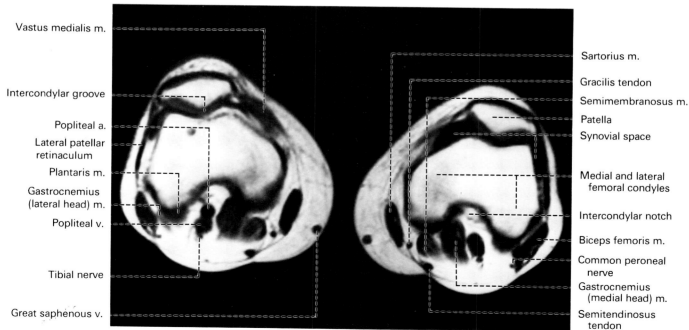

Vastus medialis m.

Intercondylar groove

Popliteal a.

Lateral patellar retinaculum

Plantaris m.

Gastrocnemius (lateral head) m.

Popliteal v.

Tibial nerve

Great saphenous v.

Sartorius m.

Gracilis tendon

Semimembranosus m.

Patella

Synovial space

Medial and lateral femoral condyles

Intercondylar notch

Biceps femoris m.

Common peroneal nerve

Gastrocnemius (medial head) m.

Semitendinosus tendon

Figure 15.1.2

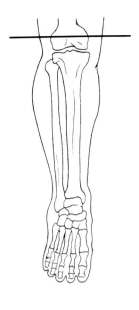

1. The lateral and medial patellar retinacula are demonstrated.

2. The posterior cruciate ligament is seen in the intercondylar notch. It attaches on the medial femoral condyle.

3. Semimembranosus becomes tendinous as it approaches its insertion onto the posteromedial aspect of the medial tibial condyle and knee joint capsule.

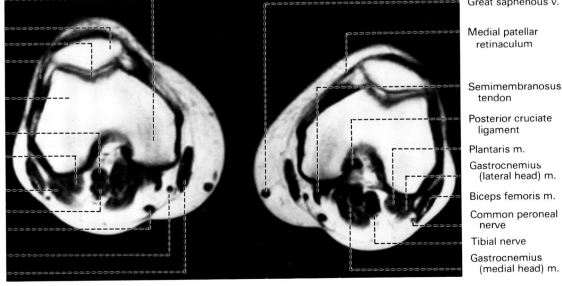

Medial femoral condyle
Patella
Intercondylar groove
Lateral patellar retinaculum
Lateral femoral condyle
Popliteal a.
Plantaris m.
Gastrocnemius (lateral head) m.
Popliteal v.
Semitendinosus tendon
Gracilis tendon
Sartorius m.

Great saphenous v.
Medial patellar retinaculum
Semimembranosus tendon
Posterior cruciate ligament
Plantaris m.
Gastrocnemius (lateral head) m.
Biceps femoris m.
Common peroneal nerve
Tibial nerve
Gastrocnemius (medial head) m.

Figure 15.1.3

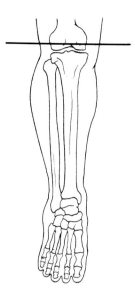

1. This section, just inferior to the patella, shows the patellar ligament and the infrapatellar fat pad posterior to it.

2. Both cruciate ligaments are demonstrated in the intercondylar notch. The anterior cruciate attaches to the medial surface of the lateral femoral condyle.

3. Both heads of gastrocnemius are enlarging as the sections move toward the calf.

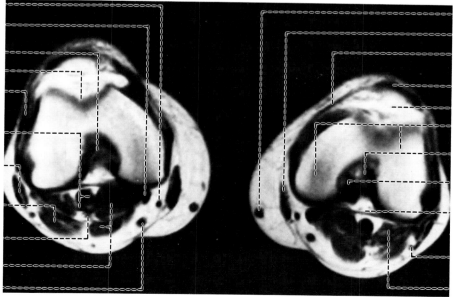

Left labels: Gracilis tendon; Semimembranosus tendon; Intercondylar notch; Intercondylar groove; Lateral patellar retinaculum; Popliteal a. and v.; Biceps femoris m.; Gastrocnemius (lateral head) m.; Tibial nerve; Gastrocnemius (medial head) m.; Semitendinosus tendon

Right labels: Great saphenous v.; Sartorius m.; Medial patellar retinaculum; Patellar ligament; Infrapatellar fat pad; Medial and lateral femoral condyles; Anterior cruciate ligament; Posterior cruciate ligament; Posterior meniscofemoral ligament; Common peroneal nerve; Plantaris m.

Figure 15.1.4

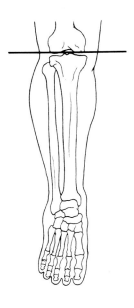

1. The medial and lateral retinacula are demonstrated on either side of the patellar ligament.

2. Biceps femoris has become tendinous as it approaches its insertion onto the fibular head.

3. The three components of the pes anserinus (sartorius, gracilis, and semitendinosus) course close together inferiorly.

4. Note the locations of the tibial and common peroneal nerves as they are about to leave the thigh.

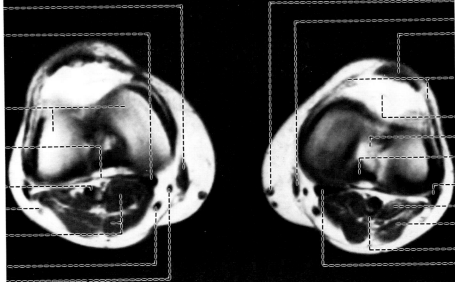

Sartorius m.

Semimembranosus tendon

Medial and lateral femoral condyles

Posterior meniscofemoral ligament

Popliteal vessels

Common peroneal nerve

Gastrocnemius (medial head) m.

Semitendinosus tendon
Gracilis tendon

Great saphenous v.

Sartorius tendon
Patellar ligament

Medial and lateral patellar retinacula

Infrapatellar fat pad

Intercondylar notch

Posterior cruciate ligament

Biceps femoris tendon

Plantaris m.

Gastrocnemius (lateral head) m.

Tibial nerve

Semimembranosus tendon

Figure 15.1.5

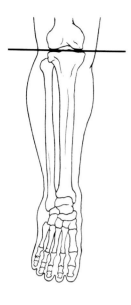

1. Note the patellar retinacula attaching to the patellar ligament.

2. Semimembranosus inserts onto the medial tibial condyle and posterior joint capsule.

3. The tibial nerve courses posterior to the popliteal artery.

4. The infrapatellar fat pad is prominent on this image.

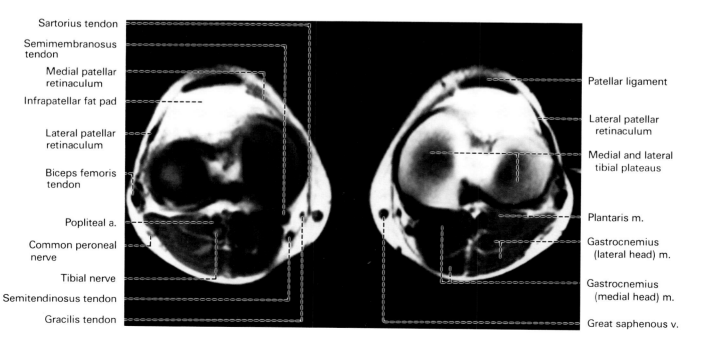

Figure 15.1.6

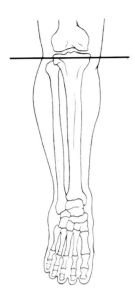

1. The image is through the tibial plateaus.

2. The popliteus muscle is seen immediately along the posterior border of the left tibia, and the popliteal vessels course on its posterior surface.

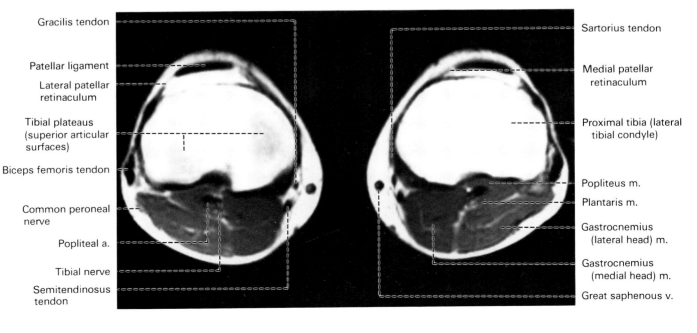

Gracilis tendon

Patellar ligament

Lateral patellar retinaculum

Tibial plateaus (superior articular surfaces)

Biceps femoris tendon

Common peroneal nerve

Popliteal a.

Tibial nerve

Semitendinosus tendon

Sartorius tendon

Medial patellar retinaculum

Proximal tibia (lateral tibial condyle)

Popliteus m.

Plantaris m.

Gastrocnemius (lateral head) m.

Gastrocnemius (medial head) m.

Great saphenous v.

Figure 15.1.7

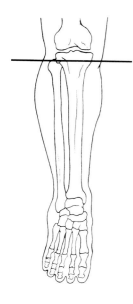

1. The patellar ligament inserts onto the anterior tibial tuberosity.

2. Immediately adjacent to the pes anserine complex the great saphenous vein is seen.

3. Note the relation of the common peroneal nerve to the fibular head.

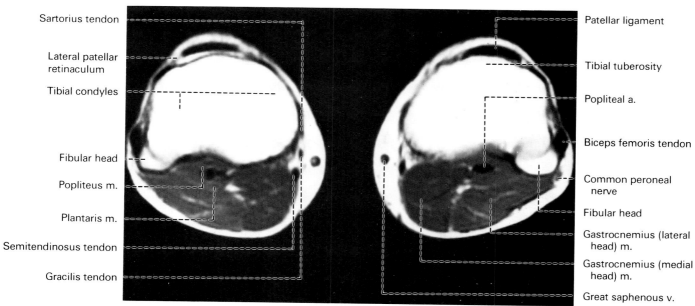

Sartorius tendon

Lateral patellar retinaculum

Tibial condyles

Fibular head

Popliteus m.

Plantaris m.

Semitendinosus tendon

Gracilis tendon

Patellar ligament

Tibial tuberosity

Popliteal a.

Biceps femoris tendon

Common peroneal nerve

Fibular head

Gastrocnemius (lateral head) m.

Gastrocnemius (medial head) m.

Great saphenous v.

Figure 15.1.8

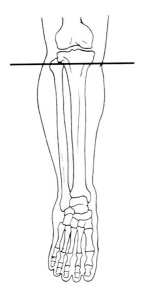

1. Note the origin of soleus, which arises in part from the head of the fibula.

2. The popliteal vessels are situated between popliteus and soleus.

3. The biceps femoris tendon is seen at its insertion on the fibular head.

4. Note the prominence in the anterolateral aspect of the tibia (Gerdy's tubercle) that functions as the insertion of the iliotibial tract.

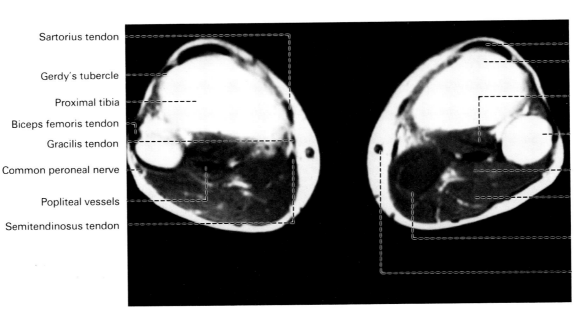

Figure 15.1.9

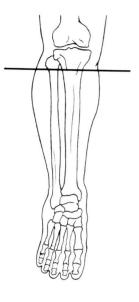

1. Two anterior compartment muscles, tibialis anterior and extensor digitorum longus, can now be seen.

2. At this level, the pes anserinus has been formed from the coalescence of sartorius, gracilis, and semitendinosus tendons.

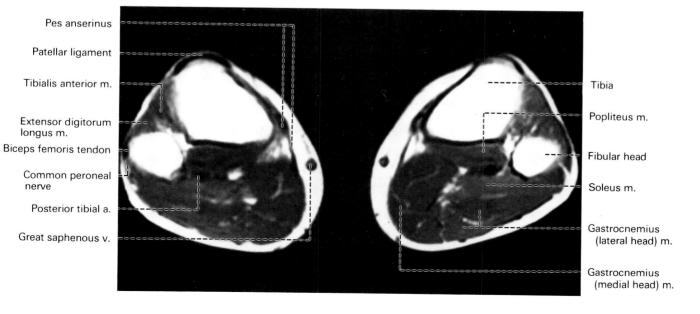

Pes anserinus

Patellar ligament

Tibialis anterior m.

Extensor digitorum longus m.

Biceps femoris tendon

Common peroneal nerve

Posterior tibial a.

Great saphenous v.

Tibia

Popliteus m.

Fibular head

Soleus m.

Gastrocnemius (lateral head) m.

Gastrocnemius (medial head) m.

Figure 15.1.10

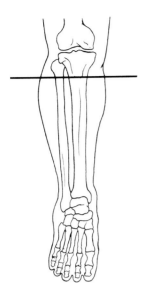

1. At this level the popliteal artery has divided giving rise to the posterior tibial and peroneal arteries.

2. Note tibialis posterior between the tibia and fibula as it arises from the interosseous membrane.

3. Peroneus longus originates from the anterolateral aspect of the shaft of the fibula.

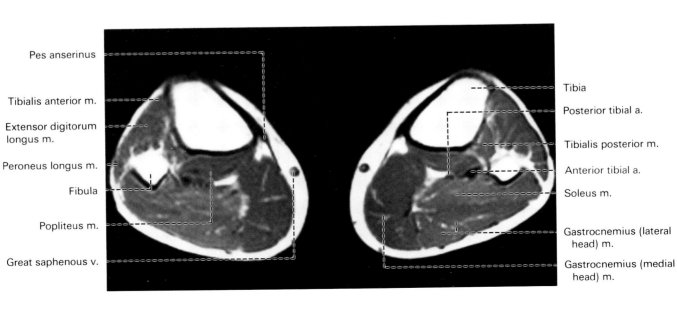

Pes anserinus

Tibialis anterior m.

Extensor digitorum longus m.

Peroneus longus m.

Fibula

Popliteus m.

Great saphenous v.

Tibia

Posterior tibial a.

Tibialis posterior m.

Anterior tibial a.

Soleus m.

Gastrocnemius (lateral head) m.

Gastrocnemius (medial head) m.

Figure 15.1.11

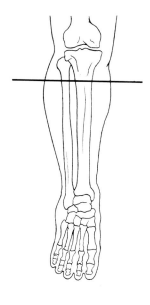

1. The calf vessels lie between the deep and superficial muscles of the posterior compartment.

2. Note the anterior tibial artery coursing horizontally over the proximal edge of the interosseous membrane to enter the anterior compartment.

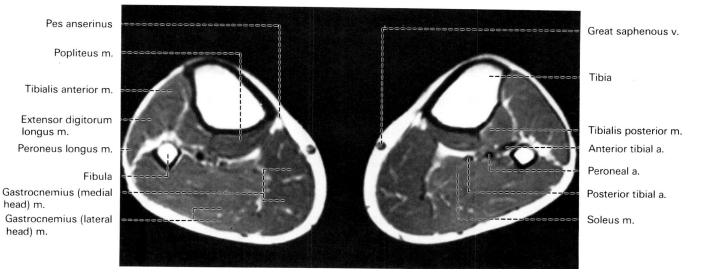

Pes anserinus

Popliteus m.

Tibialis anterior m.

Extensor digitorum longus m.

Peroneus longus m.

Fibula

Gastrocnemius (medial head) m.

Gastrocnemius (lateral head) m.

Great saphenous v.

Tibia

Tibialis posterior m.

Anterior tibial a.

Peroneal a.

Posterior tibial a.

Soleus m.

Figure 15.1.12

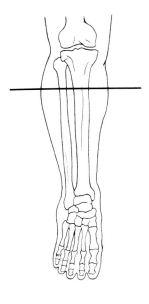

1. The anterior tibial artery lies on the interosseous membrane in the anterior compartment.

2. The anterior compartment muscles are distinguishable as tibialis anterior, extensor hallucis longus, and extensor digitorum longus.

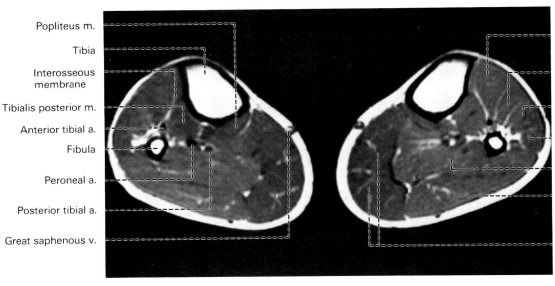

Popliteus m.

Tibia

Interosseous membrane

Tibialis posterior m.

Anterior tibial a.

Fibula

Peroneal a.

Posterior tibial a.

Great saphenous v.

Tibialis anterior m.

Extensor hallucis longus m.

Extensor digitorum longus m.

Peroneus longus m.

Soleus m.

Gastrocnemius (lateral head) m.

Gastrocnemius (medial head) m.

Figure 15.1.13

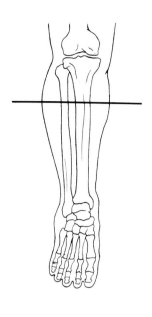

1. The gastrocnemius and soleus form the bulk of the muscles of the calf at this level.

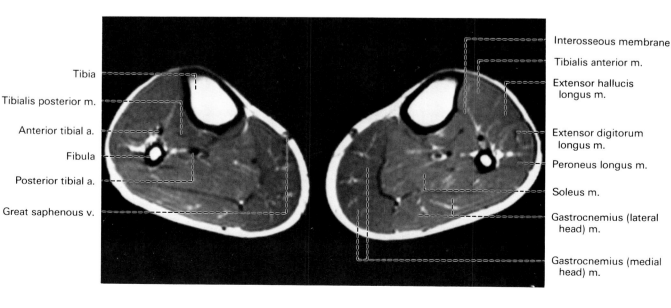

Tibia

Tibialis posterior m.

Anterior tibial a.

Fibula

Posterior tibial a.

Great saphenous v.

Interosseous membrane

Tibialis anterior m.

Extensor hallucis longus m.

Extensor digitorum longus m.

Peroneus longus m.

Soleus m.

Gastrocnemius (lateral head) m.

Gastrocnemius (medial head) m.

Figure 15.1.14

1. Note that the interosseous membrane is well-defined and bows anteriorly.

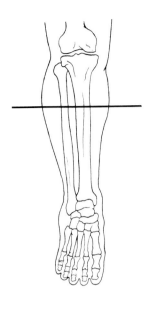

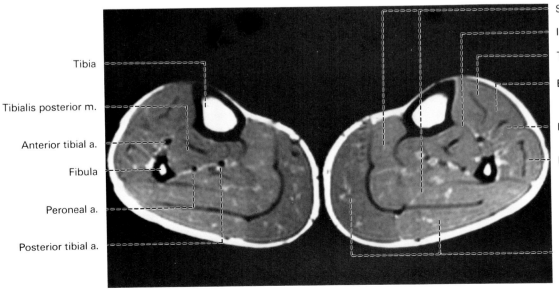

Figure 15.1.15

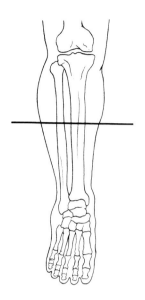

1. Of the long flexors of the foot, the two that are identified at this level are flexor digitorum longus and tibialis posterior.

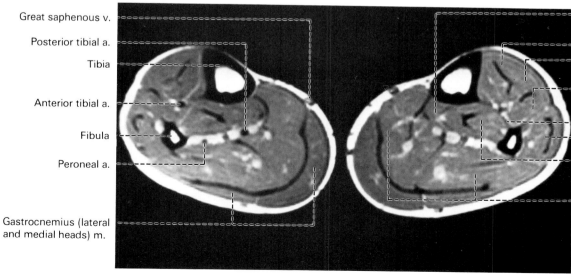

Great saphenous v.

Posterior tibial a.

Tibia

Anterior tibial a.

Fibula

Peroneal a.

Gastrocnemius (lateral and medial heads) m.

Flexor digitorum longus m.

Tibialis anterior m.

Extensor hallucis longus m.

Extensor digitorum longus m.

Interosseous membrane

Peroneus longus m.

Tibialis posterior m.

Soleus m.

Figure 15.1.16

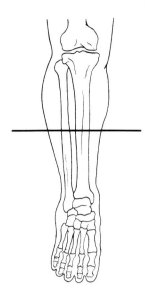

1. Note that the peroneus longus muscle and tendon lie superficial to the peroneus brevis muscle. These muscles are separated from the anterior compartment by an intermuscular septum.

2. All three long flexor muscles of the foot are identified on this section. These are the tibialis posterior, flexor digitorum longus, and flexor hallucis longus.

3. The gastrocnemius tendon is becoming more prominent.

4. Extensor hallucis longus is covered on its anterior surface by tibialis anterior.

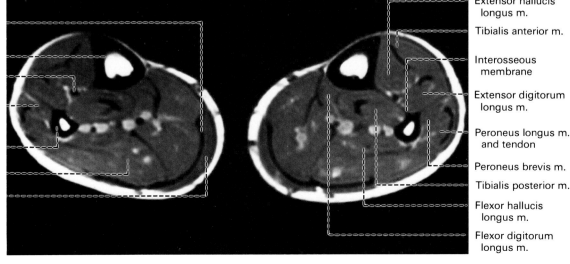

Figure 15.1.17

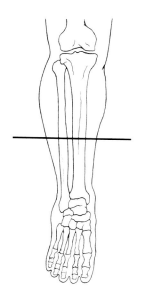

1. At this level gastrocnemius continues as the gastrocnemius tendon.

2. Also of note at this level is the prominent tibial nutrient artery.

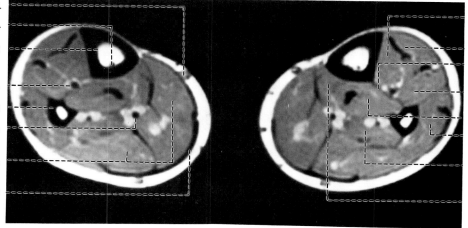

Great saphenous v.
Tibial nutrient a.
Tibia
Anterior tibial a.
Fibula
Posterior tibial a.
Soleus m.
Gastrocnemius tendon

Extensor hallucis longus m.
Tibialis anterior m.
Interosseous membrane
Extensor digitorum longus m.
Tibialis posterior m.
Peroneus longus and brevis mm.
Flexor hallucis longus m.
Flexor digitorum longus m.

Figure 15.1.18

1. In cross section both the tibia and fibula appear triangular at this level.

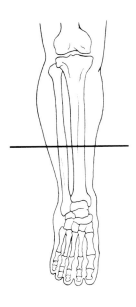

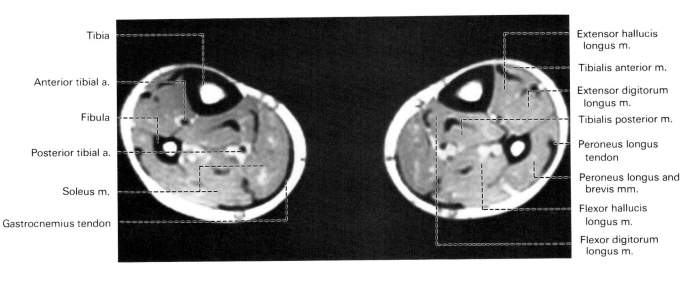

Tibia

Anterior tibial a.

Fibula

Posterior tibial a.

Soleus m.

Gastrocnemius tendon

Extensor hallucis longus m.

Tibialis anterior m.

Extensor digitorum longus m.

Tibialis posterior m.

Peroneus longus tendon

Peroneus longus and brevis mm.

Flexor hallucis longus m.

Flexor digitorum longus m.

Figure 15.1.19

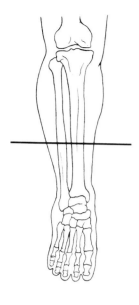

1. Most muscles at this level have developed a tendinous component that becomes more prominent distally.

2. Note that the anterior tibial artery remains on the anterior surface of the interosseous membrane.

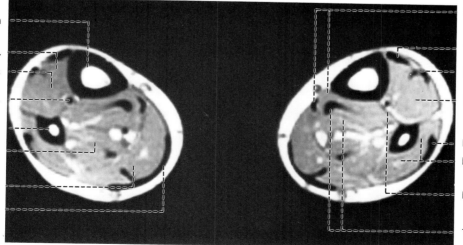

Tibia

Tibialis anterior m.

Extensor hallucis longus m.

Anterior tibial a.

Fibula

Flexor hallucis longus m.

Soleus m.

Gastrocnemius tendon

Flexor digitorum longus m. and tendon

Tibialis anterior tendon

Extensor hallucis longus tendon

Extensor digitorum longus m.

Peroneus longus tendon

Peroneus longus and brevis mm.

Interosseous membrane

Tibialis posterior m. and tendon

Figure 15.1.20

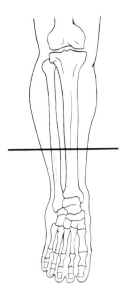

1. The soleus muscle diminishes in size as the sections approach the ankle.

2. The gastrocnemius tendon thickens and narrows prior to becoming the calcaneal (Achilles) tendon.

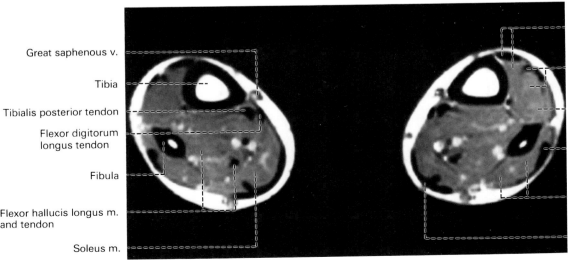

Great saphenous v.

Tibia

Tibialis posterior tendon

Flexor digitorum longus tendon

Fibula

Flexor hallucis longus m. and tendon

Soleus m.

Tibialis anterior m. and tendon

Extensor hallucis longus m. and tendon

Extensor digitorum longus m.

Peroneus longus and brevis tendons

Peroneus longus and brevis mm.

Gastrocnemius tendon

Figure 15.1.21

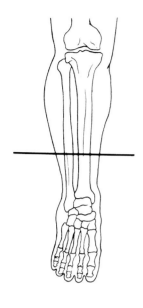

1. Tibialis anterior is completely tendinous at this level.

2. Note that the tibialis posterior tendon has crossed in front of flexor digitorum longus at this level. It will remain in this position throughout the rest of its course in the ankle.

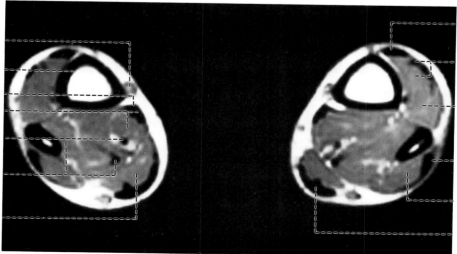

Great saphenous v.

Tibia

Tibialis posterior tendon

Flexor digitorum longus tendon

Posterior tibial a.

Flexor hallucis longus m. and tendon

Soleus m.

Tibialis anterior tendon

Extensor hallucis longus m. and tendon

Extensor digitorum longus m.

Peroneus longus and brevis tendons

Peroneus brevis m.

Calcaneal (Achilles) tendon

Figure 15.1.22

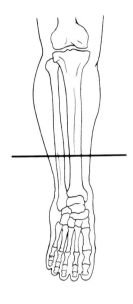

1. Soleus has nearly completed its insertion into the calcaneal (Achilles) tendon.

2. Note that the tibial cortex is thinning.

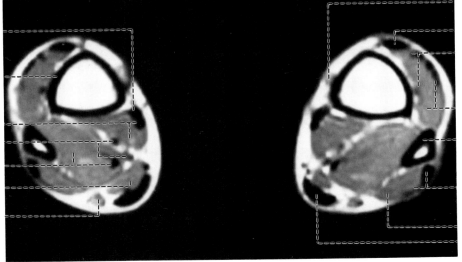

Tibialis posterior tendon

Tibia

Flexor digitorum longus m. and tendon

Posterior tibial vessels

Flexor hallucis longus m. and tendon

Soleus m.

Small saphenous v.

Great saphenous v.

Tibialis anterior tendon

Extensor hallucis longus m. and tendon

Extensor digitorum longus m. and tendon

Fibula

Peroneus longus and brevis mm. and tendons

Peroneus brevis m.

Calcaneal (Achilles) tendon

CORONAL

Figure 15.2.1

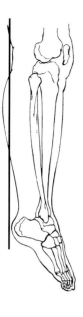

1. The medial and lateral heads of gastrocnemius are separated by a median raphe.

2. Soleus is partially demonstrated in this section.

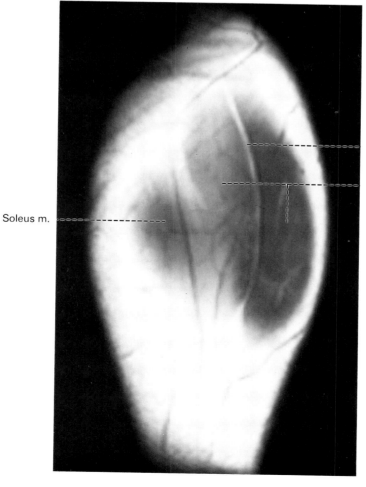

Small saphenous v.

Gastrocnemius (lateral and medial heads) m.

Soleus m.

Figure 15.2.2

1. This section passes through the gastrocnemius and soleus muscles.

2. The bulk of gastrocnemius is on the medial side of the calf.

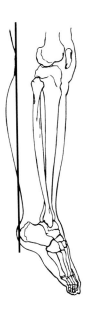

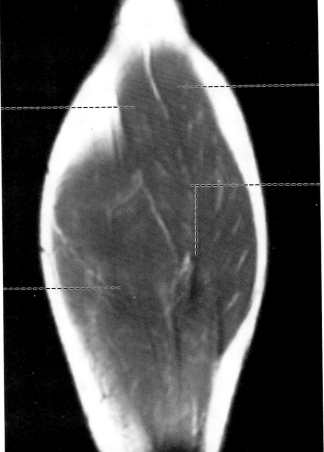

Gastrocnemius (lateral head) m.

Gastrocnemius (medial head) m.

Tendinous raphe between gastrocnemius m. heads

Soleus m.

Figure 15.2.3

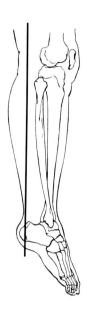

1. This section passes through both heads of the gastrocnemius and soleus muscles.

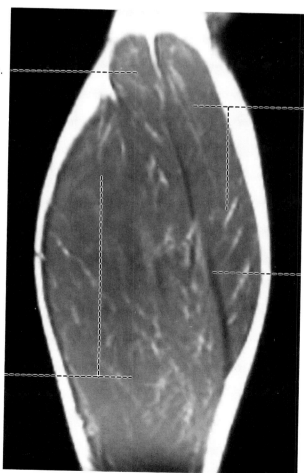

Gastrocnemius (lateral head) m.

Gastrocnemius (medial head) m.

Tendinous raphe between gastrocnemius m. heads

Soleus m.

Figure 15.2.4

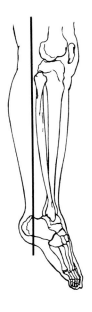

1. The size and extent of soleus is appreciated in this section.

2. The small saphenous vein courses superiorly to drain into the popliteal vein.

3. Note the semimembranosus muscle and tendon on the posteromedial aspect of the knee.

4. Plantaris is seen at its origin on the lateral femoral condyle along with the lateral head of gastrocnemius.

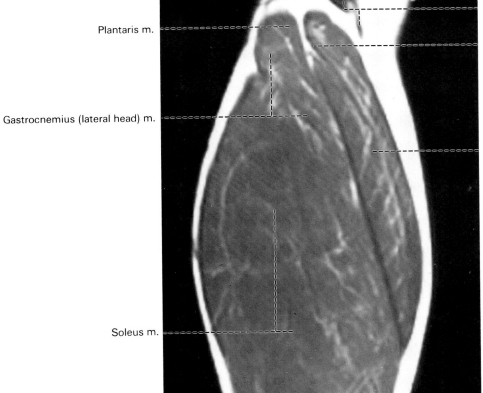

Figure 15.2.5

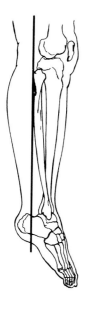

1. Note the size and extent of the soleus muscle.

2. Some of the deep veins of the calf are depicted in this section.

3. The popliteal vessels course between the two heads of gastrocnemius.

4. The peroneal muscles are demonstrated immediately lateral to the fibula.

5. The biceps femoris tendon courses inferiorly toward its insertion on the head of the fibula.

6. Gracilis and semitendinosus (components of pes anserinus) are seen medial to the knee. Sartorius forms the third component of the pes anserinus anteriorly.

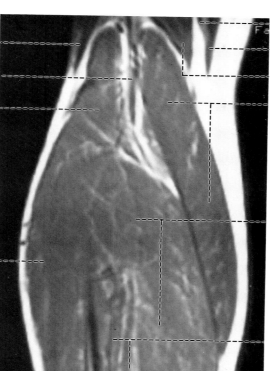

Biceps femoris tendon

Popliteal vessels

Gastrocnemius (lateral head) m.

Peroneus longus m.

Peroneus brevis m.

Fibula

Semitendinosus tendon

Gracilis tendon

Semimembranosus m.

Gastrocnemius (medial head) m.

Soleus m.

Deep vv. of calf

Figure 15.2.6

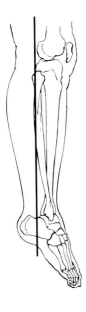

1. Note the common peroneal nerve descending behind biceps femoris.

2. Gastrocnemius covers soleus and soleus in turn covers the long flexors of the foot.

3. The popliteal vessels are seen between the two heads of gastrocnemius.

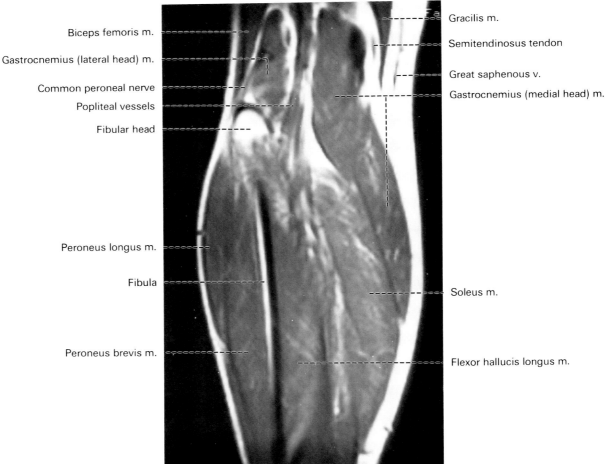

Figure 15.2.7

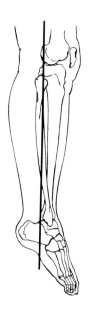

1. The biceps femoris tendon inserts onto the head of the fibula.

2. Note the origins of the medial and lateral heads of gastrocnemius just proximal to the medial and lateral femoral condyles.

3. The gracilis tendon crosses the joint as it descends to join the other components of pes anserinus, the sartorius and semitendinosus tendons.

4. The anterior tibial artery crosses above the interosseous membrane to enter the anterior compartment.

5. Peroneus longus and brevis muscles are demonstrated against the lateral surface of the fibula.

6. The great saphenous vein courses superiorly in the subcutaneous tissues of the calf medially.

7. Of the long flexors of the foot, the flexor hallucis longus and tibialis posterior muscles are seen at this level.

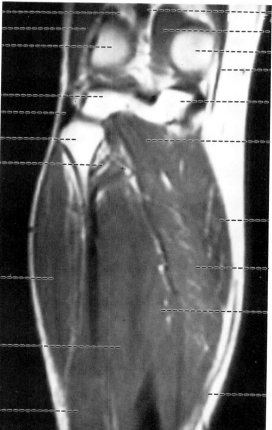

Gastrocnemius (lateral head) m.
Biceps femoris m.
Lateral femoral condyle

Lateral tibial condyle
Biceps femoris tendon

Fibular head

Anterior tibial a.

Peroneus longus m.

Flexor hallucis longus m.

Peroneus brevis m.

Popliteal vessels
Gastrocnemius (medial head) m.
Medial femoral condyle
Gracilis tendon

Medial tibial condyle

Popliteus m.

Gastrocnemius (medial head) m.

Soleus m.

Tibialis posterior m.

Great saphenous v.

Tibia

Figure 15.2.8

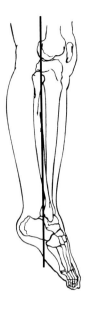

1. The lateral (fibular) collateral ligament is demonstrated in this section.

2. Popliteus originates from the posterior surface of the proximal tibia. The tibial artery trifurcates on the posterior surface of this muscle.

3. Note that the posterior cruciate ligament is fixed distally to the posterior intercondylar area of the tibia and extends to attach to the lateral surface of the medial femoral condyle.

4. A nutrient vessel is identified in the medullary space of the tibia along the posterior cortex (also seen on axial images).

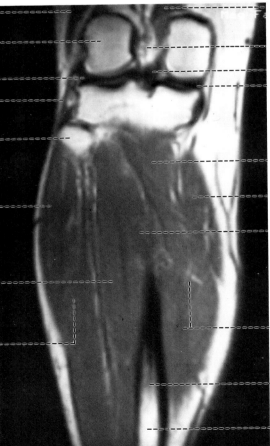

Biceps femoris m.

Lateral femoral condyle

Lateral meniscus (posterior horn)

Lateral collateral ligament

Fibular head

Peroneus longus m.

Flexor hallucis longus m.

Extensor digitorum longus m.

Gastrocnemius (medial head) m.

Intercondylar notch

Posterior cruciate ligament

Medial meniscus (posterior horn)

Popliteus m.

Gastrocnemius (medial head) m.

Tibialis posterior m.

Flexor digitorum longus m.

Nutrient vessel

Tibia

Figure 15.2.9

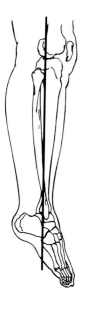

1. The anterior cruciate ligament attaches to the medial surface of the lateral femoral condyle. The posterior cruciate attaches to the lateral surface of the medial femoral condyle.

2. Peroneus longus is seen anterolateral to the fibula.

3. All the long extensors of the foot seen in this section are anterolateral to the tibia.

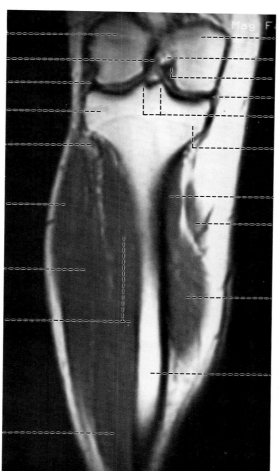

Lateral femoral condyle
Anterior cruciate ligament
Lateral meniscus (body)
Lateral tibial condyle
Fibular head
Peroneus longus m.
Extensor digitorum longus m.
Tibialis anterior m.
Extensor hallucis longus m.

Medial femoral condyle
Intercondylar notch
Posterior cruciate ligament
Medial meniscus (body)
Intercondylar eminence (medial and lateral tubercles)
Medial tibial condyle
Tibialis posterior m.
Gastrocnemius (medial head) m.
Flexor digitorum longus m.
Tibia

Figure 15.2.10

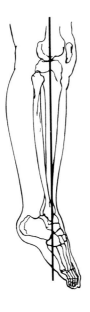

1. This section passes through the anterior portion of the intercondylar notch and intercondylar eminence.

2. The anterior cruciate originates from the nonarticular surface of the tibia just anterior to the intercondylar eminence.

3. The anterior horns of the medial and lateral menisci are depicted in this section as small triangles.

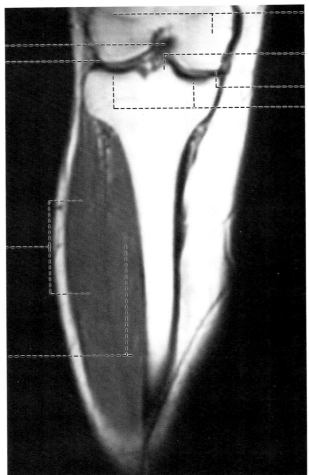

Anterior cruciate ligament
Lateral meniscus (anterior horn)

Medial and lateral femoral condyles

Medial tubercle of intercondylar eminence

Medial meniscus (anterior horn)

Medial and lateral plateaus

Extensor digitorum longus m.

Tibialis anterior m.

Figure 15.2.11

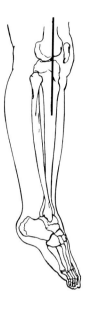

1. This section passes through the medial (tibial) collateral ligament.

2. Note that the medial meniscus is adherent to the medial (tibial) collateral ligament.

3. The lateral patellar retinaculum is seen on the lateral aspect of the knee.

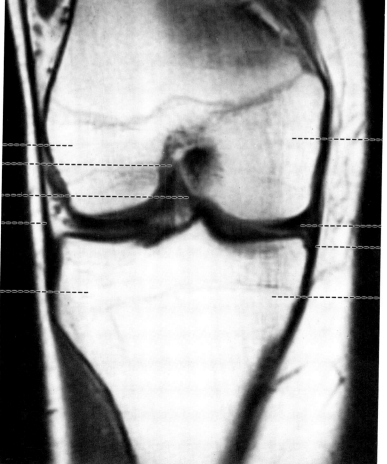

Lateral femoral condyle

Intercondylar notch

Anterior cruciate ligament

Iliotibial tract

Lateral tibial condyle

Medial tibial condyle

Medial meniscus

Medial (tibial) collateral ligament

Medial femoral condyle

Figure 15.2.12

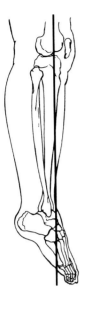

1. The iliotibial tract is seen on this section. It inserts on the anteromedial aspect of the lateral tibial condyle (Gerdy's tubercle).

2. Extensor digitorum longus and tibialis anterior are seen lateral to the tibia. These two muscles cover the anterior surface of extensor hallucis longus.

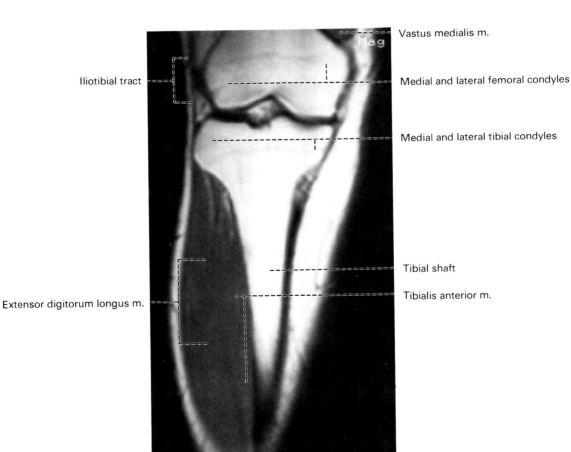

Figure 15.2.13

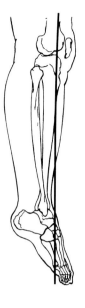

1. The iliotibial tract is seen coursing inferiorly anterolateral to the knee joint.

2. Tibialis anterior lies against the lateral surface of the tibia.

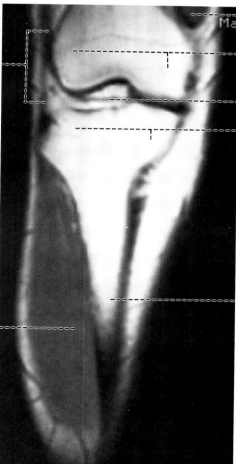

Vastus medialis m.

Medial and lateral femoral condyles

Iliotibial tract

Transverse genicular ligament

Medial and lateral tibial condyles

Tibial shaft

Tibialis anterior m.

Figure 15.2.14

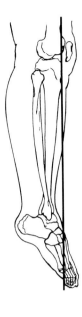

1. Vastus medialis inserts on the medial patellar retinaculum.

2. The iliotibial tract courses distally to insert on the anteromedial surface of the lateral tibial condyle (Gerdy's tubercle).

3. Tibialis anterior is partially demonstrated against the lateral surface of the tibia, which acts, in part, as the origin for this muscle.

Lateral patellar retinaculum

Iliotibial tract

Tibialis anterior m.

Vastus medialis m.

Medial patellar retinaculum

Medial and lateral femoral condyles

Tibia

Figure 15.2.15

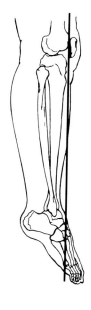

1. On either side of the patella the medial and lateral patellar retinacula are demonstrated.

2. The femoral condyles are partially outlined; inferior to the condyles the infrapatellar fat pad is seen.

3. The patella tracks in the shallow intercondylar sulcus during flexion and extension of the knee.

4. The patellar ligament inserts onto the tibial tubercle.

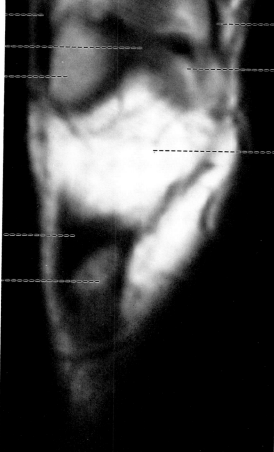

Figure 15.2.16

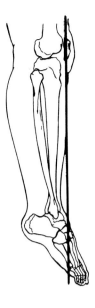

1. This anterior coronal section passes superficially through the patella.

2. The patellar ligament is partially demonstrated inferior to the patella.

3. Superficial veins are noted medial to the patella.

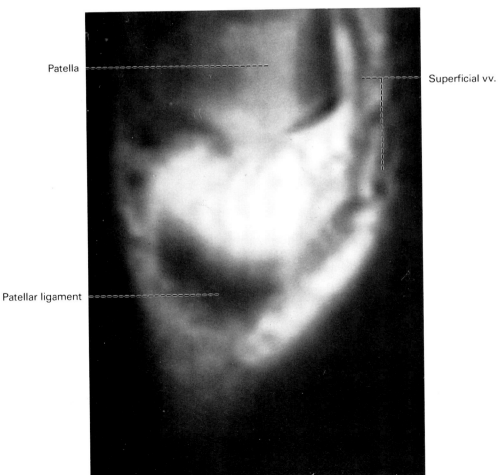

Figure 15.3.1

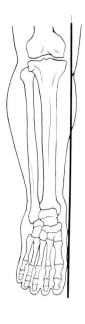

1. This is the most medial section of the calf and it passes through the medial head of gastrocnemius.

2. The great saphenous vein is seen in the subcutaneous tissues.

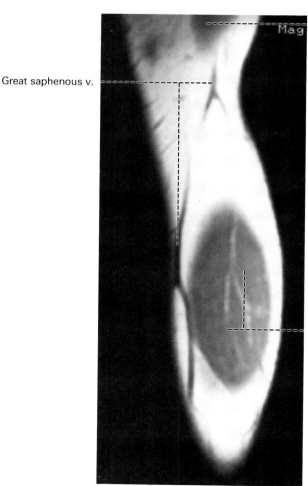

Semimembranosus m.

Great saphenous v.

Gastrocnemius (medial head) m.

Figure 15.3.2

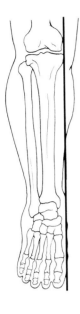

1. In the distal thigh the semitendinosus tendon is seen posterior to the semimembranosus muscle.

2. Soleus is partially demonstrated deep to gastrocnemius.

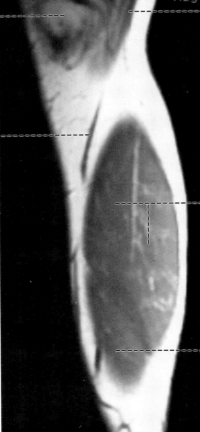

Figure 15.3.3

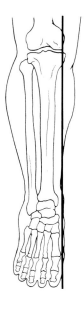

1. The insertion of semimembranosus to the posteromedial aspect of the medial tibial condyle is demonstrated.

2. The semitendinosus tendon courses distal and more anterior to the semimembranosus insertion to become the posterior component of a combined three-tendon insertion named the pes anserinus.

3. Note the gastrocnemius tendon between the bellies of the soleus and gastrocnemius muscles.

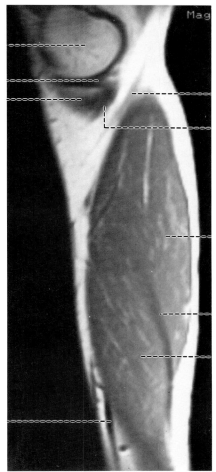

Figure 15.3.4

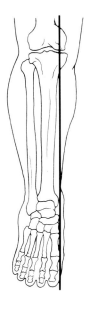

1. The typical "bow-tie" appearance of the medial meniscus is depicted in this section.

2. Note the semimembranosus tendon coursing inferiorly toward its insertion on the tibia.

3. The medial head of gastrocnemius originates from the posterior surface of the distal femur above the femoral condyle.

4. The semitendinosus tendon is imaged close to its insertion on the tibia anteromedially just distal to the medial tibial condyle.

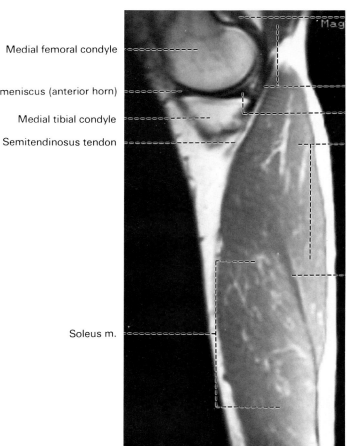

Medial femoral condyle

Medial meniscus (anterior horn)

Medial tibial condyle

Semitendinosus tendon

Soleus m.

Gastrocnemius (medial head) m.

Semimembranosus m. and tendon

Medial meniscus (posterior horn)

Gastrocnemius (medial head) m.

Gastrocnemius tendon

Figure 15.3.5

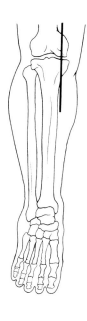

1. This section is through the medial meniscus.

2. The low signal triangular structures are the anterior and posterior horns of the medial meniscus.

3. The posterior horn of the medial meniscus is larger than the anterior horn.

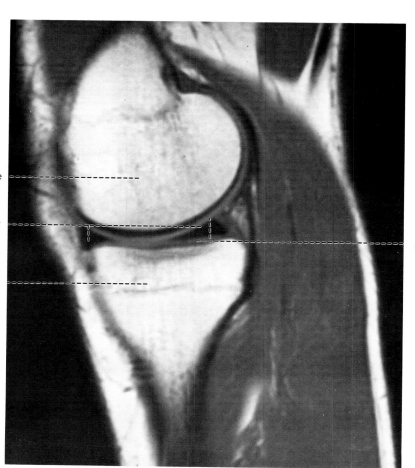

Medial femoral condyle

Medial meniscus (anterior and posterior horns)

Medial tibial condyle

Articular cartilage

Figure 15.3.6

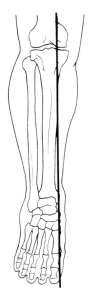

1. Note the size and extent of the soleus muscle. It extends from the soleal line on the posterior surface of the tibia to just above the ankle inferiorly.

2. Both the soleus and gastrocnemius tendons join to form the calcaneal (Achilles) tendon.

3. The insertion of the pes anserinus tendon onto the tibia is demonstrated.

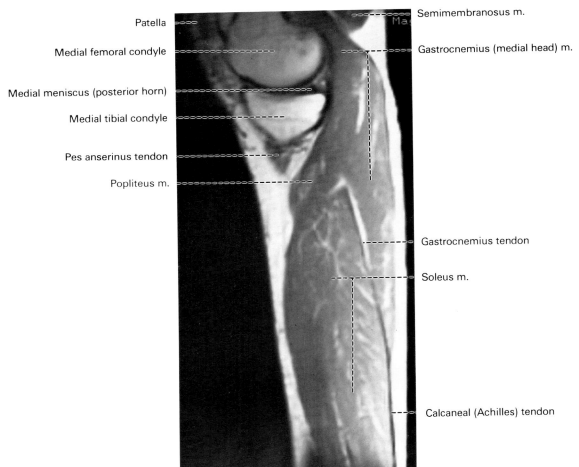

Patella
Medial femoral condyle
Medial meniscus (posterior horn)
Medial tibial condyle
Pes anserinus tendon
Popliteus m.

Semimembranosus m.
Gastrocnemius (medial head) m.
Gastrocnemius tendon
Soleus m.
Calcaneal (Achilles) tendon

Figure 15.3.7

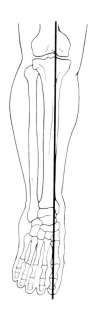

1. The posterior cruciate ligament is seen within the intercondylar notch.

2. Note the fleshy origin of the popliteus muscle from the posterior surface of the proximal tibia.

3. The patellar ligament and infrapatellar fat pad are seen inferior to the patella.

4. Flexor digitorum longus is deep to soleus, originating from the tibial shaft posteriorly.

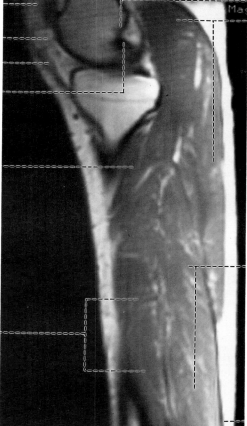

Patella — Intercondylar notch — Gastrocnemius (medial head) m. — Infrapatellar fat pad — Patellar tendon — Posterior cruciate ligament — Popliteus m. — Soleus m. — Flexor digitorum longus m. — Calcaneal (Achilles) tendon — Tibial shaft

Figure 15.3.8

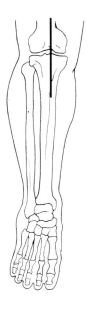

1. This section illustrates the size and course of the posterior cruciate ligament.

2. It has a slightly curved course and is completely devoid of signals.

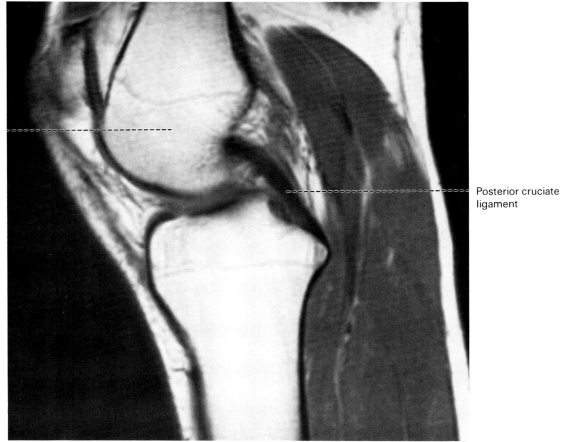

Medial femoral condyle

Posterior cruciate ligament

Figure 15.3.9

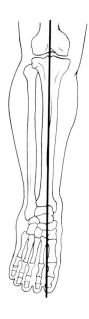

1. This section shows both the anterior and posterior cruciate ligaments.

2. Popliteus courses superolaterally to become intra-articular.

3. Note the patellar ligament and its attachment to the tibial tubercle.

4. The infrapatellar fat pad is demonstrated anterior to the joint.

5. The posterior tibial artery courses distally between soleus and the long flexors of the foot.

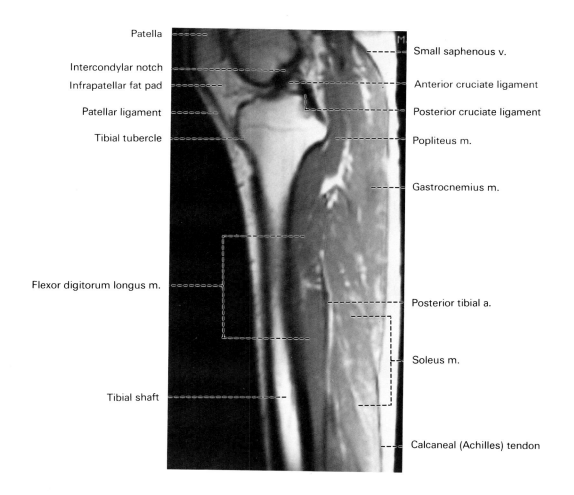

Patella
Intercondylar notch
Infrapatellar fat pad
Patellar ligament
Tibial tubercle

Flexor digitorum longus m.

Tibial shaft

Small saphenous v.
Anterior cruciate ligament
Posterior cruciate ligament
Popliteus m.

Gastrocnemius m.

Posterior tibial a.

Soleus m.

Calcaneal (Achilles) tendon

Figure 15.3.10

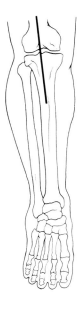

1. This section passes through the anterior cruciate ligament.

2. Note that the anterior cruciate is smaller in diameter than the posterior cruciate ligament.

3. There are typically more signals from the anterior cruciate than the posterior cruciate ligament.

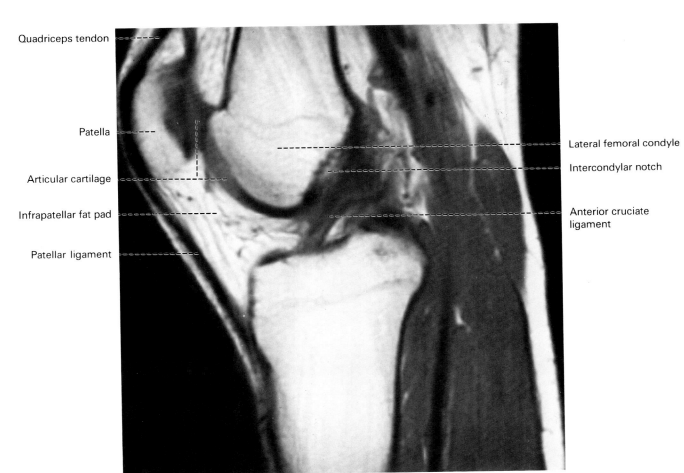

Quadriceps tendon

Patella

Articular cartilage

Infrapatellar fat pad

Patellar ligament

Lateral femoral condyle

Intercondylar notch

Anterior cruciate ligament

Figure 15.3.11

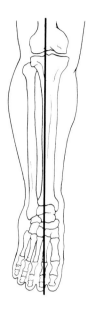

1. The posterior cruciate is again demonstrated on this section because it is larger than the anterior cruciate.

2. The popliteal vessels course distal to the knee on the surface of the popliteus muscle where the popliteal artery trifurcates, with some variation, into the anterior tibial, posterior tibial, and peroneal arteries.

3. Tibialis posterior and flexor hallucis longus are demonstrated deep to soleus.

4. The patella, patellar ligament, infrapatellar fat pad, and tibial tubercle are all seen on this section.

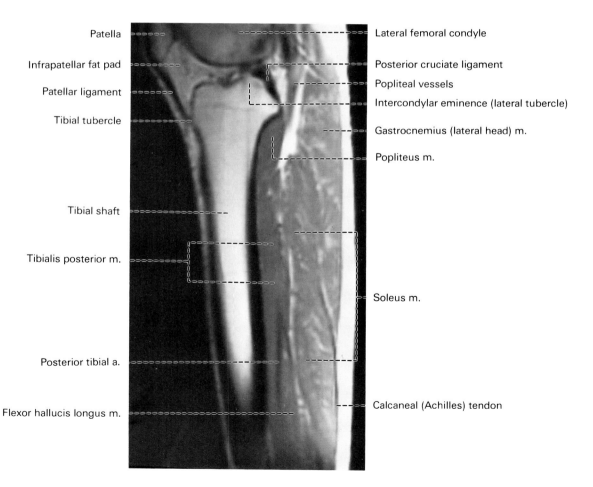

Patella — Lateral femoral condyle
Infrapatellar fat pad — Posterior cruciate ligament
Patellar ligament — Popliteal vessels
Tibial tubercle — Intercondylar eminence (lateral tubercle)
Gastrocnemius (lateral head) m.
Popliteus m.
Tibial shaft
Tibialis posterior m.
Soleus m.
Posterior tibial a.
Calcaneal (Achilles) tendon
Flexor hallucis longus m.

Figure 15.3.12

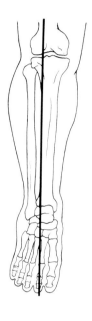

1. Note the popliteal artery as it divides on the surface of the popliteus muscle.

2. The lateral head of gastrocnemius, which is smaller than the medial, is seen close to its origin just proximal to the lateral femoral condyle.

3. Inferiorly this section passes just lateral to the tibia where tibialis anterior is imaged.

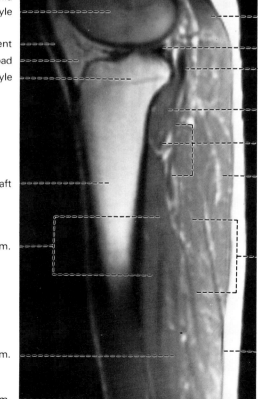

Patella
Lateral femoral condyle

Patellar ligament
Infrapatellar fat pad
Lateral tibial condyle

Tibial shaft

Tibialis posterior m.

Flexor hallucis longus m.

Tibialis anterior m.

Gastrocnemius (lateral head) m

Lateral meniscus (posterior horn)
Popliteal a.

Popliteus m.

Popliteal a., trifurcation

Gastrocnemius (lateral head) m.

Soleus m.

Calcaneal (Achilles) tendon

Figure 15.3.13

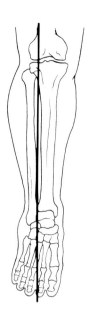

1. Note the relation of the popliteal artery to the popliteus muscle.

2. Tibialis posterior is partially demonstrated. It originates from the fibula, interosseous membrane, and tibia.

3. The anterior and posterior horns of the lateral meniscus are seen.

4. In the anterior compartment, all three long extensors are demonstrated in this section.

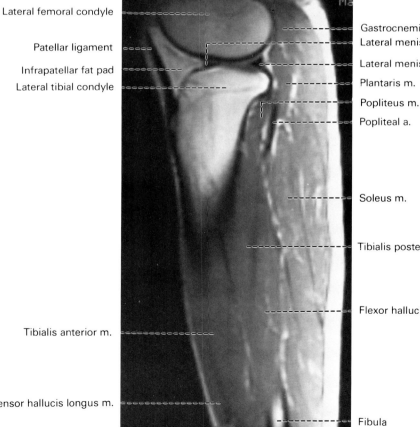

Lateral femoral condyle
Patellar ligament
Infrapatellar fat pad
Lateral tibial condyle

Gastrocnemius (lateral head) m.
Lateral meniscus (anterior horn)
Lateral meniscus (posterior horn)
Plantaris m.
Popliteus m.
Popliteal a.

Soleus m.

Tibialis posterior m.

Flexor hallucis longus m.

Tibialis anterior m.

Extensor hallucis longus m.

Extensor digitorum longus m.

Fibula

Figure 15.3.14

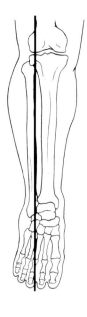

1. The plantaris muscle originates in close proximity to the origin of the lateral head of gastrocnemius.

2. The popliteus tendon courses superolaterally and becomes intra-articular prior to its insertion on the lateral femoral condyle.

3. The typical bow-tie appearance of the meniscus is demonstrated in this sagittal section.

4. Flexor hallucis longus, which originates from the posterior and distal half of the fibula, is seen deep to the soleus muscle.

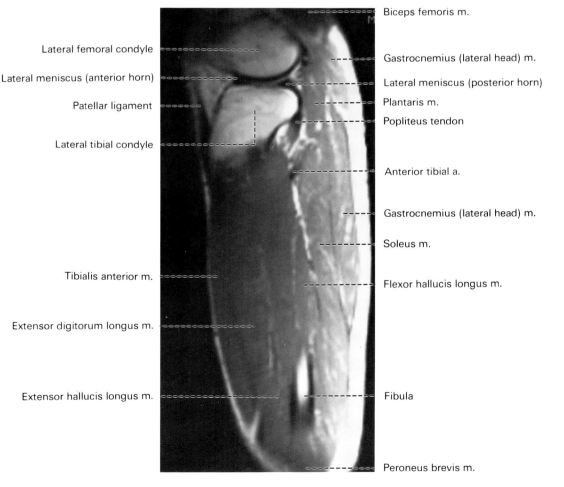

Biceps femoris m.

Lateral femoral condyle

Gastrocnemius (lateral head) m.

Lateral meniscus (anterior horn)

Lateral meniscus (posterior horn)

Patellar ligament

Plantaris m.

Popliteus tendon

Lateral tibial condyle

Anterior tibial a.

Gastrocnemius (lateral head) m.

Soleus m.

Tibialis anterior m.

Flexor hallucis longus m.

Extensor digitorum longus m.

Extensor hallucis longus m.

Fibula

Peroneus brevis m.

Figure 15.3.15

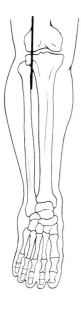

1. This section is through the lateral meniscus.

2. Note the triangular shape of the meniscus in cross section.

3. The hyaline cartilage covering the articular surfaces has more signals than the fibrocartilage in the menisci.

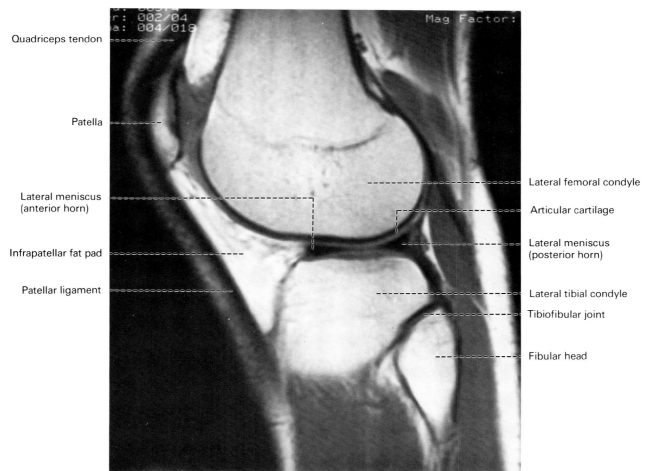

Figure 15.3.16

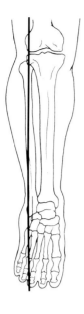

1. The posterior horn of the lateral meniscus is demonstrated in this section.

2. The anterior tibial artery is seen crossing to the anterior compartment above the upper end of the interosseous membrane.

3. In the anterior compartment, extensor digitorum longus covers extensor hallucis longus.

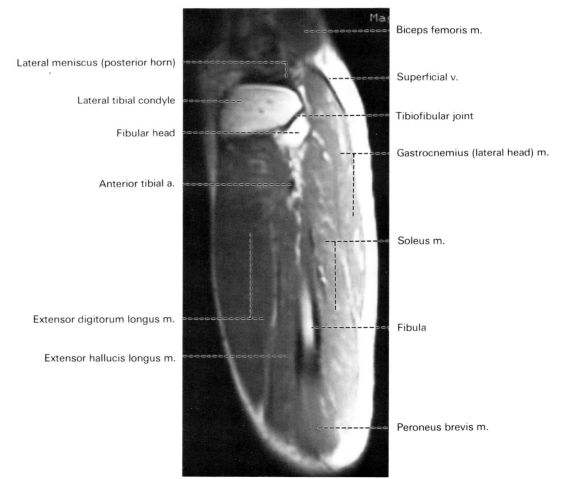

Lateral meniscus (posterior horn)

Lateral tibial condyle

Fibular head

Anterior tibial a.

Extensor digitorum longus m.

Extensor hallucis longus m.

Biceps femoris m.

Superficial v.

Tibiofibular joint

Gastrocnemius (lateral head) m.

Soleus m.

Fibula

Peroneus brevis m.

Figure 15.3.17

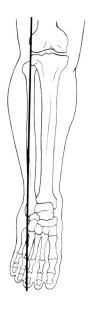

1. This section passes through the tibiofibular joint, which is a synovial joint.

2. The peroneus brevis tendon is slightly anterior to the peroneus longus tendon.

3. Biceps femoris crosses the knee joint laterally to insert on the fibular head.

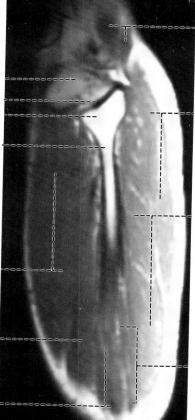

Figure 15.3.18

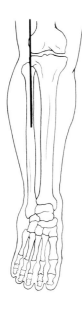

1. This section demonstrates the insertion of the biceps femoris tendon on the fibular head.

2. The lateral meniscus and articular cartilage on the femoral condyle are distinctly seen.

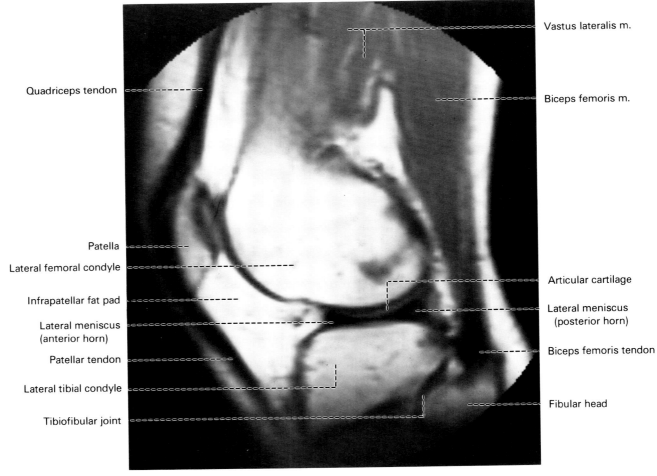

Quadriceps tendon

Patella

Lateral femoral condyle

Infrapatellar fat pad

Lateral meniscus (anterior horn)

Patellar tendon

Lateral tibial condyle

Tibiofibular joint

Vastus lateralis m.

Biceps femoris m.

Articular cartilage

Lateral meniscus (posterior horn)

Biceps femoris tendon

Fibular head

Figure 15.3.19

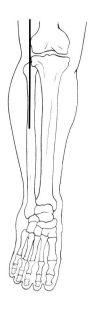

1. This section is through the lateral (fibular) collateral ligament.

2. The course of the lateral collateral ligament is oblique in the sagittal plane.

3. The biceps femoris tendon and lateral collateral ligament both insert on the fibular head.

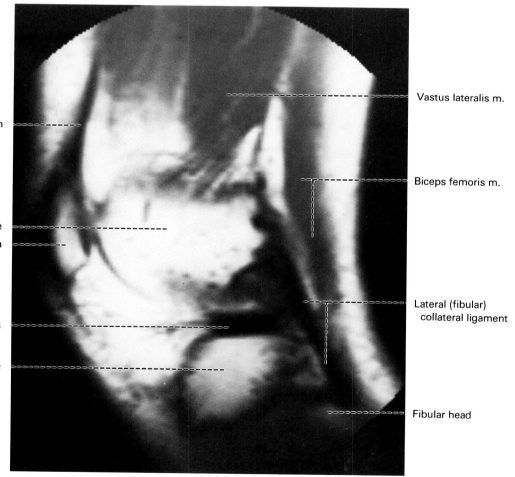

Quadriceps tendon

Lateral femoral condyle

Patella

Body of lateral meniscus

Lateral tibial condyle

Vastus lateralis m.

Biceps femoris m.

Lateral (fibular) collateral ligament

Fibular head

Figure 15.3.20

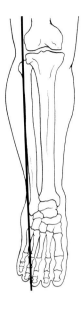

1. Note the insertion of the biceps femoris tendon and fibular collateral ligament to the fibular head.

2. The posterior aspect of soleus is covered partially by gastrocnemius.

3. Extensor digitorum longus lies anterior to extensor hallucis longus.

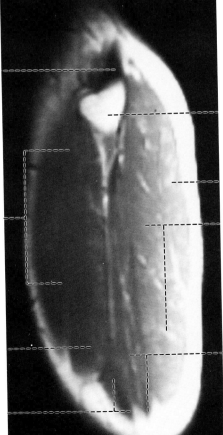

Biceps femoris tendon and lateral (fibular) collateral ligament

Fibular head

Extensor digitorum longus m.

Gastrocnemius (lateral head) m.

Soleus m.

Extensor hallucis longus m.

Peroneus longus m. and tendon

Peroneus brevis m. and tendon

Figure 15.3.21

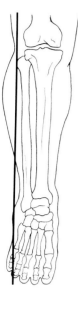

1. The common peroneal nerve descends posterior to the fibular head and then divides into the superficial and deep peroneal nerves (not seen in this section).

2. The tendinous portions of the peroneal muscles are demonstrated in the lower part of this image.

3. Extensor digitorum longus is partially demonstrated.

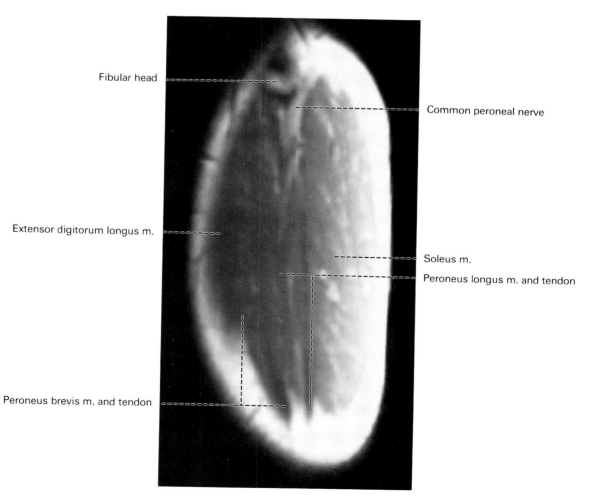

Figure 15.3.22

1. This section delineates the posterior intermuscular septum separating peroneus longus anteriorly from soleus posteriorly.

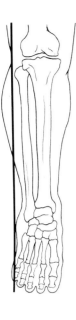

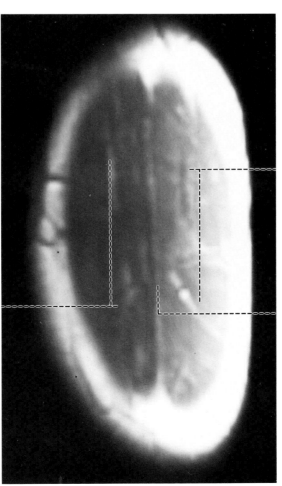

Peroneus longus m.

Soleus m.

Posterior crural intermuscular septum

Figure 15.3.23

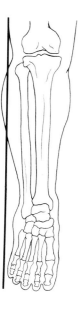

1. This lateral section of the calf passes through soleus posteriorly and peroneus longus anteriorly. These two muscles are separated by the posterior intermuscular septum.

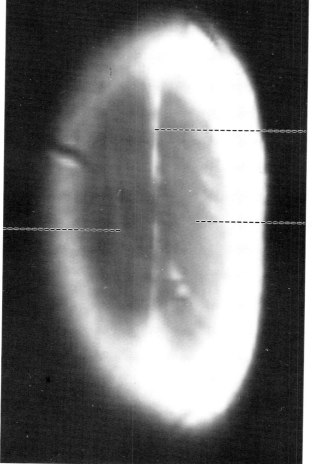

Posterior crural intermuscular septum

Peroneus longus m.

Soleus m.

Chapter 16

ANKLE

AXIAL

Figure 16.1.1

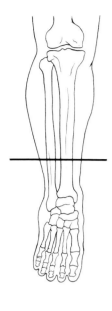

1. Flexor hallucis longus is interposed between tibialis posterior and the fibula; its tendinous portion can be noted centrally.

2. The peroneals, composed of peroneus longus and peroneus brevis, lie posterior to the fibula and are contiguous with flexor hallucis longus.

3. The tendinous portion of peroneus longus is anterolateral to peroneus brevis.

4. The calcaneal (Achilles) tendon is seen posteriorly, and immediately lateral to it is the small saphenous vein.

5. The great saphenous vein is situated medial to the tibia.

6. The tibialis anterior tendon lies immediately anterior to the tibia.

7. The long extensors are lateral to the tibia. Their tendons are partially formed.

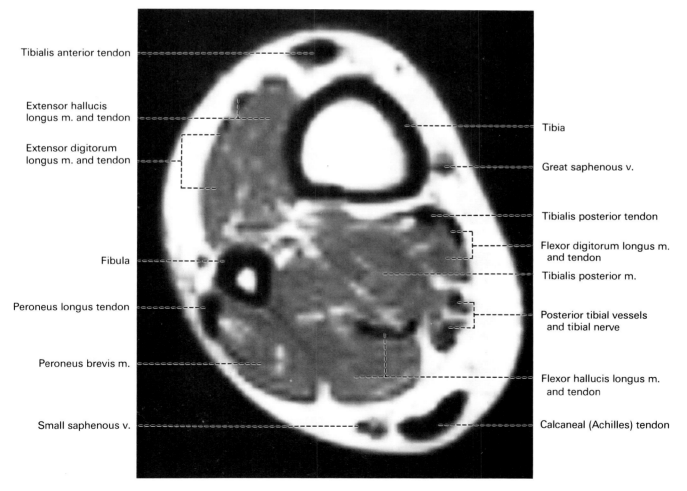

Figure 16.1.2

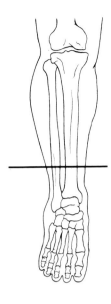

1. The tendon of tibialis posterior is anterior to the tendon of flexor digitorum longus.

2. Immediately posterior to the above structures lie the posterior tibial vessels and tibial nerve.

3. Flexor hallucis longus is largely muscular at this level.

4. The intermuscular septum between the lateral compartment and the posterior compartment is seen at the junction between peroneus brevis and flexor hallucis longus.

5. The interosseous membrane separates the anterior compartment from the posterior compartment.

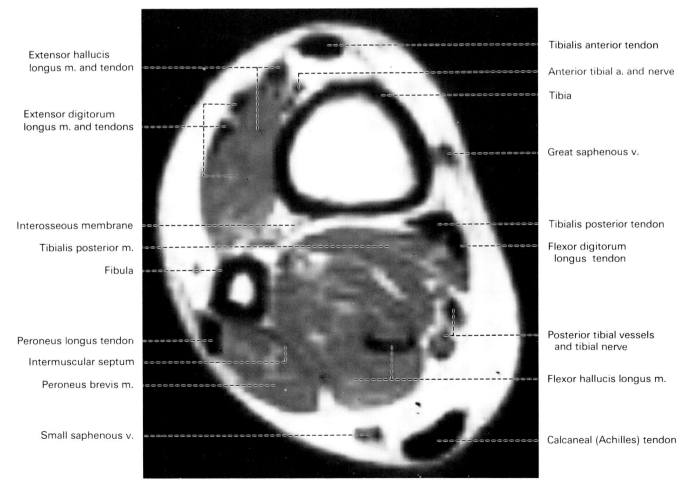

Extensor hallucis longus m. and tendon

Extensor digitorum longus m. and tendons

Interosseous membrane

Tibialis posterior m.

Fibula

Peroneus longus tendon

Intermuscular septum

Peroneus brevis m.

Small saphenous v.

Tibialis anterior tendon

Anterior tibial a. and nerve

Tibia

Great saphenous v.

Tibialis posterior tendon

Flexor digitorum longus tendon

Posterior tibial vessels and tibial nerve

Flexor hallucis longus m.

Calcaneal (Achilles) tendon

Figure 16.1.3

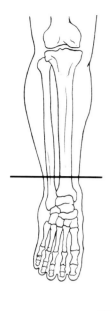

1. Peroneus brevis remains posterior and medial to peroneus longus. Both of these structures are posterior to the fibula.

2. The great saphenous vein remains immediately adjacent to the medial tibial cortex.

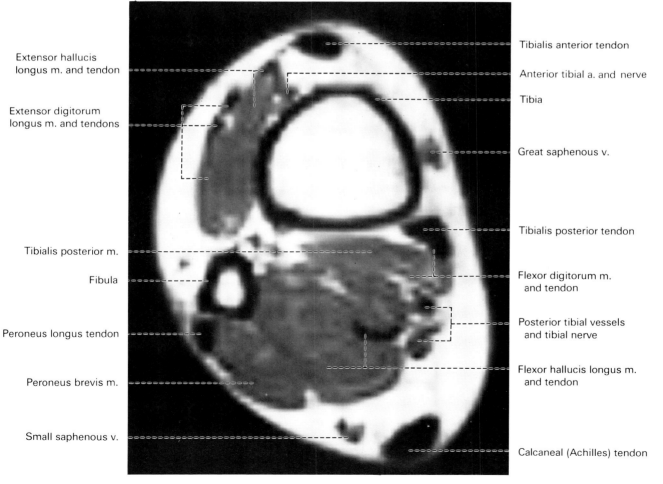

Extensor hallucis longus m. and tendon

Extensor digitorum longus m. and tendons

Tibialis posterior m.

Fibula

Peroneus longus tendon

Peroneus brevis m.

Small saphenous v.

Tibialis anterior tendon

Anterior tibial a. and nerve

Tibia

Great saphenous v.

Tibialis posterior tendon

Flexor digitorum m. and tendon

Posterior tibial vessels and tibial nerve

Flexor hallucis longus m. and tendon

Calcaneal (Achilles) tendon

Figure 16.1.4

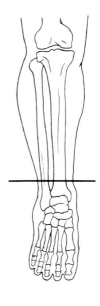

1. The anterior tibial vessels are deep to extensor hallucis longus.

2. The fibular notch starts to form at this level.

3. Note the relationship between the tibialis posterior tendon, flexor digitorum longus tendon, the posterior neurovascular bundle, and the tendon of flexor hallucis longus. A helpful mnemonic used by medical students to remember this sequence is "*Tom, Dick, and Nervous Harry.*"

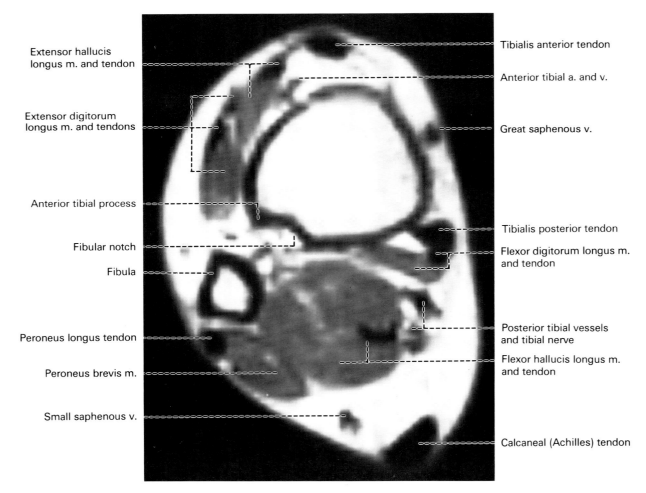

Extensor hallucis longus m. and tendon

Extensor digitorum longus m. and tendons

Anterior tibial process

Fibular notch

Fibula

Peroneus longus tendon

Peroneus brevis m.

Small saphenous v.

Tibialis anterior tendon

Anterior tibial a. and v.

Great saphenous v.

Tibialis posterior tendon

Flexor digitorum longus m. and tendon

Posterior tibial vessels and tibial nerve

Flexor hallucis longus m. and tendon

Calcaneal (Achilles) tendon

Figure 16.1.5

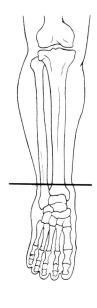

1. At this level the only muscular component in the posterior compartment is flexor hallucis longus.

2. Peroneus brevis is composed of its tendinous and muscular portions and remains posterior and medial to the peroneus longus tendon.

3. The muscles in the anterior compartment are diminishing in size.

Extensor hallucis longus m. and tendon

Extensor digitorum longus m. and tendons

Anterior tibial process

Fibular notch

Fibula

Peroneus longus tendon

Peroneus brevis m. and tendon

Small saphenous v.

Tibialis anterior tendon

Anterior tibial a. and nerve

Great saphenous v.

Tibia

Tibialis posterior tendon

Flexor digitorum longus tendon

Posterior tibial vessels and tibial nerve

Flexor hallucis longus m. and tendon

Calcaneal (Achilles) tendon

Figure 16.1.6

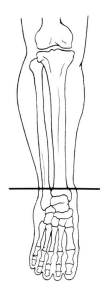

1. Note the close proximity of the posterior tibial tendon and flexor digitorum longus tendon.

2. The posterior boundary of the fibular notch forms the posterior malleolus.

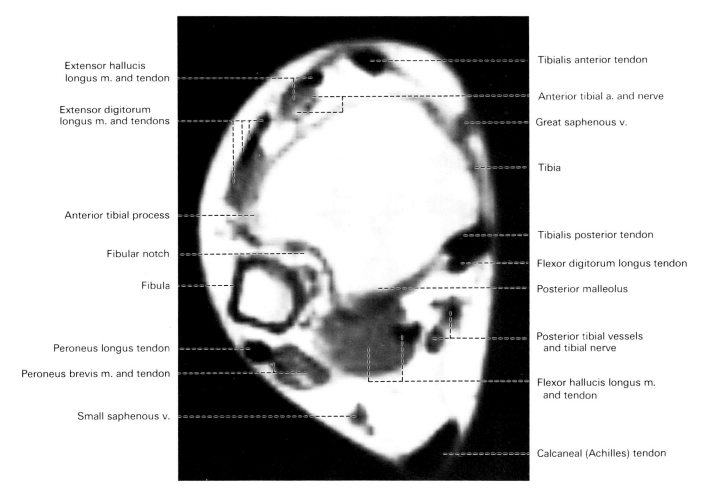

Extensor hallucis longus m. and tendon

Extensor digitorum longus m. and tendons

Anterior tibial process

Fibular notch

Fibula

Peroneus longus tendon

Peroneus brevis m. and tendon

Small saphenous v.

Tibialis anterior tendon

Anterior tibial a. and nerve

Great saphenous v.

Tibia

Tibialis posterior tendon

Flexor digitorum longus tendon

Posterior malleolus

Posterior tibial vessels and tibial nerve

Flexor hallucis longus m. and tendon

Calcaneal (Achilles) tendon

Figure 16.1.7

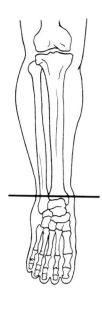

1. The anterior tibial process forms the anterior boundary of the fibular notch.

2. Note the tibiofibular syndesmosis in this section.

3. Observe the relationship between the distal portion of flexor hallucis longus and the posterior malleolus.

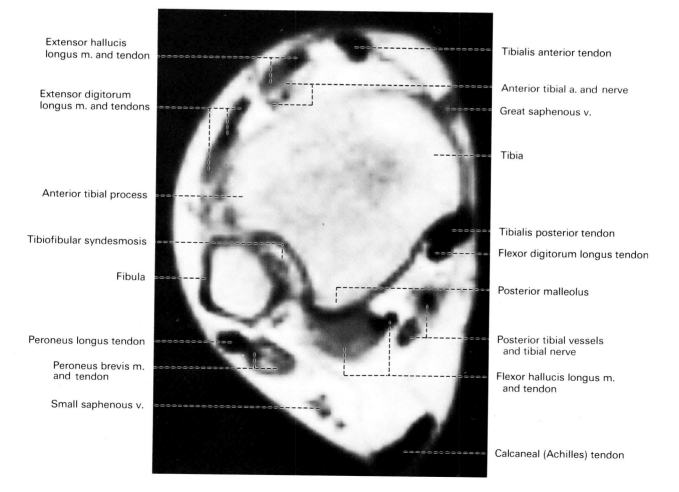

Extensor hallucis longus m. and tendon

Extensor digitorum longus m. and tendons

Anterior tibial process

Tibiofibular syndesmosis

Fibula

Peroneus longus tendon

Peroneus brevis m. and tendon

Small saphenous v.

Tibialis anterior tendon

Anterior tibial a. and nerve

Great saphenous v.

Tibia

Tibialis posterior tendon

Flexor digitorum longus tendon

Posterior malleolus

Posterior tibial vessels and tibial nerve

Flexor hallucis longus m. and tendon

Calcaneal (Achilles) tendon

Figure 16.1.8

1. In this section all three malleoli are demonstrated.

2. The posterior malleolus forms the posterior lip of the plafond.

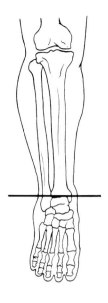

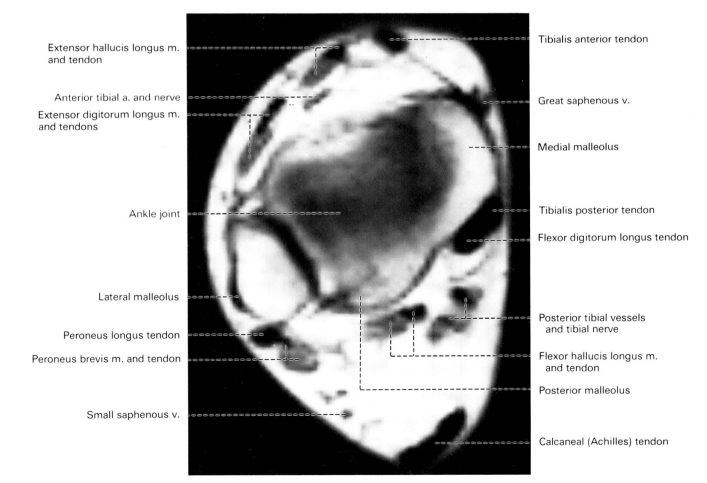

Extensor hallucis longus m. and tendon

Anterior tibial a. and nerve

Extensor digitorum longus m. and tendons

Ankle joint

Lateral malleolus

Peroneus longus tendon

Peroneus brevis m. and tendon

Small saphenous v.

Tibialis anterior tendon

Great saphenous v.

Medial malleolus

Tibialis posterior tendon

Flexor digitorum longus tendon

Posterior tibial vessels and tibial nerve

Flexor hallucis longus m. and tendon

Posterior malleolus

Calcaneal (Achilles) tendon

Figure 16.1.9

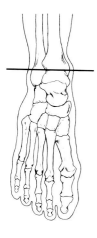

1. This section is through the dome of the talus.

2. The tibialis posterior and flexor digitorum longus tendons, in their course toward the foot, pass posterior and inferior to the medial malleolus.

3. Peroneus brevis and longus pass posterior and inferior to the lateral malleolus.

4. Some of the ligaments of the ankle are clearly delineated in this section.

Extensor hallucis longus tendon

Anterior tibial a. and nerve

Extensor digitorum longus m. and tendon

Anterior tibiotalar ligament

Lateral malleolus

Peroneus brevis tendon

Peroneus longus tendon

Small saphenous v.

Tibialis anterior tendon

Tibionavicular and anterior tibiotalar ligaments

Medial malleolus

Talar dome

Tibialis posterior tendon

Flexor digitorum longus tendon

Posterior tibial a. and nerve

Flexor hallucis longus tendon

Calcaneal (Achilles) tendon

Figure 16.1.10

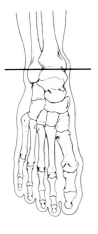

1. The calcaneal (Achilles) tendon inserts into the calcaneal tuberosity.

2. The anterior talofibular and posterior tibiotalar ligaments are demonstrated.

3. Note that the body of the talus is wider anteriorly than posteriorly.

4. The flexor hallucis longus tendon lies in a sulcus over the posterior aspect of the talus.

Extensor hallucis longus tendon

Anterior tibial a. and nerve

Extensor digitorum longus tendon

Anterior tibiotalar ligament

Talus, body

Lateral malleolus

Talus, posterior process

Peroneus longus and brevis tendons

Small saphenous v.

Tibialis anterior tendon

Tibionavicular and anterior tibiotalar ligaments

Medial malleolus

Posterior tibiotalar ligament

Tibialis posterior tendon

Flexor digitorum longus tendon

Sulcus for flexor hallucis longus tendon

Posterior tibial a. and nerve

Flexor hallucis longus tendon

Calcaneal tuberosity

Calcaneal (Achilles) tendon

Figure 16.1.11

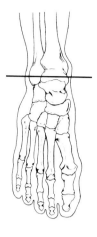

1. The great saphenous vein is seen subcutaneously in the anteromedial aspect of the ankle.

2. The small saphenous vein ascends posterior to the peroneal tendons.

3. Note the position of the anterior tibial artery and nerve between the extensor hallucis longus and flexor digitorum longus tendons.

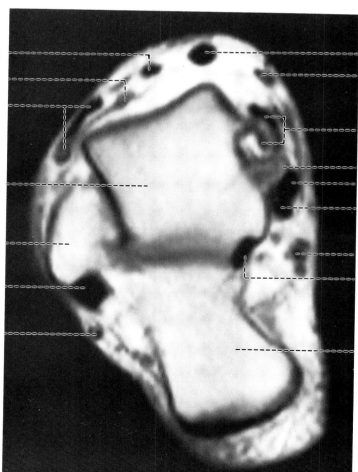

Extensor hallucis longus tendon

Anterior tibial a. and nerve

Flexor digitorum longus tendon

Talus, body

Lateral malleolus

Peroneus longus and brevis tendons

Small saphenous v.

Tibialis anterior tendon

Great saphenous v.

Tibionavicular and anterior tibiotalar ligaments

Medial malleolus

Tibialis posterior tendon

Flexor digitorum longus tendon

Posterior tibial a. and nerve

Flexor hallucis longus m.

Calcaneal tuberosity

Figure 16.1.12

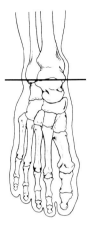

1. The extensor digitorum longus tendon divides into five separate tendons before it inserts.

2. A portion of the flexor retinaculum is demonstrated covering the medial surface of the flexor digitorum longus and tibialis posterior tendons.

3. The superior peroneal retinaculum forms at this level.

4. The posterior (lateral) subtalar joint is demonstrated in this section.

Extensor hallucis longus tendon

Anterior tibial a. and nerve

Extensor digitorum longus tendon

Tibialis posterior tendon

Posterior subtalar joint

Lateral malleolus

Superior peroneal retinaculum

Peroneus longus and brevis tendons

Small saphenous v.

Talus, body

Tibialis anterior tendon

Great saphenous v.

Tibionavicular and anterior tibiotalar ligaments

Flexor retinaculum

Flexor digitorum longus tendon

Flexor hallucis longus tendon

Posterior tibial a. and nerve

Calcaneal tuberosity

Figure 16.1.13

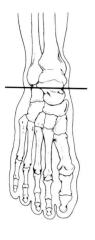

1. Note the superior peroneal retinaculum and its relationship to the peroneal tendons.

2. The posterior (lateral) subtalar joint is well defined in this section.

3. The abductor hallucis muscle originates from the calcaneal tuberosity.

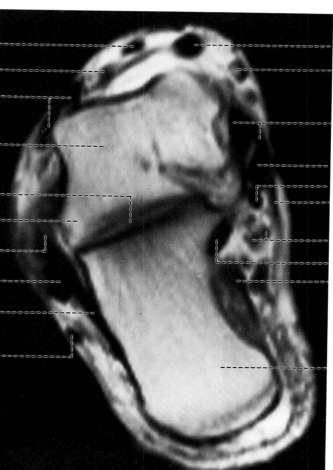

Extensor hallucis longus tendon

Anterior tibial a. and nerve

Extensor digitorum longus tendon

Talus

Posterior subtalar joint

Talus, lateral process

Peroneus brevis tendon

Peroneus longus tendon

Superior peroneal retinaculum

Small saphenous v.

Tibialis anterior tendon

Great saphenous v.

Tibionavicular and anterior tibiotalar ligaments

Tibialis posterior tendon

Flexor digitorum longus tendon

Flexor retinaculum

Posterior tibial a. and nerve

Flexor hallucis longus tendon

Abductor hallucis m.

Calcaneus

Figure 16.1.14

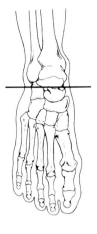

1. Flexor hallucis longus courses distally under the sustentaculum tali.

2. The middle (medial) subtalar joint forms between the sustentaculum tali and the inferior and medial aspect of the talus.

3. The tarsal sinus is demonstrated in this section.

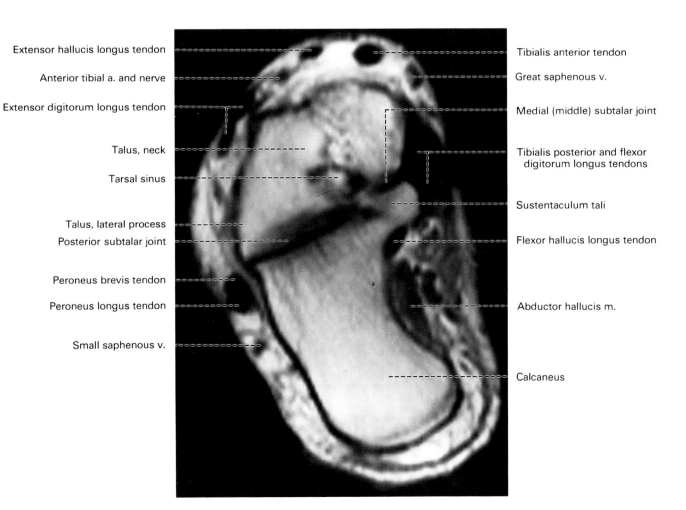

Extensor hallucis longus tendon — Tibialis anterior tendon

Anterior tibial a. and nerve — Great saphenous v.

Extensor digitorum longus tendon — Medial (middle) subtalar joint

Talus, neck — Tibialis posterior and flexor digitorum longus tendons

Tarsal sinus — Sustentaculum tali

Talus, lateral process — Flexor hallucis longus tendon

Posterior subtalar joint —

Peroneus brevis tendon —

Peroneus longus tendon — Abductor hallucis m.

Small saphenous v. — Calcaneus

Figure 16.1.15

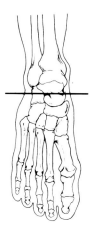

1. This section passes through the head of the talus.

2. The middle (medial) subtalar joint is clearly demonstrated in this section.

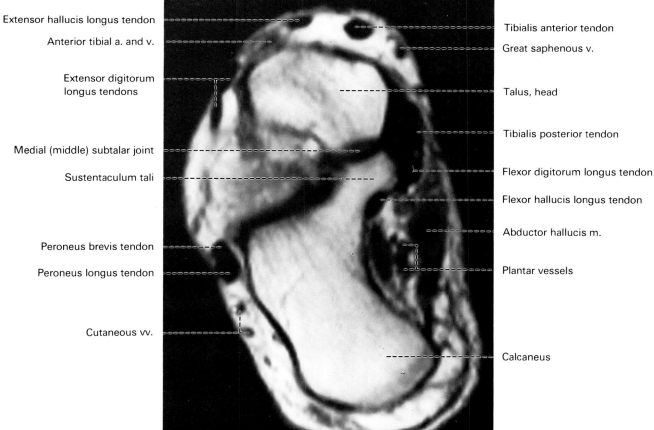

Extensor hallucis longus tendon

Anterior tibial a. and v.

Extensor digitorum longus tendons

Medial (middle) subtalar joint

Sustentaculum tali

Peroneus brevis tendon

Peroneus longus tendon

Cutaneous vv.

Tibialis anterior tendon

Great saphenous v.

Talus, head

Tibialis posterior tendon

Flexor digitorum longus tendon

Flexor hallucis longus tendon

Abductor hallucis m.

Plantar vessels

Calcaneus

Figure 16.1.16

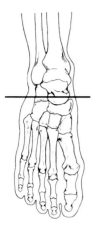

1. Extensor digitorum longus has divided into smaller individual tendons.

2. The posterior tibial artery divides into the medial and lateral plantar arteries on the surface of the abductor hallucis muscle.

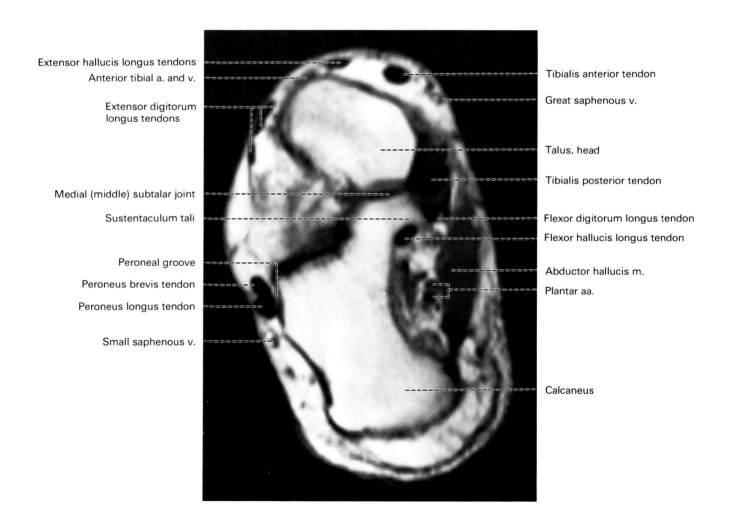

Extensor hallucis longus tendons

Anterior tibial a. and v.

Extensor digitorum longus tendons

Medial (middle) subtalar joint

Sustentaculum tali

Peroneal groove

Peroneus brevis tendon

Peroneus longus tendon

Small saphenous v.

Tibialis anterior tendon

Great saphenous v.

Talus, head

Tibialis posterior tendon

Flexor digitorum longus tendon

Flexor hallucis longus tendon

Abductor hallucis m.

Plantar aa.

Calcaneus

Figure 16.1.17

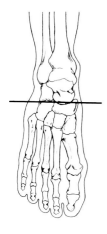

1. This section passes through the distal portion of the talus and calcaneus. The navicular tuberosity is also partially demonstrated.

2. Note the origin of the extensor digitorum brevis muscle from the antero-superior aspect of the calcaneus.

3. The peroneal tendons are demonstrated on the lateral aspect of the calcaneus in the peroneal groove.

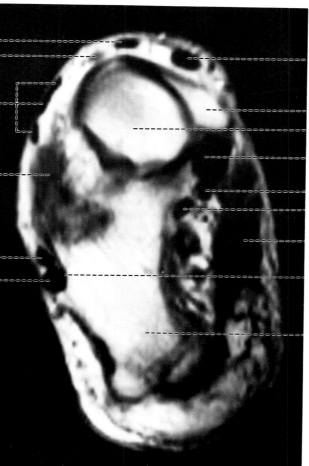

Extensor hallucis longus tendon
Dorsalis pedis a.
Extensor digitorum longus tendons
Extensor digitorum brevis m.
Peroneus brevis tendon
Peroneus longus tendon

Tibialis anterior tendon
Navicular tuberosity
Talus, head
Tibialis posterior tendon
Flexor digitorum longus tendon
Flexor hallucis longus tendon
Abductor hallucis m.
Peroneal groove
Calcaneus

Figure 16.2.1

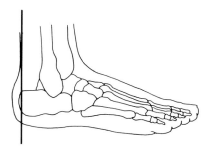

1. This posterior section passes through the calcaneal (Achilles) tendon, which inserts on the calcaneal tuberosity.

2. The fat pad of the heel is demonstrated inferior to the calcaneus.

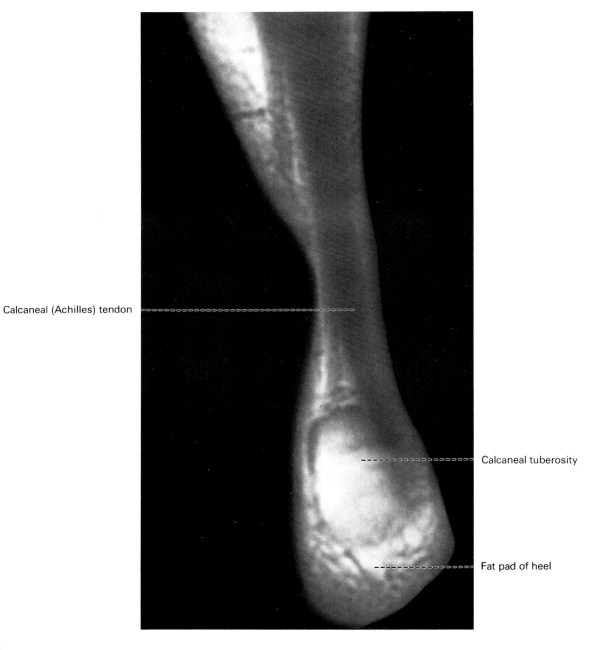

Calcaneal (Achilles) tendon

Calcaneal tuberosity

Fat pad of heel

Figure 16.2.2

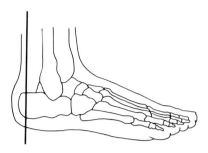

1. Soleus inserts into the calcaneal (Achilles) tendon.

2. Note the thick fibrous septa within the fat pad of the heel.

3. The split appearance of the calcaneal (Achilles) tendon is due to its concave configuration prior to its insertion.

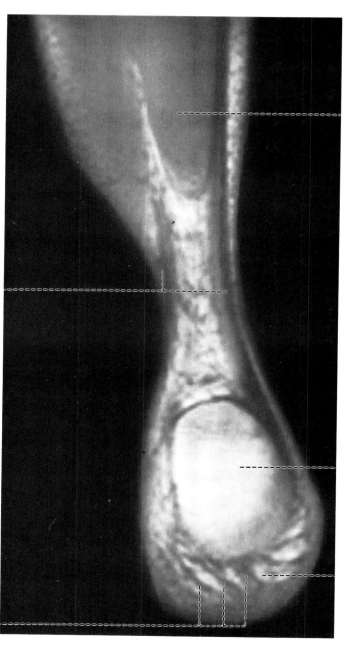

Soleus m.

Calcaneal (Achilles) tendon

Calcaneal tuberosity

Fat pad of heel

Fibrous septa

Figure 16.2.3

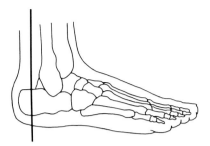

1. Peroneus brevis and flexor hallucis longus originate on the posterolateral and posterior aspect of the fibula, respectively.

2. Note the small saphenous vein ascending superficially posterior to the lateral malleolus.

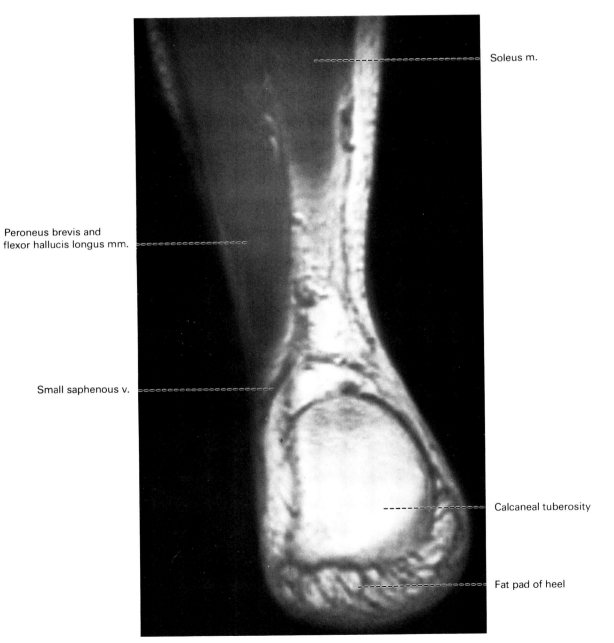

Soleus m.

Peroneus brevis and flexor hallucis longus mm.

Small saphenous v.

Calcaneal tuberosity

Fat pad of heel

Figure 16.2.4

1. Note the relationship of the peroneal muscles and tendons to the fibula.

2. This section goes through the long flexor muscles of the foot.

3. Note the prominent fibrous septa in the fat pad of the heel.

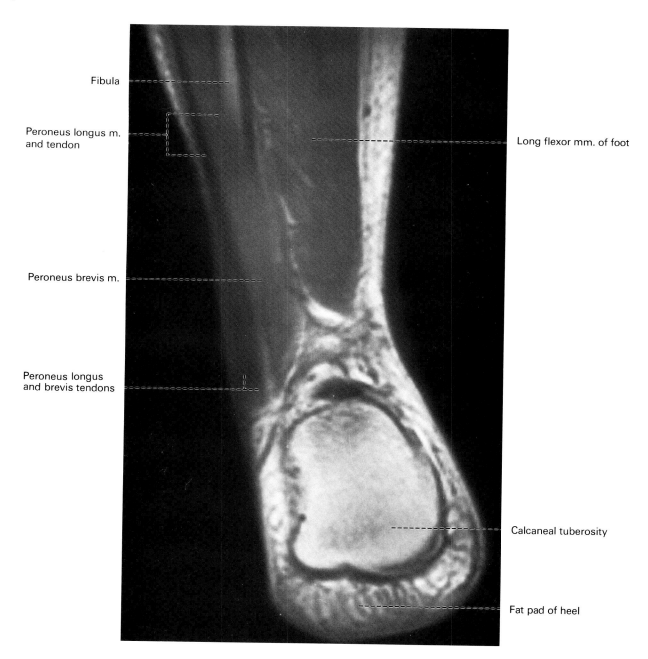

Fibula

Peroneus longus m.
and tendon

Long flexor mm. of foot

Peroneus brevis m.

Peroneus longus
and brevis tendons

Calcaneal tuberosity

Fat pad of heel

Figure 16.2.5

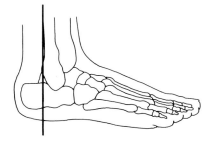

1. The flexor digitorum longus muscle and tendon as well as the tibialis posterior muscle and tendon are clearly demonstrated.

2. Just above the ankle the tibialis posterior tendon crosses anterior to the flexor digitorum longus tendon.

3. Note the origins of abductor hallucis, flexor digitorum brevis, and abductor digiti minimi from the calcaneal tuberosity.

4. The low signal intensity structure inferior to the lateral malleolus represents the peroneus longus and brevis tendons.

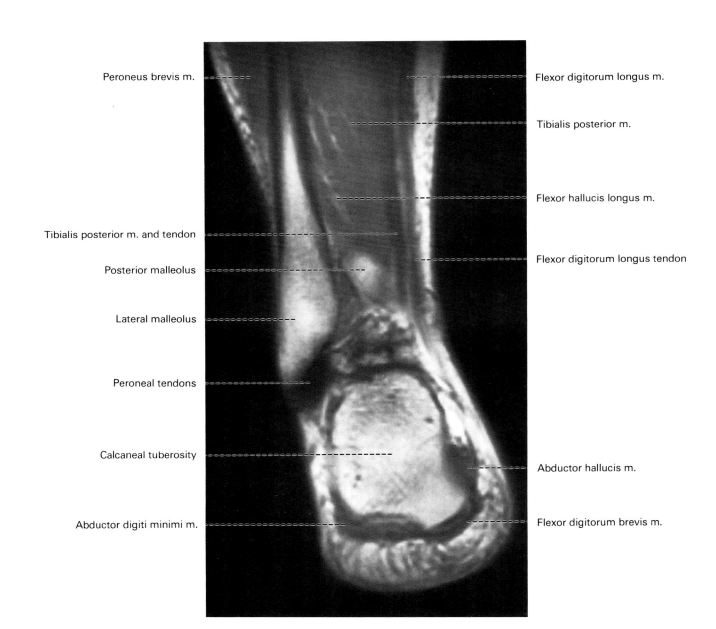

Peroneus brevis m.

Flexor digitorum longus m.

Tibialis posterior m.

Flexor hallucis longus m.

Tibialis posterior m. and tendon

Flexor digitorum longus tendon

Posterior malleolus

Lateral malleolus

Peroneal tendons

Calcaneal tuberosity

Abductor hallucis m.

Abductor digiti minimi m.

Flexor digitorum brevis m.

Figure 16.2.6

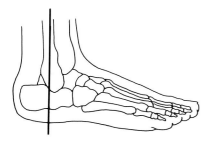

1. Muscle fibers originating from the distal third of the fibula belong to the flexor hallucis longus muscle.

2. The flexor digitorum longus and tibialis posterior tendons are demonstrated.

3. Because of its fibrous composition the plantar aponeurosis appears as a low signal intensity structure. It is seen superficial to flexor digitorum brevis.

4. The peroneal tendons course inferior to the lateral malleolus.

5. Note the posterior process of the talus immediately superior to the calcaneus.

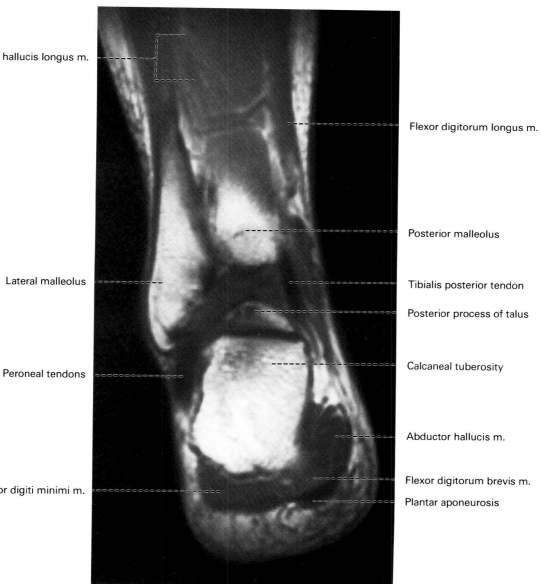

Flexor hallucis longus m.

Flexor digitorum longus m.

Posterior malleolus

Lateral malleolus

Tibialis posterior tendon

Posterior process of talus

Calcaneal tuberosity

Peroneal tendons

Abductor hallucis m.

Flexor digitorum brevis m.

Abductor digiti minimi m.

Plantar aponeurosis

Figure 16.2.7

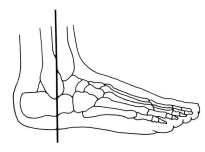

1. This section passes through the posterior process of the talus.

2. Note the origin of the quadratus plantae muscle from the calcaneal tuberosity deep to the flexor digitorum brevis muscle.

3. The thick plantar aponeurosis is seen in this section.

4. The calcaneofibular ligament extends from the lateral malleolus to the calcaneus.

5. Muscles of the anterior compartment are situated between the tibia and fibula.

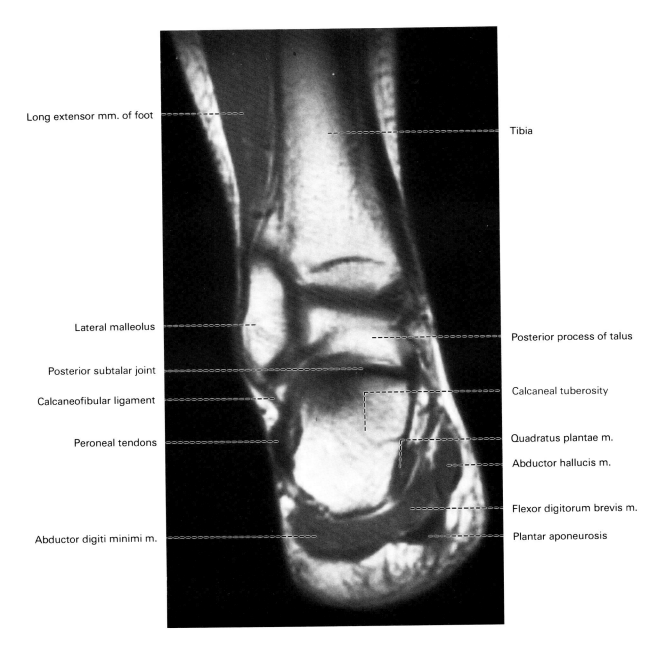

Long extensor mm. of foot

Lateral malleolus

Posterior subtalar joint

Calcaneofibular ligament

Peroneal tendons

Abductor digiti minimi m.

Tibia

Posterior process of talus

Calcaneal tuberosity

Quadratus plantae m.

Abductor hallucis m.

Flexor digitorum brevis m.

Plantar aponeurosis

Figure 16.2.8

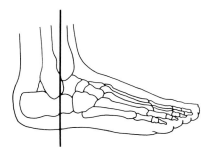

1. All the intrinsic muscles of the foot originate from the calcaneus.

2. The subtalar joint is in reality three joints; the posterior (lateral) subtalar joint is the most posterior and is demonstrated in this section.

Long extensor mm. of foot

Tibia

Ankle joint

Talus

Lateral process of talus

Sustentaculum tali

Posterior subtalar joint

Peroneus brevis tendon

Abductor hallucis m.

Quadratus plantae m.

Peroneus longus tendon

Flexor digitorum brevis m.

Abductor digiti minimi m.

Plantar aponeurosis

Figure 16.2.9

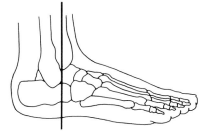

1. The flexor hallucis longus tendon courses toward the forefoot inferior to the sustentaculum tali, whereas the tendons of tibialis posterior and flexor digitorum longus, in this section, are situated superiorly.

2. The inferior medial surface of the talus and the sustentaculum tali form the middle (medial) subtalar joint.

3. Note the peroneal tendons diverging on the surface of the peroneal groove.

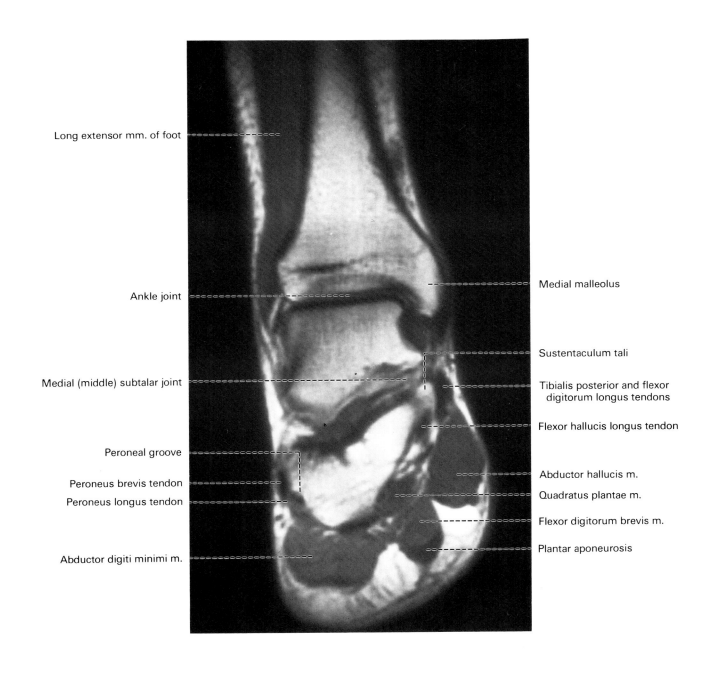

Long extensor mm. of foot

Ankle joint

Medial (middle) subtalar joint

Peroneal groove

Peroneus brevis tendon
Peroneus longus tendon

Abductor digiti minimi m.

Medial malleolus

Sustentaculum tali

Tibialis posterior and flexor digitorum longus tendons

Flexor hallucis longus tendon

Abductor hallucis m.

Quadratus plantae m.

Flexor digitorum brevis m.

Plantar aponeurosis

Figure 16.2.10

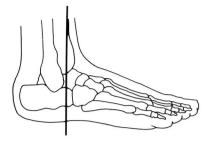

1. In the midfoot the flexor digitorum longus tendon crosses the flexor hallucis longus tendon and continues superficial (inferior) to it.

2. The peroneus longus tendon courses medial to the peroneus brevis tendon before it enters the cuboid sulcus.

3. Note extensor digitorum longus descending anterolaterally toward the foot.

4. The deltoid ligament is seen connecting the talus to the medial malleolus.

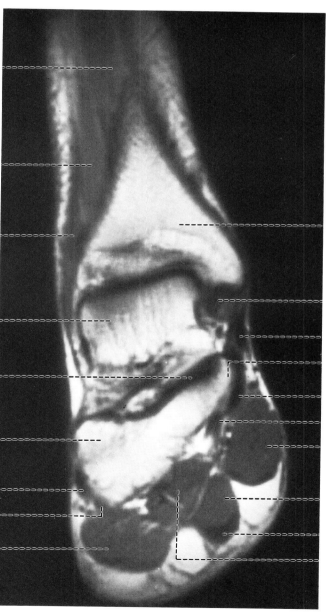

Tibialis anterior m.

Extensor hallucis longus m.

Extensor digitorum longus m.

Talus

Medial (middle) subtalar joint

Calcaneus

Peroneus brevis tendon

Peroneus longus tendon

Abductor digiti minimi m.

Tibia

Deltoid ligament

Tibialis posterior tendon

Sustentaculum tali

Flexor digitorum longus tendon

Flexor hallucis longus tendon

Abductor hallucis m.

Flexor digitorum brevis m.

Plantar aponeurosis

Quadratus plantae m.

Figure 16.2.11

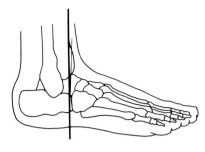

1. In this section the flexor digitorum longus tendon has crossed the flexor hallucis longus tendon to become superficial to it.

2. Extensor digitorum brevis is partially demonstrated as it originates from the anterior superior aspect of the calcaneus laterally.

3. The long extensor tendons of the foot (tibialis anterior, extensor hallucis longus, and extensor digitorum longus) are clearly depicted on the anterior surface of the distal tibia.

4. Note the anterior tibiotalar portion of the deltoid ligament medial to the talus.

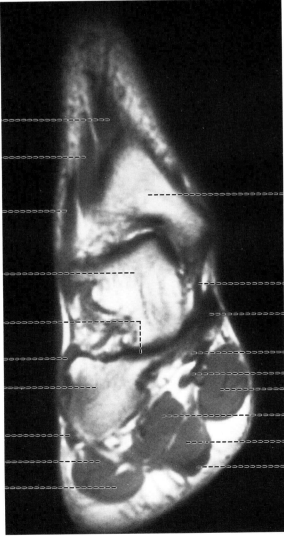

Tibialis anterior tendon

Extensor hallucis longus tendon

Extensor digitorum longus tendon — Tibia

Talus — Deltoid ligament (anterior tibiotalar part)

Tibialis posterior tendon

Anterior subtalar joint

Extensor digitorum brevis m. — Flexor hallucis longus tendon

Calcaneus (anterior process) — Flexor digitorum longus tendon
Abductor hallucis m.

Quadratus plantae m.

Peroneal tendons — Flexor digitorum brevis m.

Flexor digiti minimi brevis m. — Plantar aponeurosis

Abductor digiti minimi m.

Figure 16.2.12

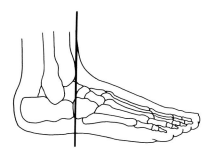

1. The tibialis posterior tendon flattens as it approaches its insertion onto the navicular tuberosity and medial cuneiform.

2. Note the location of flexor hallucis longus and flexor digitorum longus tendons between abductor hallucis and quadratus plantae muscles.

3. The peroneus longus tendon courses deep in the plantar surface of the foot within the cuboid sulcus.

4. Extensor digitorum brevis is the only muscle on the dorsum of the foot.

5. The long extensor tendons of the foot are seen anterior to the tibia.

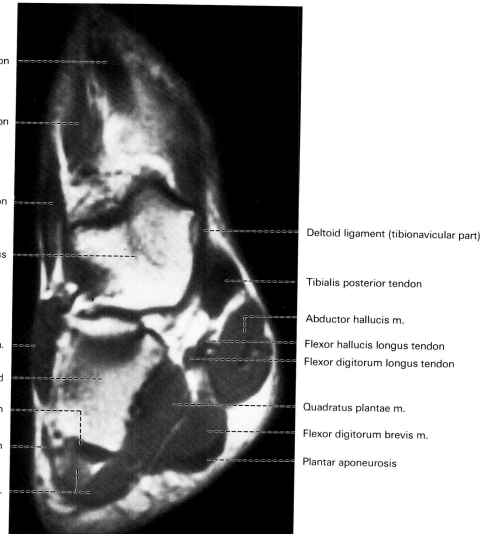

Tibialis anterior tendon

Extensor hallucis longus tendon

Extensor digitorum longus tendon

Talus

Deltoid ligament (tibionavicular part)

Tibialis posterior tendon

Abductor hallucis m.

Extensor digitorum brevis m.

Flexor hallucis longus tendon

Flexor digitorum longus tendon

Cuboid

Peroneus longus tendon

Quadratus plantae m.

Peroneus brevis tendon

Flexor digitorum brevis m.

Plantar aponeurosis

Flexor and abductor digiti minimi mm.

Figure 16.3.1

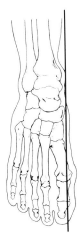

1. This medial section shows the abductor hallucis muscle and tendon.

2. Note flexor hallucis brevis inferior to the first metatarsal.

3. The great saphenous vein forms and ascends on the medial side of the foot.

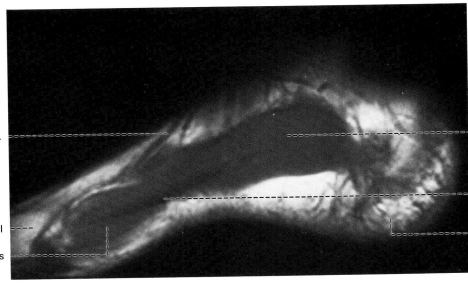

Great saphenous v.

Abductor hallucis m.

Abductor hallucis tendon

First metatarsal

Fat pad of heel

Flexor hallucis brevis m.

Figure 16.3.2

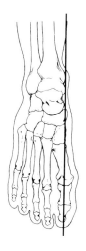

1. The tibialis posterior tendon is seen coursing anteriorly and inferiorly to insert on the plantar surface of the navicular tuberosity and medial cuneiform.

2. The flexor digitorum longus tendon descends posterior to the tibialis posterior tendon.

3. The tibialis anterior tendon is partially outlined at its insertion onto the plantar surface of the medial cuneiform and base of the first metatarsal.

4. Flexor digitorum brevis is seen at its origin from the calcaneal tuberosity.

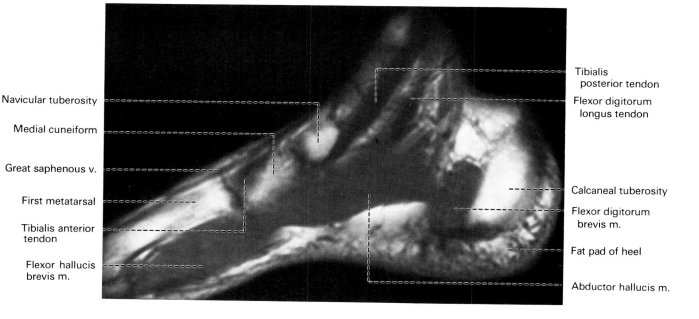

Figure 16.3.3

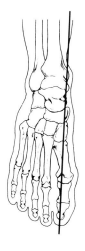

1. The long flexor tendons are located posterior to the medial malleolus and are arranged from anterior to posterior in the following order: (1) tibialis posterior tendon, (2) flexor digitorum longus tendon, and (3) flexor hallucis longus tendon.

2. The flexor hallucis longus tendon courses inferior to the sustentaculum tali.

3. Distally the flexor hallucis longus tendon is seen surrounded by flexor hallucis brevis (medial and lateral heads).

4. Note the posterior tibial artery and nerve crossing flexor hallucis longus as they enter the foot.

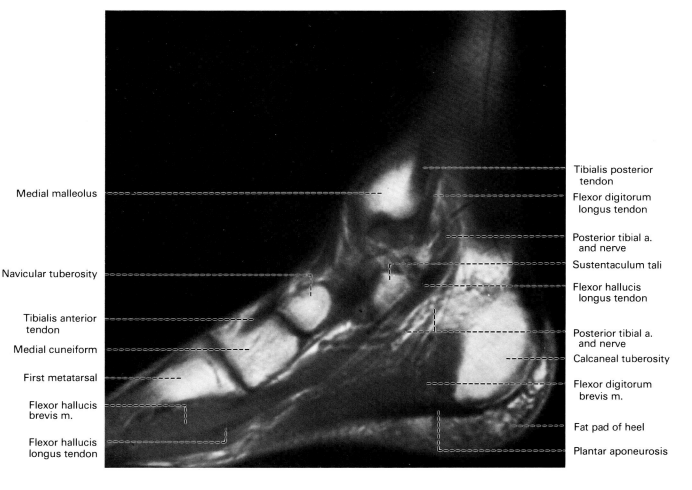

Medial malleolus

Navicular tuberosity

Tibialis anterior tendon

Medial cuneiform

First metatarsal

Flexor hallucis brevis m.

Flexor hallucis longus tendon

Tibialis posterior tendon

Flexor digitorum longus tendon

Posterior tibial a. and nerve

Sustentaculum tali

Flexor hallucis longus tendon

Posterior tibial a. and nerve

Calcaneal tuberosity

Flexor digitorum brevis m.

Fat pad of heel

Plantar aponeurosis

Figure 16.3.4

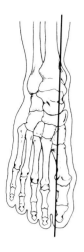

1. The calcaneal (Achilles) tendon is partially demonstrated in this section.

2. The flexor digitorum brevis and quadratus plantae are closely related and difficult to separate.

3. The course of flexor hallucis longus in the midfoot is well demonstrated.

4. The thick muscle lateral to the first metatarsal is the oblique head of the adductor hallucis.

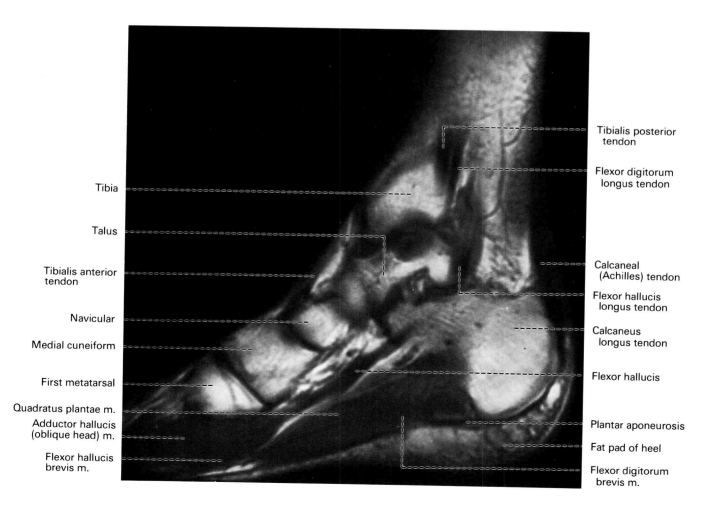

Figure 16.3.5

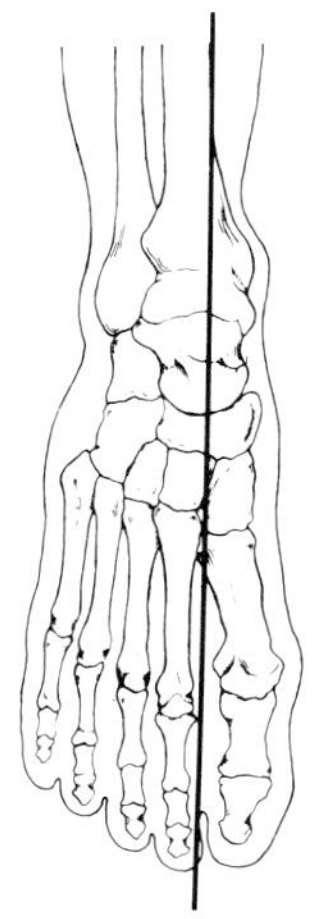

1. The calcaneal (Achilles) tendon is outlined in its entirety.
2. All three long flexor tendons are seen posterior to the distal tibia.
3. The posterior (lateral) and middle (medial) subtalar joints are demonstrated in this section.
4. Note the tibialis anterior tendon coursing obliquely anterior to the talus.

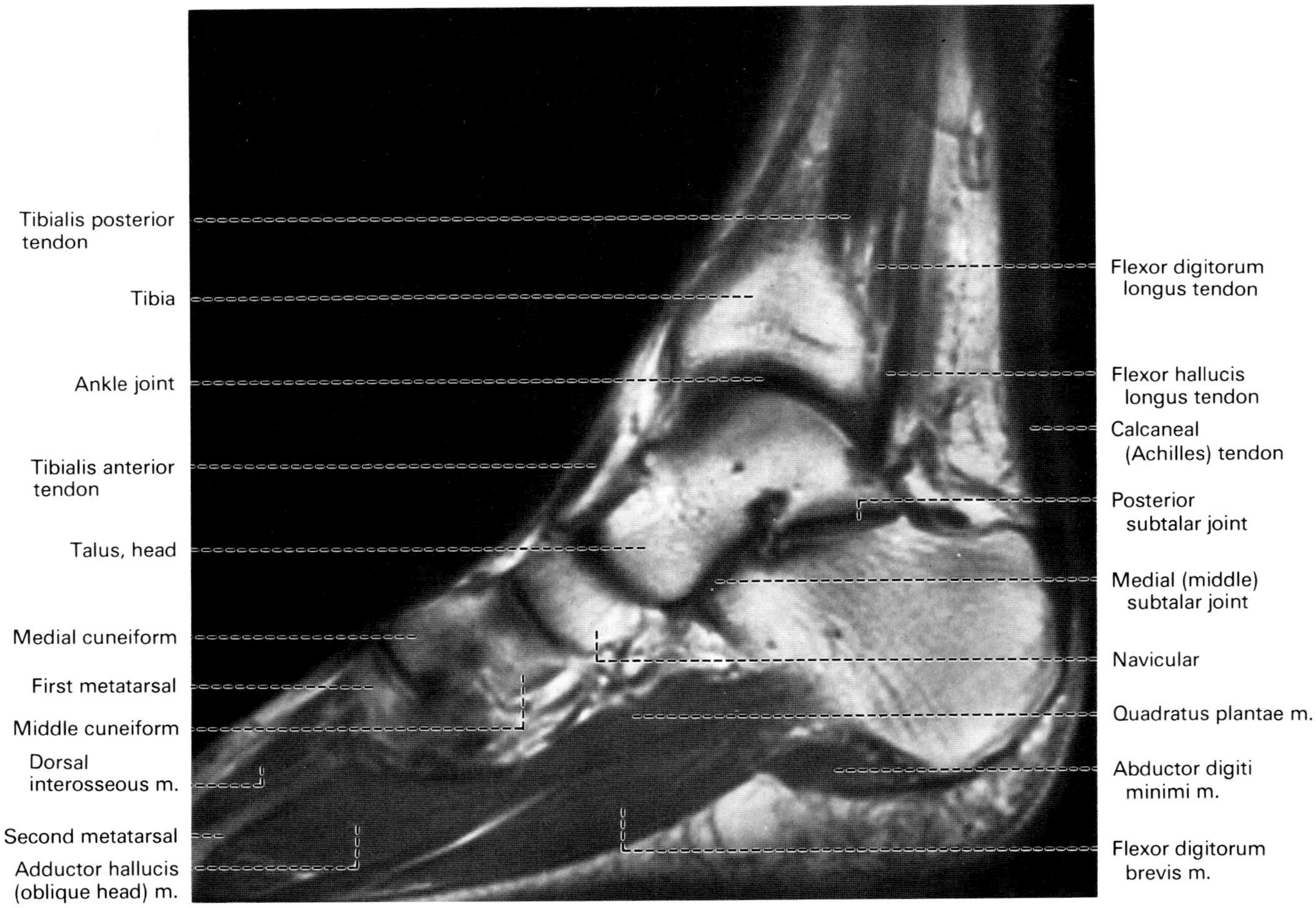
Tibialis posterior tendon
Tibia
Ankle joint
Tibialis anterior tendon
Talus, head
Medial cuneiform
First metatarsal
Middle cuneiform
Dorsal interosseous m.
Second metatarsal
Adductor hallucis (oblique head) m.
Flexor digitorum longus tendon
Flexor hallucis longus tendon
Calcaneal (Achilles) tendon
Posterior subtalar joint
Medial (middle) subtalar joint
Navicular
Quadratus plantae m.
Abductor digiti minimi m.
Flexor digitorum brevis m.

Figure 16.3.6

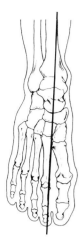

1. Note the position of the long flexor muscles posterior to the distal tibia.

2. The tarsal sinus is seen separating the posterior (lateral) and middle (medial) subtalar joints.

3. The soleus muscle is situated between the long flexor muscles and the calcaneal (Achilles) tendon.

4. Peroneus longus courses deep in the foot toward its insertion at the plantar aspect of the medial cuneiform and base of the first metatarsal.

5. Note the rich vascular network deep in the arch of the foot between quadratus plantae and the tarsal bones.

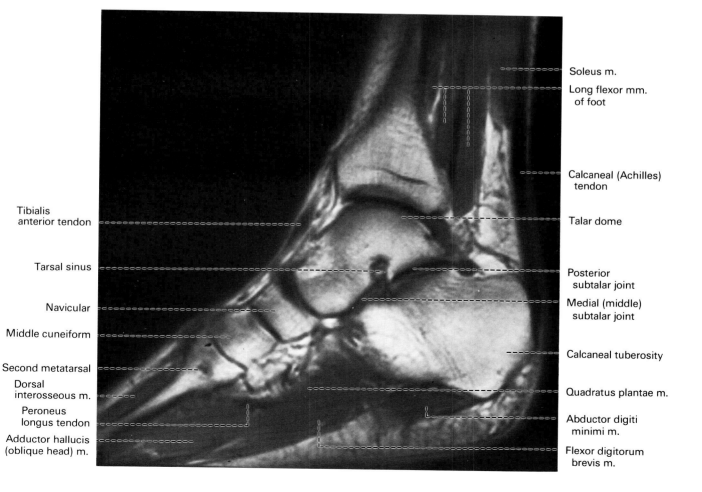

Figure 16.3.7

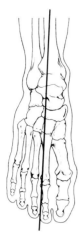

1. As the sections move laterally, the cuboid and abductor digiti minimi muscles can be seen.

2. Note the peroneus longus tendon as it exits the cuboid sulcus and proceeds medially.

3. In this ankle an os trigonum is demonstrated posterior to the talus.

4. Note the superficial position of the tibialis anterior tendon that can normally be palpated under the skin.

5. The small anterior subtalar joint is depicted in this section. In some individuals this joint is nonexistent or incorporated with the middle (medial) subtalar joint.

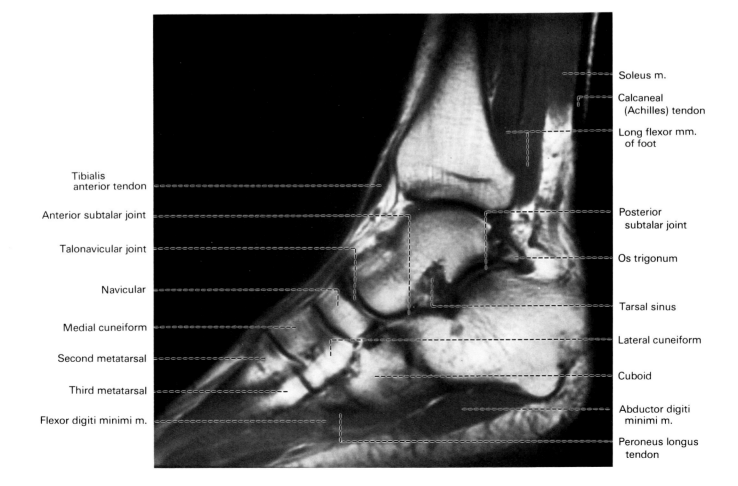

Figure 16.3.8

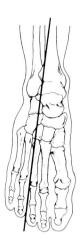

1. The anterior and posterior subtalar joints are demonstrated on this section.

2. The peroneus longus tendon is seen within the cuboid sulcus.

3. Anterior to the ankle joint, extensor hallucis longus and tibialis anterior tendons are both outlined.

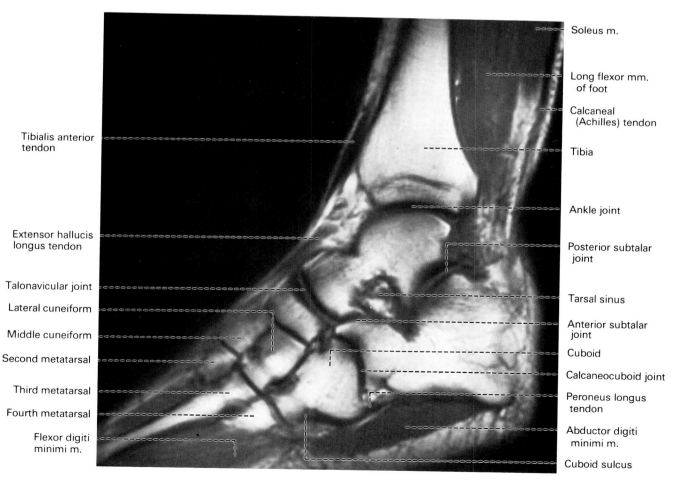

Tibialis anterior tendon

Extensor hallucis longus tendon

Talonavicular joint

Lateral cuneiform

Middle cuneiform

Second metatarsal

Third metatarsal

Fourth metatarsal

Flexor digiti minimi m.

Soleus m.

Long flexor mm. of foot

Calcaneal (Achilles) tendon

Tibia

Ankle joint

Posterior subtalar joint

Tarsal sinus

Anterior subtalar joint

Cuboid

Calcaneocuboid joint

Peroneus longus tendon

Abductor digiti minimi m.

Cuboid sulcus

Figure 16.3.9

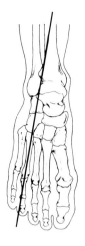

1. Flexor hallucis longus originates on the posteromedial surface of the fibula. Adjacent to it is peroneus brevis, which originates on the posterolateral surface of the fibula.

2. This section passes through the lateral process of the talus.

3. The peroneus longus tendon is seen within the cuboid sulcus.

4. Extensor digitorum brevis is seen on the dorsum of the foot.

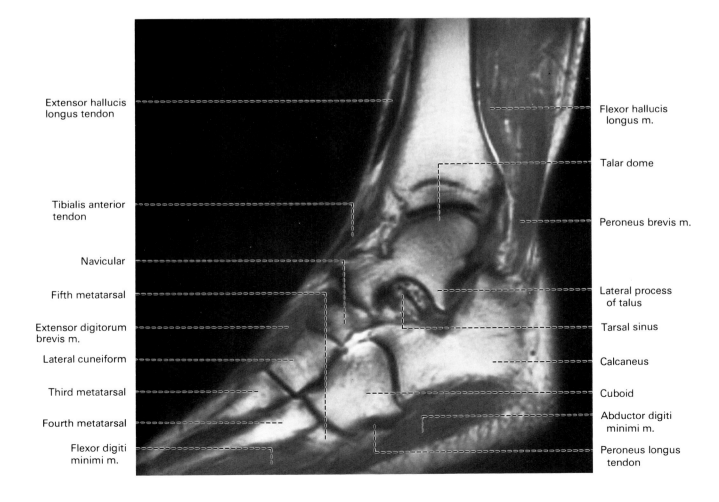

Extensor hallucis longus tendon

Tibialis anterior tendon

Navicular

Fifth metatarsal

Extensor digitorum brevis m.

Lateral cuneiform

Third metatarsal

Fourth metatarsal

Flexor digiti minimi m.

Flexor hallucis longus m.

Talar dome

Peroneus brevis m.

Lateral process of talus

Tarsal sinus

Calcaneus

Cuboid

Abductor digiti minimi m.

Peroneus longus tendon

Figure 16.3.10

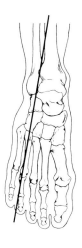

1. The peroneal tendons course posterior and inferior to the lateral malleolus.

2. In the midfoot the peroneus longus tendon is seen entering the cuboid sulcus.

3. The interosseous talocalcaneal ligament is demonstrated connecting the two bones.

4. The muscles of the anterior compartment begin to appear in this section.

5. A portion of the bifurcate ligament is shown as it extends from the calcaneus to insert on the navicular.

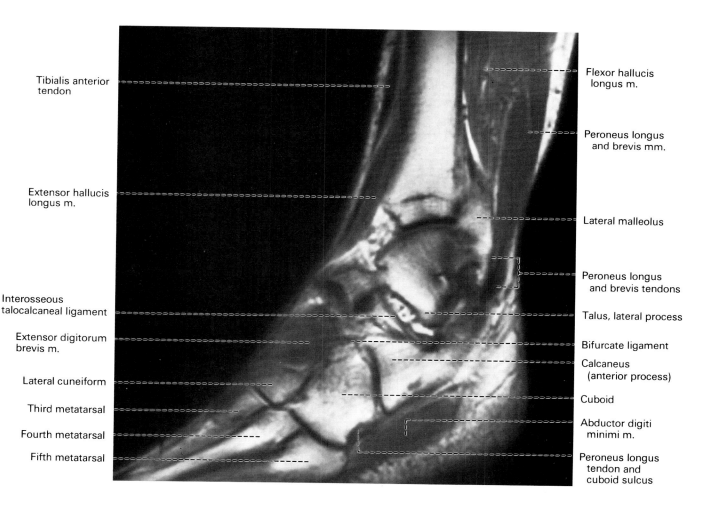

Tibialis anterior tendon

Extensor hallucis longus m.

Interosseous talocalcaneal ligament

Extensor digitorum brevis m.

Lateral cuneiform

Third metatarsal

Fourth metatarsal

Fifth metatarsal

Flexor hallucis longus m.

Peroneus longus and brevis mm.

Lateral malleolus

Peroneus longus and brevis tendons

Talus, lateral process

Bifurcate ligament

Calcaneus (anterior process)

Cuboid

Abductor digiti minimi m.

Peroneus longus tendon and cuboid sulcus

Figure 16.3.11

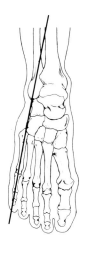

1. The peroneus longus and brevis muscles are closely related and difficult to separate.

2. The peroneus longus tendon courses posterior and inferior to the peroneus brevis tendon.

3. The peroneus longus tendon disappears from this section at the level of the calcaneus as it courses medially to enter the cuboid sulcus.

4. Peroneus brevis continues distally to insert onto the tuberosity of the fifth metatarsal.

5. Note the origin of the extensor digitorum brevis muscle from the anterior superior aspect of the calcaneus.

6. The long extensors of the foot are situated in the anterior compartment of the leg between the tibia and fibula.

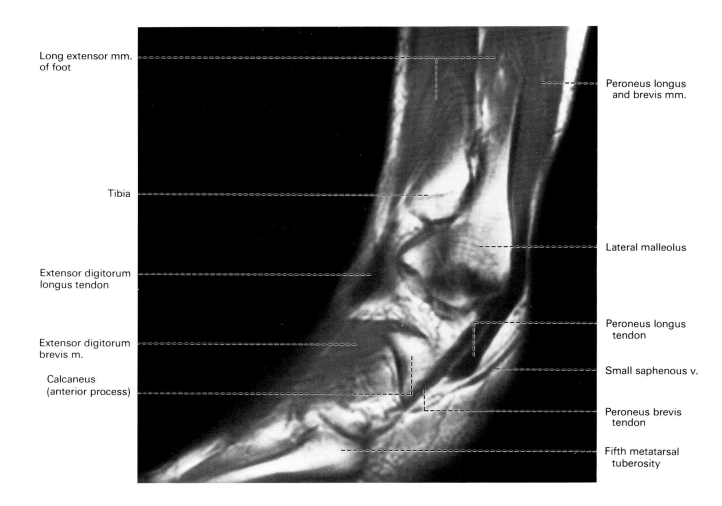

Figure 16.3.12

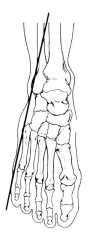

1. Note the relation of the peroneal muscles and tendons to the fibula and lateral malleolus.

2. The extensor digitorum longus tendon starts in the lower end of the anterior compartment, courses over the anterolateral aspect of the ankle, and divides into four smaller tendons on the dorsolateral aspect of the foot.

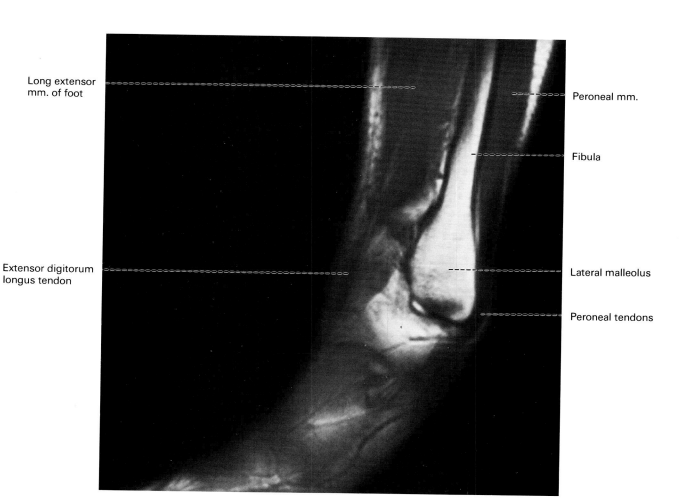

Long extensor mm. of foot

Extensor digitorum longus tendon

Peroneal mm.

Fibula

Lateral malleolus

Peroneal tendons

Chapter 17

FOOT

Figure 17.1.1

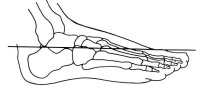

1. This section is toward the dorsum of the foot and shows the origin of the extensor digitorum brevis muscle from the anterolateral and superior aspect of the calcaneus.

2. Flexor hallucis longus and flexor digitorum longus tendons are seen as they course distally. At this level, which is superior to their crossing, the flexor hallucis longus tendon is lateral to the flexor digitorum longus tendon.

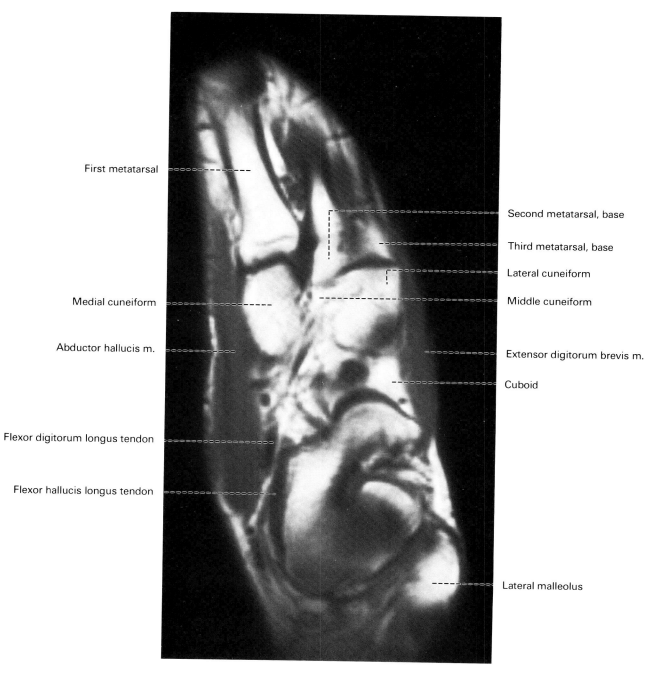

First metatarsal

Medial cuneiform

Abductor hallucis m.

Flexor digitorum longus tendon

Flexor hallucis longus tendon

Second metatarsal, base

Third metatarsal, base

Lateral cuneiform

Middle cuneiform

Extensor digitorum brevis m.

Cuboid

Lateral malleolus

Figure 17.1.2

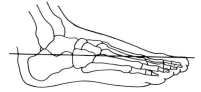

1. Note the origin of the extensor digitorum brevis muscle from the antero-superior aspect of the calcaneus.

2. The flexor hallucis longus tendon is seen crossing the flexor digitorum longus tendon.

3. The abductor hallucis muscle and tendon are demonstrated.

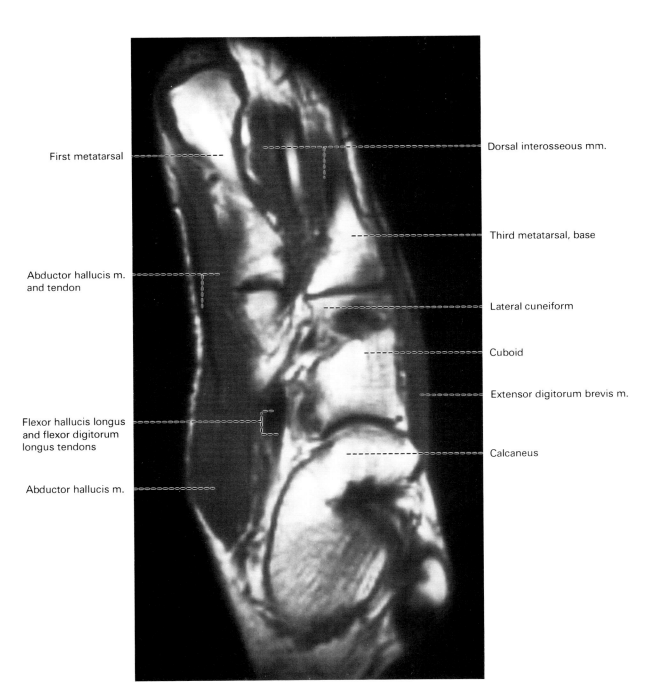

First metatarsal

Abductor hallucis m. and tendon

Flexor hallucis longus and flexor digitorum longus tendons

Abductor hallucis m.

Dorsal interosseous mm.

Third metatarsal, base

Lateral cuneiform

Cuboid

Extensor digitorum brevis m.

Calcaneus

Figure 17.1.3

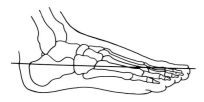

1. The lateral and medial heads of flexor hallucis brevis are demonstrated.

2. The flexor hallucis longus tendon courses distally between the medial and lateral heads of flexor hallucis brevis.

3. The fleshy muscle on the medial side of the heel is abductor hallucis.

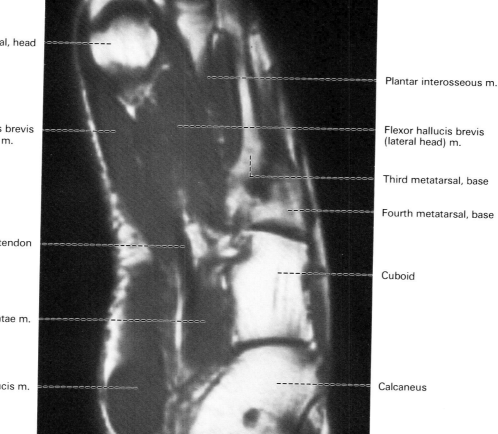

First metatarsal, head

Flexor hallucis brevis (medial head) m.

Flexor hallucis longus tendon

Quadratus plantae m.

Abductor hallucis m.

Plantar interosseous m.

Flexor hallucis brevis (lateral head) m.

Third metatarsal, base

Fourth metatarsal, base

Cuboid

Calcaneus

Peroneal tendons

Figure 17.1.4

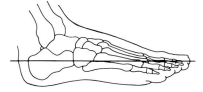

1. Note the relationship of the plantar interosseous muscles to the third and fourth metatarsals.

2. The thick fleshy muscle in the center of the foot is the oblique head of adductor hallucis.

3. The flexor hallucis longus tendon is embedded between the medial and lateral heads of flexor hallucis brevis.

4. Lateral to the flexor hallucis longus tendon is the flexor digitorum longus tendon.

5. Abductor hallucis is partially seen at its origin from the calcaneal tuberosity.

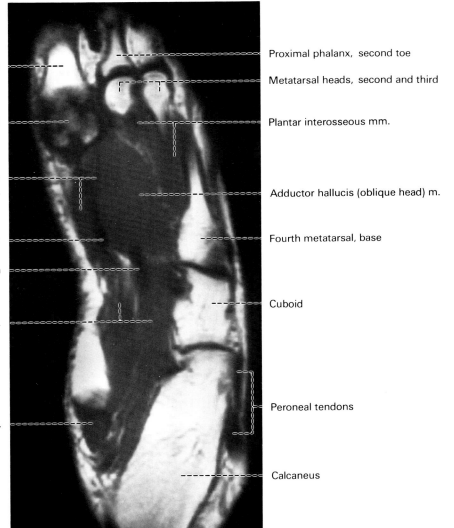

Figure 17.1.5

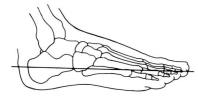

1. The peroneus longus tendon is demonstrated coursing in the direction of the cuboid sulcus.

2. The peroneus brevis tendon inserts onto the tuberosity of the fifth metatarsal.

3. Note that quadratus plantae and flexor digitorum brevis muscles end in the midfoot.

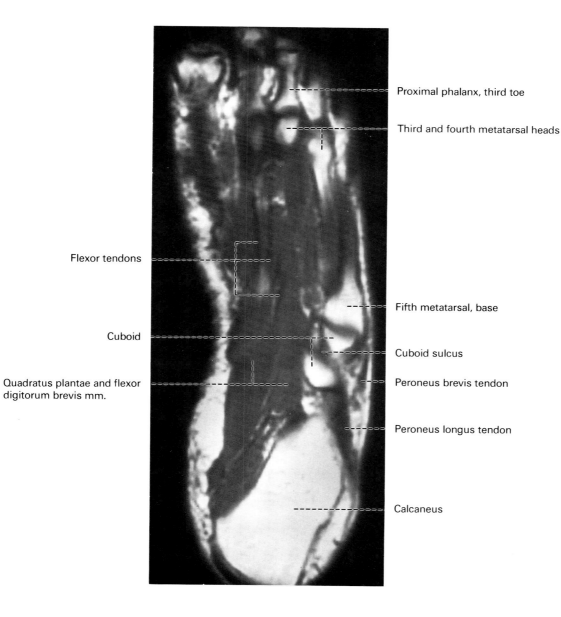

Proximal phalanx, third toe

Third and fourth metatarsal heads

Flexor tendons

Fifth metatarsal, base

Cuboid

Cuboid sulcus

Quadratus plantae and flexor digitorum brevis mm.

Peroneus brevis tendon

Peroneus longus tendon

Calcaneus

Figure 17.1.6

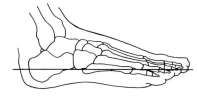

1. The flexor digitorum brevis muscle ends in the midfoot and divides into the short flexor tendons. The tendons of the short and long flexors are difficult to distinguish.

2. Flexor digitorum brevis is seen at its origin from the calcaneal tuberosity and in the midfoot immediately before it divides into its tendons.

3. Immediately medial to the origin of flexor digitorum brevis the medial head of quadratus plantae is demonstrated.

4. Flexor digiti minimi is seen medial to the fifth metatarsal.

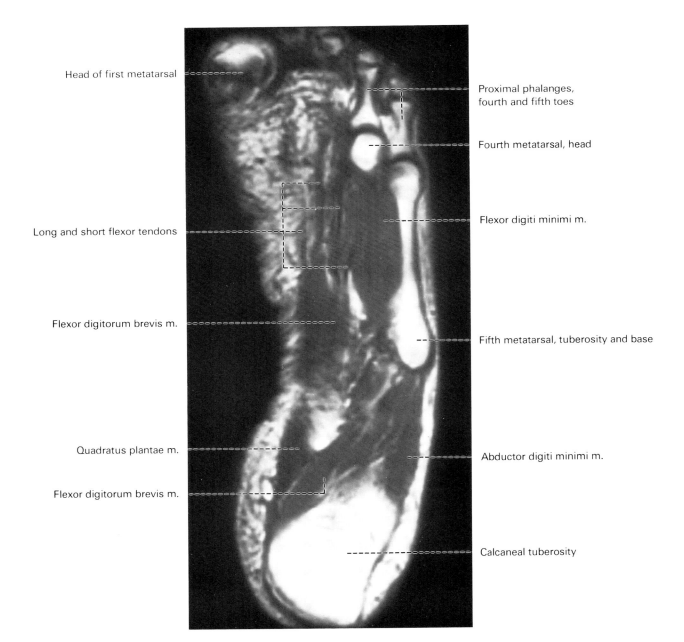

Head of first metatarsal

Long and short flexor tendons

Flexor digitorum brevis m.

Quadratus plantae m.

Flexor digitorum brevis m.

Proximal phalanges, fourth and fifth toes

Fourth metatarsal, head

Flexor digiti minimi m.

Fifth metatarsal, tuberosity and base

Abductor digiti minimi m.

Calcaneal tuberosity

Figure 17.1.7

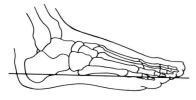

1. This section is through the fifth ray; the other rays are located superiorly.

2. Flexor digiti minimi, abductor digiti minimi, and flexor digitorum brevis muscles are partially demonstrated.

3. Both the longitudinal and transverse arches of the foot can be appreciated in this section.

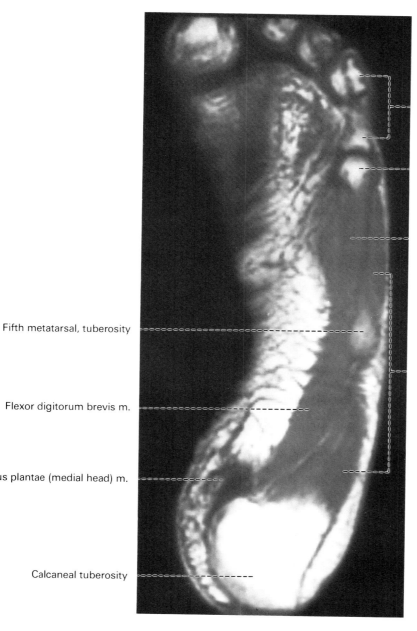

Fifth digit, phalanges

Fifth metatarsal, head

Flexor digiti minimi m.

Fifth metatarsal, tuberosity

Abductor digiti minimi m.

Flexor digitorum brevis m.

Quadratus plantae (medial head) m.

Calcaneal tuberosity

Figure 17.1.8

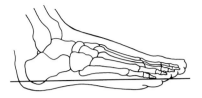

1. The lateral aspect of the foot is inferior to the medial aspect because of the presence of a transverse arch that is more pronounced at the midfoot.

2. Note the origin of abductor digiti minimi from the tuberosity of the calcaneus.

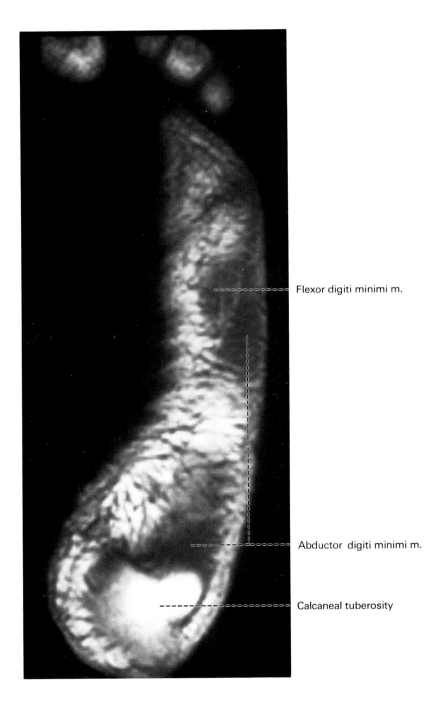

Flexor digiti minimi m.

Abductor digiti minimi m.

Calcaneal tuberosity

CORONAL

Figure 17.2.1

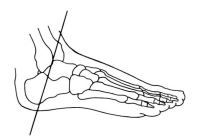

1. On the medial side, flexor digitorum longus and tibialis posterior tendons are identified inferior to the medial malleolus.

2. The peroneus longus and brevis tendons are situated inferior to the lateral malleolus.

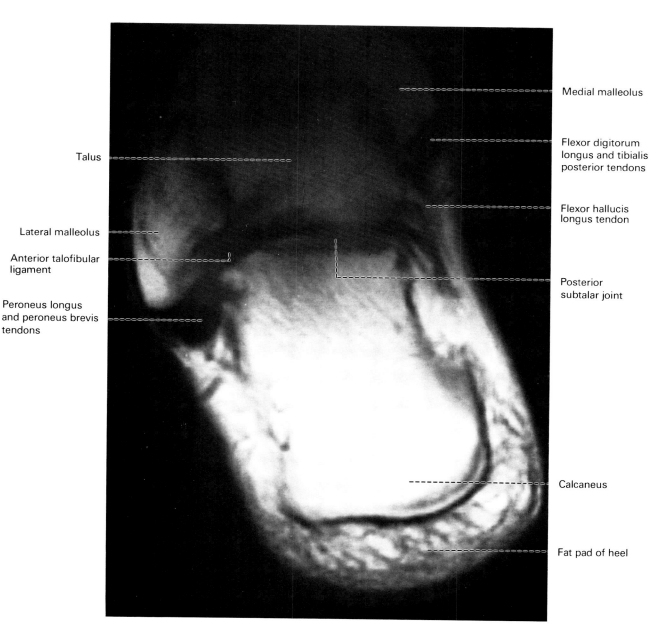

Talus

Lateral malleolus

Anterior talofibular ligament

Peroneus longus and peroneus brevis tendons

Medial malleolus

Flexor digitorum longus and tibialis posterior tendons

Flexor hallucis longus tendon

Posterior subtalar joint

Calcaneus

Fat pad of heel

Figure 17.2.2

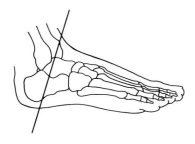

1. The tibialis posterior, flexor digitorum longus, and flexor hallucis longus tendons are identified on the medial side of the ankle.

2. The posterior tibial nerve and artery course between flexor digitorum longus and flexor hallucis longus tendons.

3. On the lateral side peroneus brevis and longus tendons are demonstrated.

4. Note the origin of the abductor hallucis muscle, flexor digitorum brevis, and plantar aponeurosis from the calcaneal tuberosity.

5. The posterior (lateral) subtalar joint is identified.

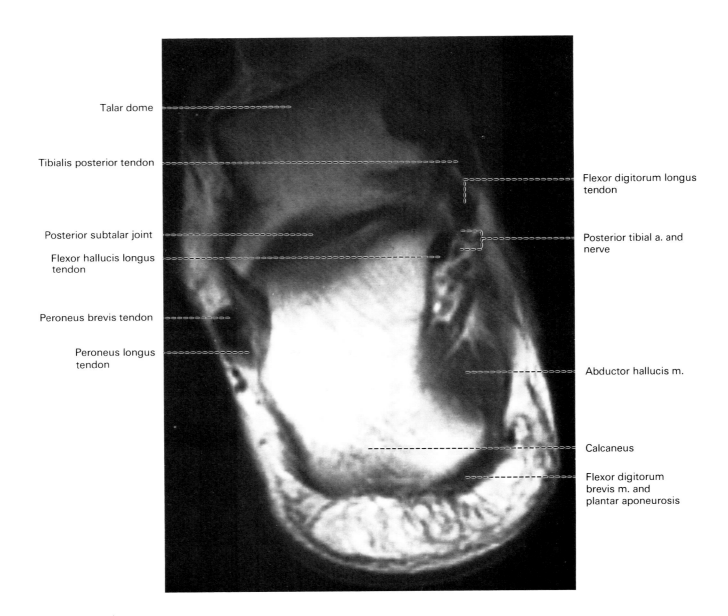

Talar dome

Tibialis posterior tendon

Flexor digitorum longus tendon

Posterior subtalar joint

Flexor hallucis longus tendon

Posterior tibial a. and nerve

Peroneus brevis tendon

Peroneus longus tendon

Abductor hallucis m.

Calcaneus

Flexor digitorum brevis m. and plantar aponeurosis

Figure 17.2.3

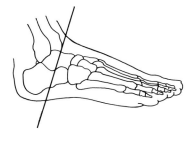

1. Anterior and superior to the talus are the tibialis anterior, extensor hallucis longus, and extensor digitorum longus tendons.

2. The middle (medial) subtalar joint is formed between the sustentaculum tali and the medial, inferior surface of the talus.

3. Some of the intrinsic muscles of the foot (abductor hallucis, flexor digitorum brevis, quadratus plantae, and abductor digiti minimi muscles) surround the inferior aspect of the calcaneus.

4. The small saphenous vein is identified inferior to the peroneal tendons.

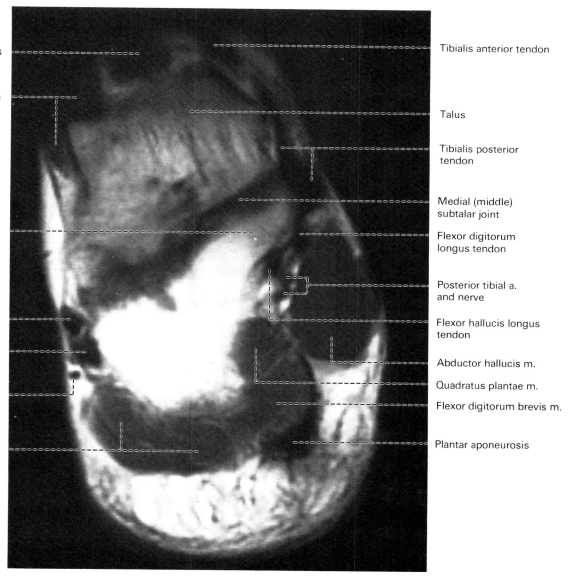

Extensor hallucis longus tendon

Extensor digitorum longus tendons

Sustentaculum tali

Peroneus brevis tendon

Peroneus longus tendon

Small saphenous v.

Abductor digiti minimi m.

Tibialis anterior tendon

Talus

Tibialis posterior tendon

Medial (middle) subtalar joint

Flexor digitorum longus tendon

Posterior tibial a. and nerve

Flexor hallucis longus tendon

Abductor hallucis m.

Quadratus plantae m.

Flexor digitorum brevis m.

Plantar aponeurosis

Figure 17.2.4

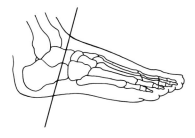

1. In the foot, the tibialis posterior tendon courses superior to both the flexor digitorum longus and flexor hallucis longus tendons.

2. The flexor digitorum longus tendon is seen crossing the flexor hallucis longus tendon to become more plantar in position.

3. The peroneus brevis and longus tendons are separating, with the latter coursing medially to reach the cuboid sulcus.

4. Note the lateral position of the extensor digitorum longus tendon with the peroneus tertius tendon branching from it.

5. The peroneus tertius tendon courses distally and inferiorly to insert onto the proximal shaft of the fifth metatarsal.

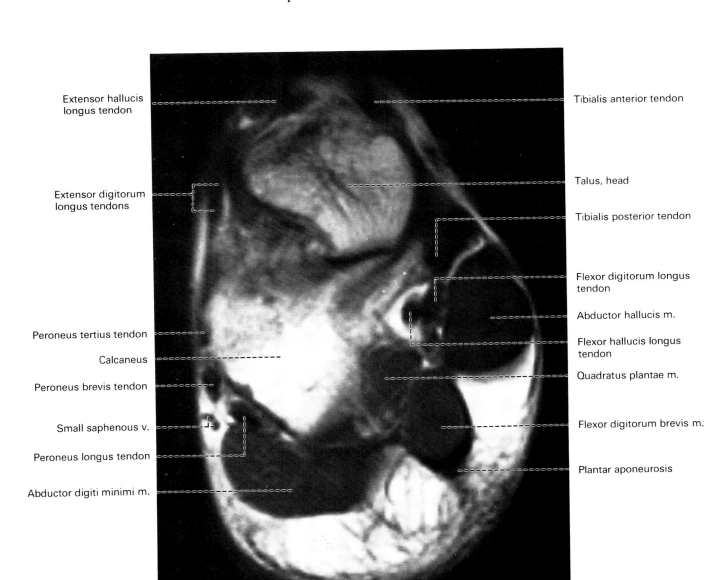

Figure 17.2.5

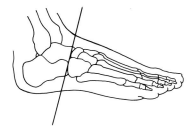

1. The tibialis posterior tendon flattens as it approaches its insertion on the plantar surface of the navicular tuberosity.

2. Note the plantar position of the flexor digitorum longus tendon in relation to the flexor hallucis longus tendon. These tendons are situated between abductor hallucis and quadratus plantae muscles.

3. The intrinsic muscles on the plantar aspect of the foot are distinctly seen.

4. Extensor digitorum brevis is identified on the superolateral aspect of the foot.

5. Extensor digitorum longus is beginning to divide into its individual digital tendons.

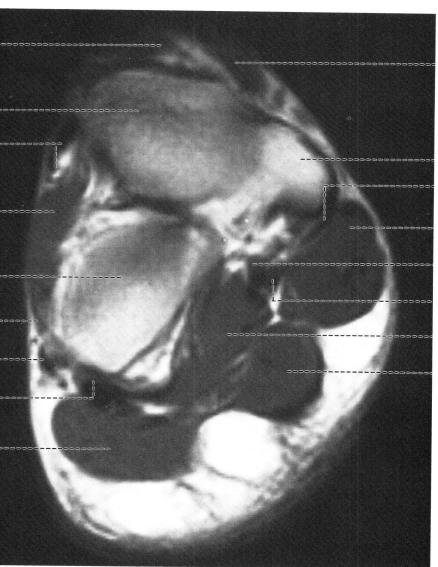

Extensor hallucis longus tendon

Talus, head

Extensor digitorum longus tendons

Extensor digitorum brevis m.

Calcaneus

Peroneus tertius tendon

Peroneus brevis tendon

Peroneus longus tendon

Abductor digiti minimi m.

Tibialis anterior tendon

Navicular tuberosity

Tibialis posterior tendon

Abductor hallucis m.

Flexor hallucis longus tendon

Flexor digitorum longus tendon

Quadratus plantae m.

Flexor digitorum brevis m.

Figure 17.2.6

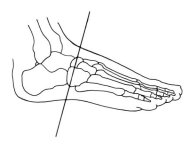

1. The peroneus longus tendon is noted in the cuboid sulcus.

2. The peroneus tertius and peroneus brevis tendons are seen to flatten prior to their insertion onto the fifth metatarsal.

3. Extensor digitorum brevis is distinctly demonstrated on the posterolateral aspect of the foot.

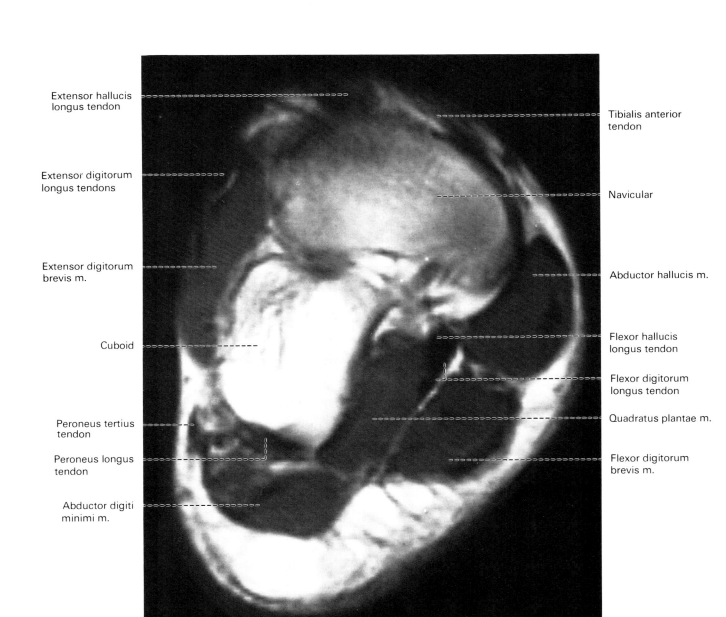

Extensor hallucis longus tendon

Extensor digitorum longus tendons

Extensor digitorum brevis m.

Cuboid

Peroneus tertius tendon

Peroneus longus tendon

Abductor digiti minimi m.

Tibialis anterior tendon

Navicular

Abductor hallucis m.

Flexor hallucis longus tendon

Flexor digitorum longus tendon

Quadratus plantae m.

Flexor digitorum brevis m.

Figure 17.2.7

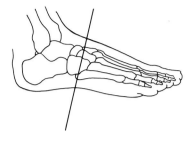

1. The tibialis anterior tendon is descending toward its insertion on the plantar aspect of the medial cuneiform and base of the first metatarsal.

2. Note the peroneus longus tendon crossing from the lateral to the medial aspect of the foot where it inserts on the plantar aspect of the medial cuneiform and base of the first metatarsal.

3. The flexor hallucis longus and flexor digitorum longus tendons are seen dorsal to the flexor digitorum brevis muscle.

4. The transverse arch is seen in this section through the midfoot.

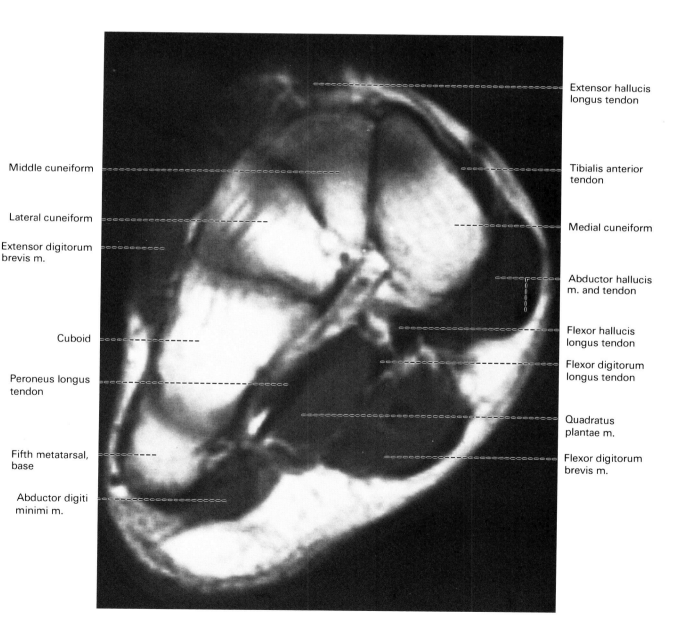

Middle cuneiform

Lateral cuneiform

Extensor digitorum brevis m.

Cuboid

Peroneus longus tendon

Fifth metatarsal, base

Abductor digiti minimi m.

Extensor hallucis longus tendon

Tibialis anterior tendon

Medial cuneiform

Abductor hallucis m. and tendon

Flexor hallucis longus tendon

Flexor digitorum longus tendon

Quadratus plantae m.

Flexor digitorum brevis m.

Figure 17.2.8

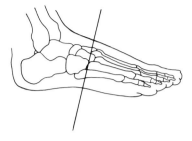

1. Abductor hallucis is tapering in size and its tendon is becoming evident.

2. Note the triangular shape of the cuneiform bones, hence their name.

3. Flexor digiti minimi is seen along the plantar aspect of the base of the fifth metatarsal near its origin.

4. The digital tendons originating from extensor digitorum longus are demonstrated.

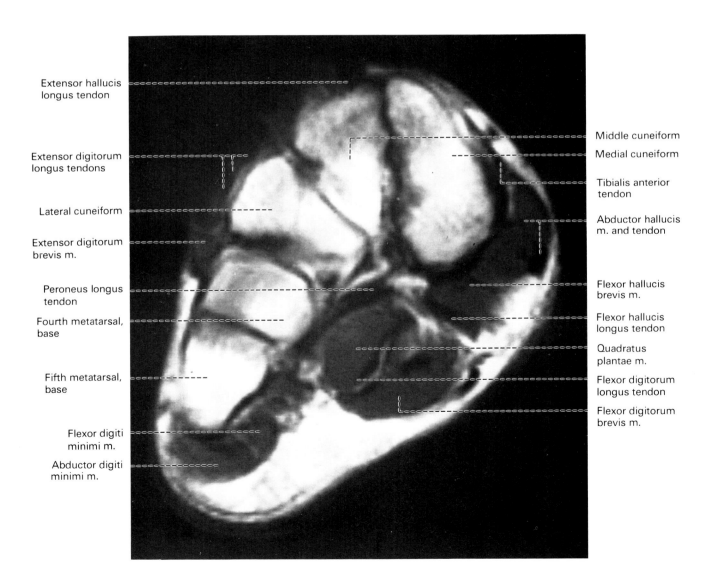

Extensor hallucis longus tendon

Extensor digitorum longus tendons

Lateral cuneiform

Extensor digitorum brevis m.

Peroneus longus tendon

Fourth metatarsal, base

Fifth metatarsal, base

Flexor digiti minimi m.

Abductor digiti minimi m.

Middle cuneiform

Medial cuneiform

Tibialis anterior tendon

Abductor hallucis m. and tendon

Flexor hallucis brevis m.

Flexor hallucis longus tendon

Quadratus plantae m.

Flexor digitorum longus tendon

Flexor digitorum brevis m.

Figure 17.2.9

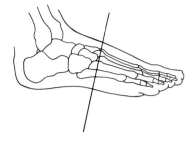

1. Note the long and short digital flexor and extensor tendons on the plantar and dorsal aspects of the foot.

2. In the center of the foot note adductor hallucis, which is a large muscle originating from the bases of the third and fourth metatarsals.

3. The flexor hallucis longus tendon is seen coursing distally along the belly of the flexor hallucis brevis muscle.

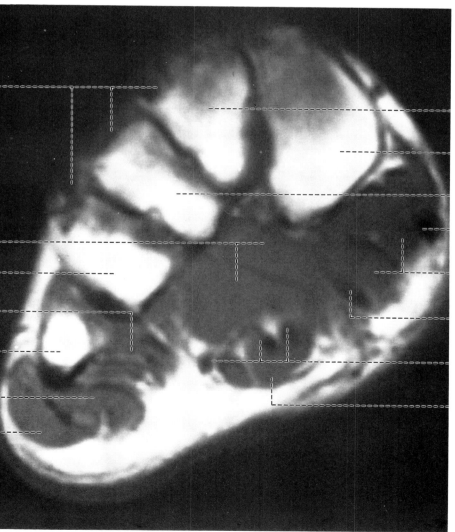

Long and short digital extensor tendons

Abductor hallucis m.

Fourth metatarsal, base

Flexor digiti minimi m.

Fifth metatarsal

Opponens digiti minimi m.

Abductor digiti minimi m.

Second metatarsal, base

First metatarsal, base

Third metatarsal, base

Abductor hallucis tendon

Flexor hallucis brevis m.

Flexor hallucis longus tendon

Long and short digital flexor tendons

Flexor digitorum brevis m.

Figure 17.2.10

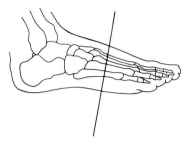

1. The tendon of abductor hallucis is seen coursing distally alongside the flexor hallucis brevis muscle.

2. Note the position of the flexor hallucis longus tendon plantar to the flexor hallucis brevis muscle.

3. The large adductor hallucis (oblique head) is seen in its central position.

4. Note the positions of the plantar and dorsal interosseous muscles and their relation to the metatarsals.

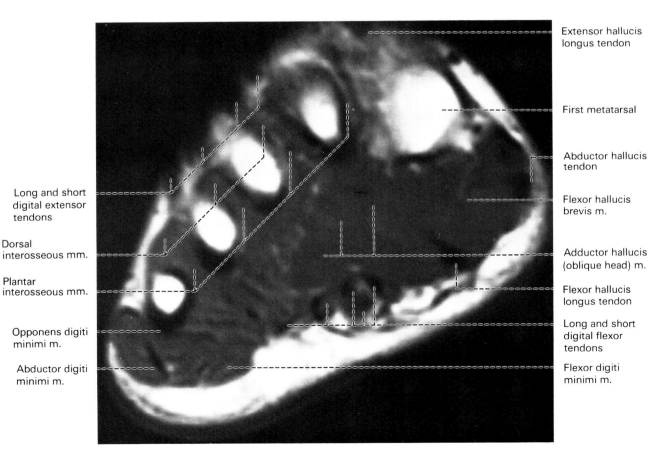

Figure 17.2.11

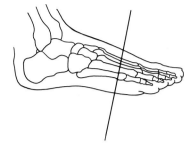

1. The extensor hallucis longus tendon is identified on the dorsum of the foot dorsal to the first metatarsal.

2. Note the relation of the lumbrical muscles to the tendons of flexor digitorum longus.

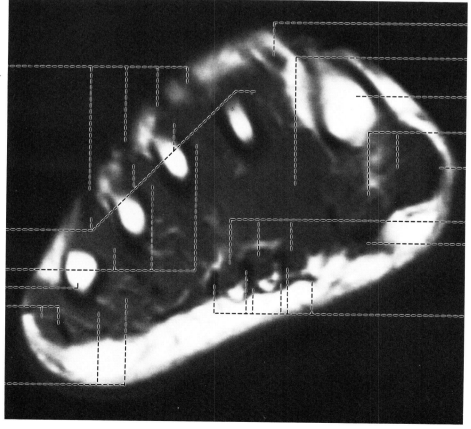

Long and short digital extensor tendons

Dorsal interosseous mm.

Plantar interosseous mm.

Fifth metatarsal

Abductor digiti minimi m. and tendon

Flexor and opponens digiti minimi mm.

Extensor hallucis longus tendon

Adductor hallucis (oblique head) m.

First metatarsal

Flexor hallucis brevis m.

Abductor hallucis tendon

Lumbrical mm.

Flexor hallucis longus tendon

Long and short digital flexor tendons

Figure 17.2.12

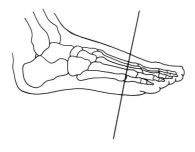

1. The medial and lateral sesamoids of the first metatarsal head are demonstrated in this section. They are located within the medial and lateral tendons of flexor hallucis brevis. The lateral sesamoid is also within the adductor hallucis tendon.

2. The flexor hallucis longus tendon passes between the two sesamoid bones.

3. Note the transversely oriented muscle fibers of adductor hallucis (transverse head).

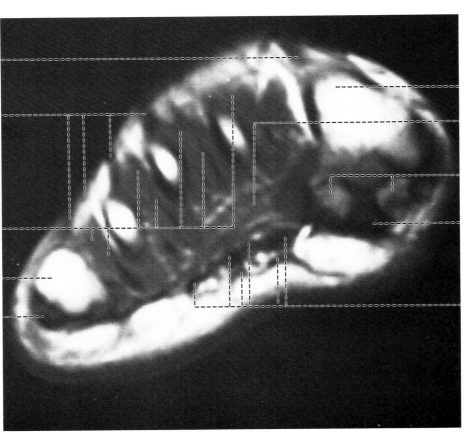

Figure 17.2.13

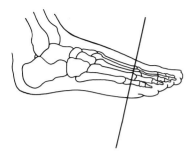

1. In this and the following sections there are no muscles, only tendons.

2. The extensor hallucis longus tendon is centrally positioned directly dorsal to the first metatarsal head.

3. The flexor hallucis longus tendon is directly inferior to the first metatarsal head.

4. The flexor and extensor tendons are well visualized.

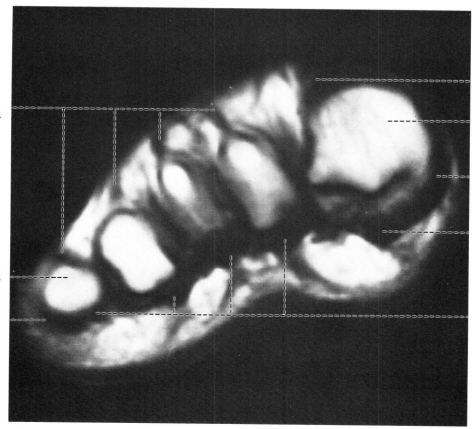

Long and short digital extensor tendons

Extensor hallucis longus tendon

First metatarsal, head

Fibrous sheath of first digit

Flexor hallucis longus tendon

Proximal phalanx, fifth toe

Fibrous sheath of fifth digit

Long and short digital flexor tendons

Figure 17.2.14

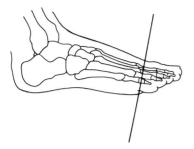

1. Note the relation of the flexor and extensor tendons to the phalanges.

2. A thick cushion of areolar connective tissue lies between the skin and the flexor tendons.

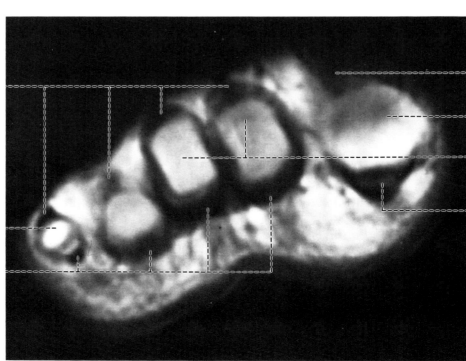

Long and short
digital extensor
tendons

Middle phalanx,
fifth toe

Long and short
digital flexor
tendons

Extensor hallucis
longus tendon

Proximal phalanx
of great toe

Proximal
phalanges, second
and third toes

Flexor hallucis
longus tendon

SAGITTAL

Figure 17.3.1

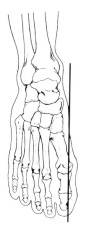

1. The abductor hallucis tendon is noted on this medial section. This tendon courses distally to insert at the base of the proximal phalanx of the great toe medially.

2. The flexor hallucis longus tendon is outlined at its insertion onto the base of the distal phalanx of the great toe.

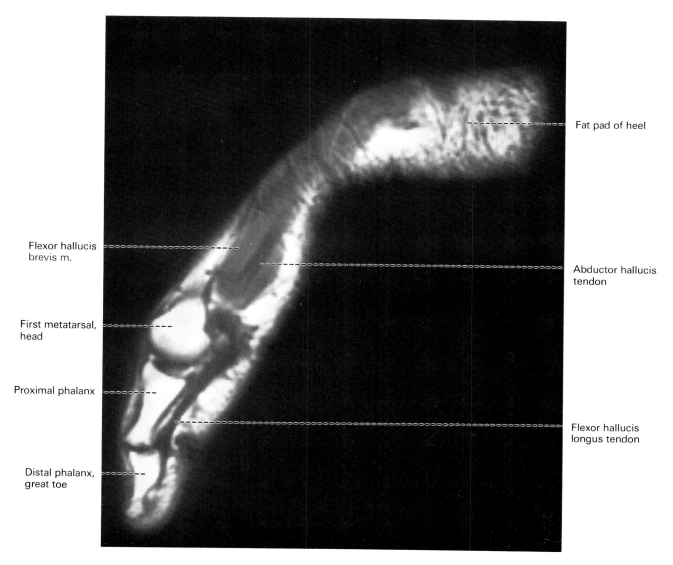

Flexor hallucis brevis m.

First metatarsal, head

Proximal phalanx

Distal phalanx, great toe

Fat pad of heel

Abductor hallucis tendon

Flexor hallucis longus tendon

Figure 17.3.2

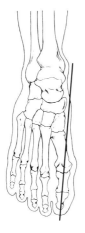

1. This medial section shows the fleshy portions of the abductor hallucis and flexor hallucis brevis muscles.

2. The medial sesamoid lies within the tendon of the medial head of flexor hallucis brevis, which inserts onto the base of the proximal phalanx.

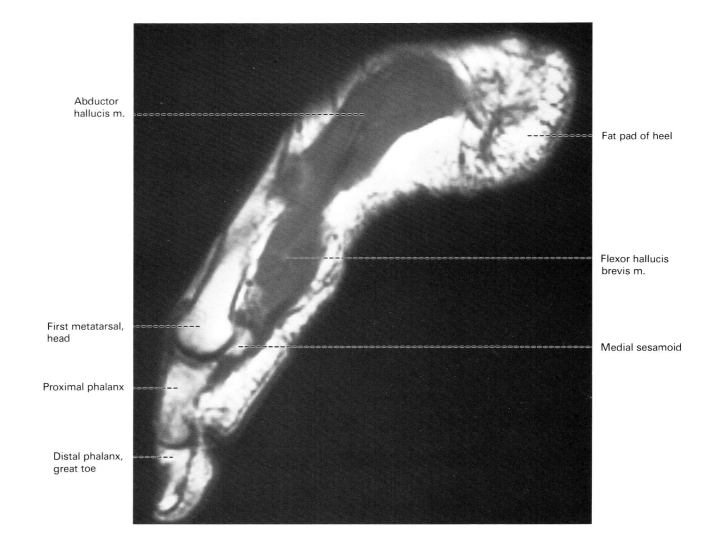

Abductor hallucis m.

Fat pad of heel

Flexor hallucis brevis m.

First metatarsal, head

Medial sesamoid

Proximal phalanx

Distal phalanx, great toe

Figure 17.3.3

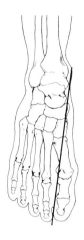

1. The tuberosity of the calcaneus is depicted. This serves as the origin of the plantar aponeurosis and the abductor hallucis, flexor digitorum brevis, quadratus plantae, and abductor digiti minimi muscles.

2. Note the insertion of the tibialis posterior tendon on the navicular and medial cuneiform.

3. The tibialis anterior tendon inserts on the medial cuneiform, and some fibers continue to insert on the base of the first metatarsal.

4. The belly of flexor hallucis brevis is also included in this section.

Tibialis posterior tendon

Navicular

Tibialis anterior tendon

Medial cuneiform

First metatarsal

Flexor hallucis brevis m.

Calcaneal tuberosity

Flexor digitorum brevis m.

Abductor hallucis m.

Plantar aponeurosis

Fat pad of heel

Figure 17.3.4

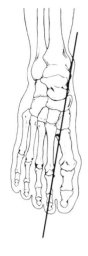

1. The course of the flexor hallucis longus tendon below the sustentaculum tali is demonstrated.

2. Note the close relation between flexor digitorum brevis and quadratus plantae muscles in the arch of the foot.

3. The adductor hallucis muscle is seen between the first and second metatarsals.

4. The distal portion of a flexor digitorum longus tendon is outlined as it courses to insert at the base of the distal phalanx of the second toe.

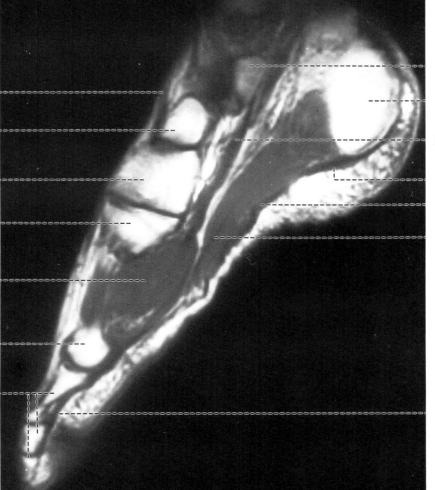

Figure 17.3.5

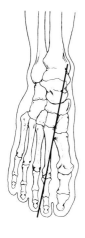

1. Note how the quadratus plantae muscle inserts on the tendon of the flexor digitorum longus.

2. In this section abductor digiti minimi originates from the inferior aspect of the calcaneal tuberosity.

3. The calcaneal (Achilles) tendon inserts on the tuberosity of the calcaneus.

4. Note the belly of the first dorsal interosseous muscle with its origin from the second metatarsal. A portion of this muscle originates from the first metatarsal.

5. Tibialis anterior crosses over the head of the talus in this section.

Tibialis anterior tendon

Talus, head

Middle subtalar joint

Navicular

Middle cuneiform

Medial cuneiform

Dorsal interosseous m.

Second metatarsal

Plantar interosseous m.

Calcaneal (Achilles) tendon

Posterior subtalar joint

Calcaneal tuberosity

Plantar aponeurosis

Abductor digiti minimi m.

Quadratus plantae m.

Flexor digitorum brevis m.

Flexor digitorum longus tendon

Adductor hallucis (oblique head) m.

Figure 17.3.6

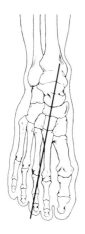

1. The posterior (lateral) subtalar joint is included in this section.

2. The flexor digitorum brevis and quadratus plantae muscles are difficult to separate in this section.

3. The tarsal sinus and head of the talus are clearly delineated.

4. Note the relation of the tibialis anterior tendon to the head of the talus as this tendon courses inferior and medially to insert on the medial surface of the medial cuneiform and base of the first metatarsal.

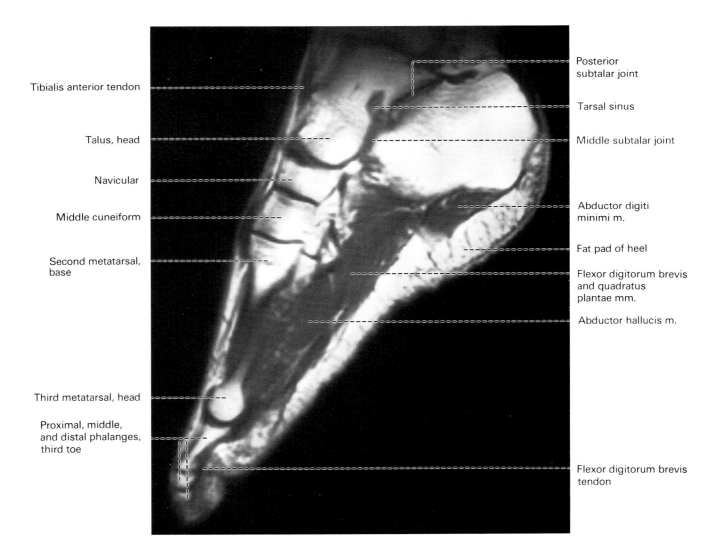

Figure 17.3.7

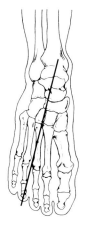

1. Both the posterior (lateral) and anterior subtalar joints are seen in this section.

2. Lumbrical and interosseous muscles can be identified.

3. Note the relation between the navicular and cuneiform bones.

4. The extensor hallucis longus tendon is seen on the dorsum of the foot.

5. The tendon of the peroneus longus is seen entering the foot inferior to the cuboid.

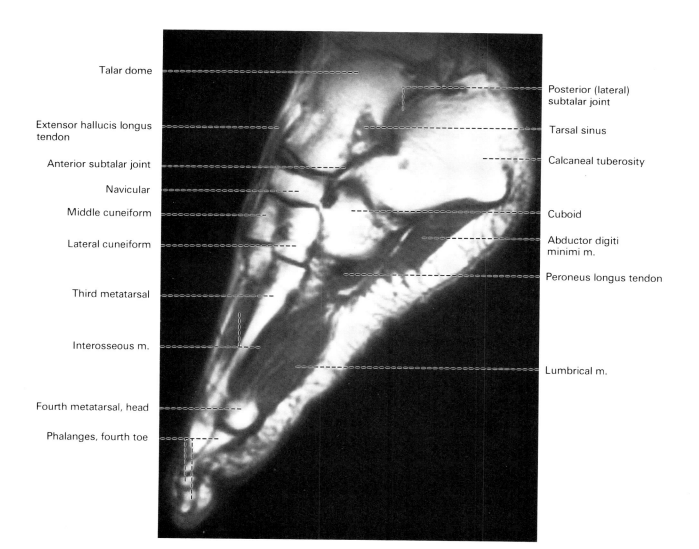

Talar dome

Extensor hallucis longus tendon

Anterior subtalar joint

Navicular

Middle cuneiform

Lateral cuneiform

Third metatarsal

Interosseous m.

Fourth metatarsal, head

Phalanges, fourth toe

Posterior (lateral) subtalar joint

Tarsal sinus

Calcaneal tuberosity

Cuboid

Abductor digiti minimi m.

Peroneus longus tendon

Lumbrical m.

Figure 17.3.8

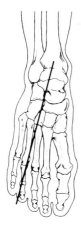

1. The lateral process of the talus and anterior process of the calcaneus are demonstrated.

2. The abductor digiti minimi and flexor digiti minimi muscles are noted over the lateral aspect of the foot.

3. Note the position of the cuboid between the calcaneus and fourth and fifth metatarsals.

4. The extensor hallucis longus tendon courses over the head of the talus.

5. The extensor digitorum brevis muscle is partially demonstrated.

6. The peroneus longus tendon is seen entering the cuboid sulcus.

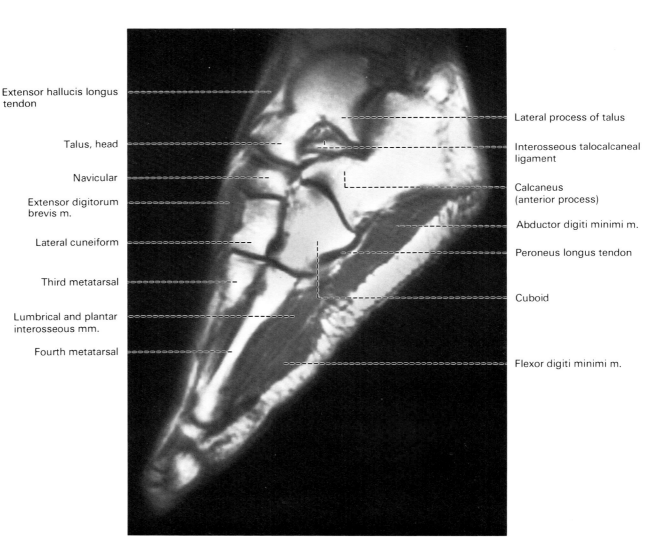

Figure 17.3.9

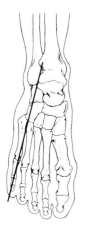

1. In this lateral section of the foot, the extensor digitorum longus tendon and extensor digitorum brevis muscle are well seen.

2. Abductor digiti minimi and flexor digiti minimi brevis muscles are situated over the lateral plantar aspect of the foot.

3. Peroneus longus is seen approaching the cuboid sulcus.

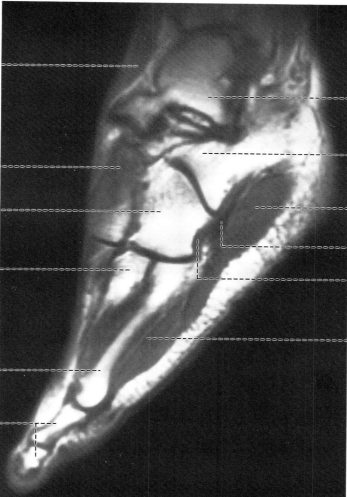

Extensor digitorum longus tendons

Extensor digitorum brevis m.

Cuboid

Fourth metatarsal

Fifth metatarsal

Phalanges, fifth toe

Lateral process of talus

Calcaneus (anterior process)

Abductor digiti minimi m.

Peroneus longus tendon

Cuboid sulcus

Flexor digiti minimi brevis m.

Figure 17.3.10

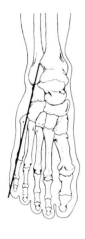

1. The peroneus longus and peroneus brevis tendons are outlined. The peroneus brevis tendon continues distally to insert onto the tuberosity of the fifth metatarsal.

2. Flexor digiti minimi brevis lies on the plantar surface of the fifth metatarsal.

3. Note the origin of extensor digitorum brevis from the superior and lateral surface of the calcaneus (anterior process).

4. Extensor digitorum longus is demonstrated.

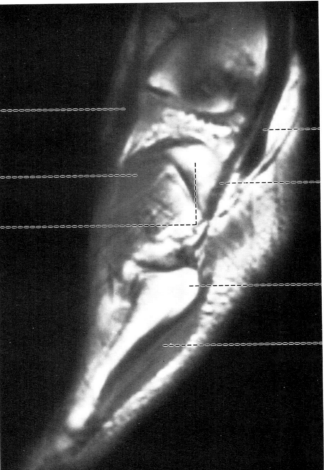

Extensor digitorum longus tendon

Extensor digitorum brevis m.

Calcaneus (anterior process)

Peroneus longus tendon

Peroneus brevis tendon

Fifth metatarsal, tuberosity

Flexor digiti minimi brevis m.

Index